AF569955

Atlas of Craniopharyngioma

Songtao Qi
Editor

Atlas of Craniopharyngioma

Pathology, Classification and Surgery

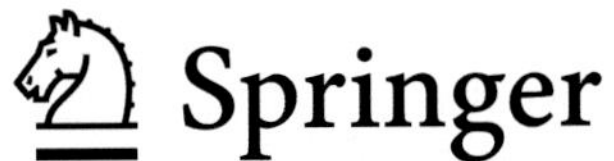

Springer

Editor
Songtao Qi
Neurosurgery Department of Nanfang Hospital
Southern Medical University
Guangzhou
Guangdong
China

ISBN 978-981-13-7324-4 ISBN 978-981-13-7322-0 (eBook)
https://doi.org/10.1007/978-981-13-7322-0

© Springer Nature Singapore Pte Ltd. 2020
This work is subject to copyright. All rights are reserved by the Publisher, whether the whole or part of the material is concerned, specifically the rights of translation, reprinting, reuse of illustrations, recitation, broadcasting, reproduction on microfilms or in any other physical way, and transmission or information storage and retrieval, electronic adaptation, computer software, or by similar or dissimilar methodology now known or hereafter developed.
The use of general descriptive names, registered names, trademarks, service marks, etc. in this publication does not imply, even in the absence of a specific statement, that such names are exempt from the relevant protective laws and regulations and therefore free for general use.
The publisher, the authors, and the editors are safe to assume that the advice and information in this book are believed to be true and accurate at the date of publication. Neither the publisher nor the authors or the editors give a warranty, expressed or implied, with respect to the material contained herein or for any errors or omissions that may have been made. The publisher remains neutral with regard to jurisdictional claims in published maps and institutional affiliations.

This Springer imprint is published by the registered company Springer Nature Singapore Pte Ltd.
The registered company address is: 152 Beach Road, #21-01/04 Gateway East, Singapore 189721, Singapore

Foreword

This is a timely book. The application of endoscopy, new advanced media in imaging, surgical preparation, intraoperative navigation, and imaging have quite literally opened up the surgical view of deep-seated lesions in critical locations. Craniopharyngiomas are the quintessential deep-seated, midline lesion surrounded by critical structures; this surgical atlas provides the necessary surgical roadmap to guide these surgical journeys.

The author group, Prof Qi and his team at Nanfang Hospital, have accumulated a unique experience with a wide range of surgical material and their insights and pearls are of immense value to those who do not have the advantage of their catchment.

It will become a valuable addition in the operative arsenal of the neurosurgeon.

Nelson M. Oyesiku
Neurosurgery and Medicine (Endocrinology)
Emory University School of Medicine
Atlanta, GA, USA

Emory Pituitary Center
Emory University School of Medicine
Atlanta, GA, USA

Department of Neurosurgery
Emory University School of Medicine
Atlanta, GA, USA

Preface

Craniopharyngioma is defined by the WHO as an intracranial benign tumor that cannot be cured due to anatomical factors. Surgery, radiotherapy, cystic aspiration, and internal irradiation or intracapsular chemotherapy are considered as "proper" treatment options for craniopharyngioma. Partial surgical resection combined with stereotactic radiotherapy is applied in many medical centers, which results in craniopharyngioma being basically incurable, and even if the patient has long-term survival, health is impaired and quality of life is low.

Since 1998, our team has treated approximately 1000 cases of primary and recurrent craniopharyngioma for curative purposes. Approximately 800 cases were admitted in our centers and received systematic clinical therapy. The total resection rate of primary craniopharyngioma from 1998 to 2003 was approximately 85%, which has reached the level reported in the Yasargil period, and the total tumor resection rate from 2004 to 2008 was nearly 90%. From 2009 to the present (2018, May), the total resection rate is higher than 95% and there were no perioperative deaths in the past three years.

We have progressed greatly in craniopharyngioma treatment in the past 20 years because we have been focusing on the effects of tumor origin and membranous structures on the tumor growth pattern through clinical, embryonic, and histological studies. The QST classification of craniopharyngioma based on tumor origin and surrounding membranous structures was established. This classification has the following advantages compared with the previous important classification. First, this classification is in line with the embryonic origin theory and is not concerned with the notion of "intra-third ventricle craniopharyngioma," which leads to the misconception that tumors can originate in the third ventricle. Second, some large and complex craniopharyngiomas can be well classified by the QST system, and this system can more accurately reflect the relationship between the tumor and important structures such as the hypothalamus, so as to facilitate the correct surgical approach. Third, the QST system is not only related to the symptoms, endocrine status, and pathological types of patients, but also reflects the difficulty of surgery in different cases and accurately determines the prognosis.

The previous classifications may have not paid sufficient attention to the origin of the tumor. Some classifications were only based on clinical observation and the experience of the surgeon that did not emphasize the embryonic origin of craniopharyngioma. Some other classifications are only based on the relative relationship between important structures and the tumor. Some are even based on the relative position of the third ventricle, which also does not emphasize the pathological relationship between the tumor and the hypothalamic tissue. These resulted in the need for a long learning curve for doctors or lead to failure in successfully treating a craniopharyngioma, and also lead to the view that craniopharyngiomas involving the third ventricle floor are not suitable for surgical resection. This is also the root cause why conservative treatments for craniopharyngioma are still advocated and the belief that this benign tumor cannot be cured.

In the past 20 years, our team carried out systematic and comprehensive research on craniopharyngioma. The chief editor of this atlas, Professor Qi Songtao, achieved a total resection rate of 97% in approximately 600 craniopharyngioma cases. Some patients can maintain functional hypothalamic-pituitary secretion and some patients even had restored fertility. The main content of this atlas includes the development of craniopharyngioma from the embryonic perspective, the microanatomy of surrounding membranous structures, the histopathological relationship between the tumor and the adjacent structures, and the QST classification and its application in transcranial and transsphenoidal approaches.

Although craniopharyngioma has become a curable intracranial tumor in the author's center, it is undeniable that it is a task for neurosurgeons to deal with this benign tumor due to its strategic location and malignant biological behavior. This is also the purpose of our atlas. We will feel gratified if more patients can safely undergo total resection, rather than partial resection plus radiotherapy, chemotherapy, or immunotherapy.

Craniopharyngioma is a long-term disease in the clinical process. We have numerous colleagues in this field and cannot list them all in this book. However, their contribution will definitely be remembered forever.

Guangzhou, China
2018-8-30

Songtao Qi

Contents

About the Editor

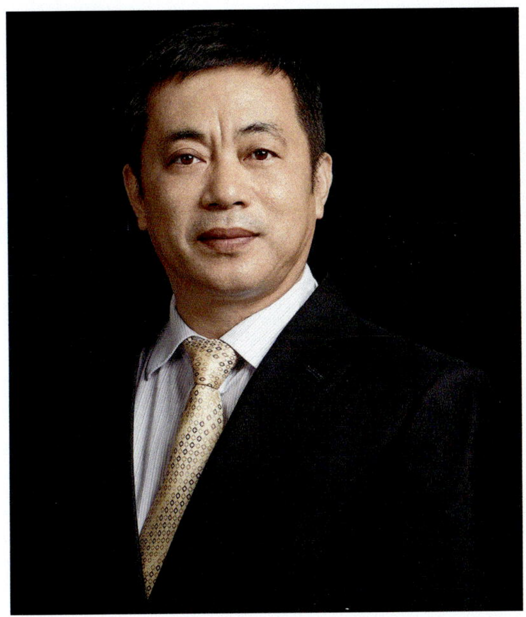

Chief editor: Songtao Qi
Associate editors: Jun Pan, Yi Liu, Xi'an Zhang, and Jun Fan

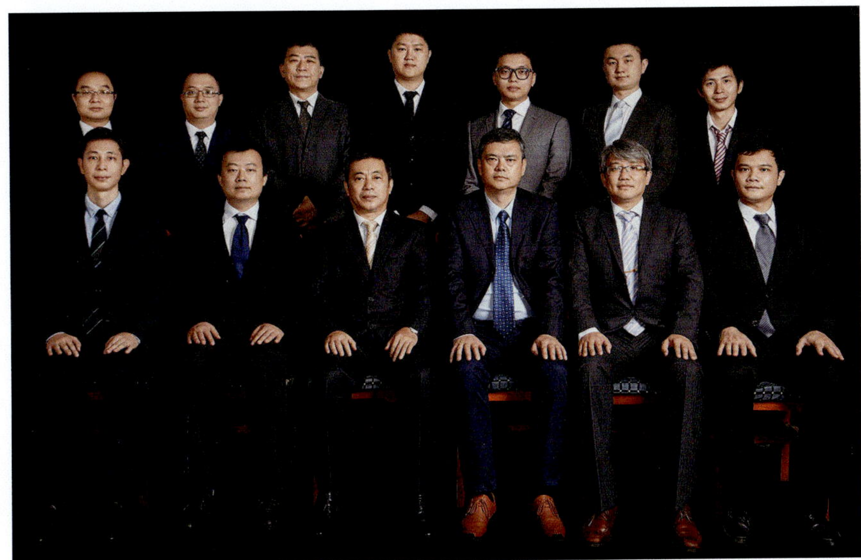

Editors: from left to right sitting in the first row: Jun Fan, Xi-an Zhang, Songtao Qi, Jun Pan, Yun-tao Lu, and Yi Liu; from left to right in the second row: Jing Nie, Jun-xiang Peng, Jin Shi, Chao-hu Wang, Zhan-peng Feng, Shi-chao Zhang, and Yun Bao

Part I

The Basics of Craniopharyngioma

Histology and Embryology Related to Craniopharyngiomas

1

Shi-chao Zhang and Chao-hu Wang

1.1 Introduction

Craniopharyngiomas are complex epithelial neoplasms of the sellar region and are divided by WHO into the adamantinomatous type (aCP) and the papillary type (pCP). It is considered that aCPs derive from neoplastic transformation of ectopic embryonic remnants of the craniopharyngeal duct and Rathke's pouch, and these tumors share features with odontogenic tumors suggesting a common origin. The pathogenesis of pCPs is less understood, but these tumors may arise from metaplastic transformation of anterior pituitary epithelial cells, especially those located in the pars tuberalis. Thus, craniopharyngiomas do not belong to neuroepithelial tumors, and embryological study is important for elucidating the features of craniopharyngioma.

The pia mater and the neural tube develop from the ectoderm. The pituitary stalk and the neurohypophysis are covered by the pia mater in continuity with the pia mater covering the nerve tissue of the third ventricle floor. Since craniopharyngioma does not originate from the neuroepithelium, it is understandable that craniopharyngioma is an extra-pia mater tumor.

1.2 Development of the Pituitary Gland

Rathke's pouch is a dorsal outgrowth of the primary oral inlet and appears at the 4th to 5th week during human embryologic development. It is also the ectodermal rudiment of the adenohypophysis (anterior lobe of the pituitary gland). The neurohypophysis (posterior lobe of the pituitary gland) arises from an evagination of neuroectoderm from the base of the diencephalon. A thickening in the wall of the diencephalon can be seen in the 5th week, and the wall continues to descend until flexing above the floor of Rathke's pouch from the 7th to 9th week (Fig. 1.1). At the same time, the oral part of Rathke's pouch is closed by mesenchymal cell differentiation. Then, the anterior wall of the pouch continues to grow and forms a cell mass, which is called the adenohypophysis primordium, and gives rise to the anterior lobe of the pituitary (Fig. 1.2). The upper part of Rathke's pouch rotates, partially wrapping the pituitary stalk leading to the formation of the pars tuberalis of the pituitary. Meanwhile, the posterior wall of the pouch remains as a tube-like structure with several layers of epithelial cells, which is the predecessor of the intermediate lobe of the pituitary.

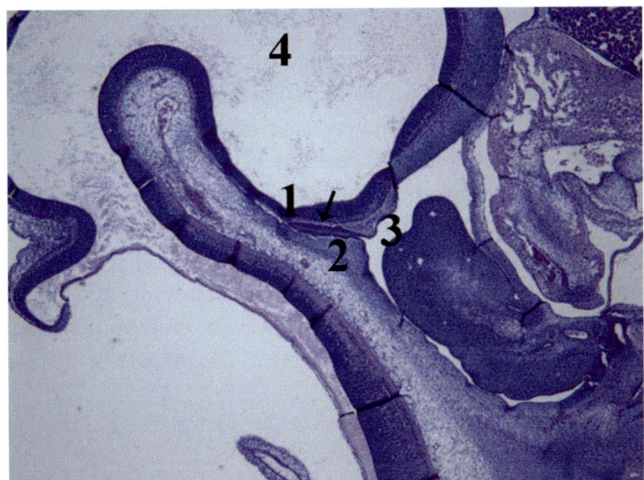

Fig. 1.1 A sagittal tissue section of a 7th week embryo (HE stain, 10 × 10). The brain vesicle can be seen, and the base of the diencephalon thickens. Meanwhile, Rathke's pouch grows into the incrassated diencephalon. A clear acidophilic stained demarcation is showed between them, which is considered to be the pia mater. (1) Diencephalon, (2) Rathke's pouch, (3) stomodeal, (4) brain vesicle. Arrow: Pia mater

S.-c. Zhang (✉) · C.-h. Wang
Department of Neurosurgery, Nanfang Hospital of Southern Medical University, Guangzhou, Guangdong, China

© Springer Nature Singapore Pte Ltd. 2020
S. Qi (ed.), *Atlas of Craniopharyngioma*, https://doi.org/10.1007/978-981-13-7322-0_1

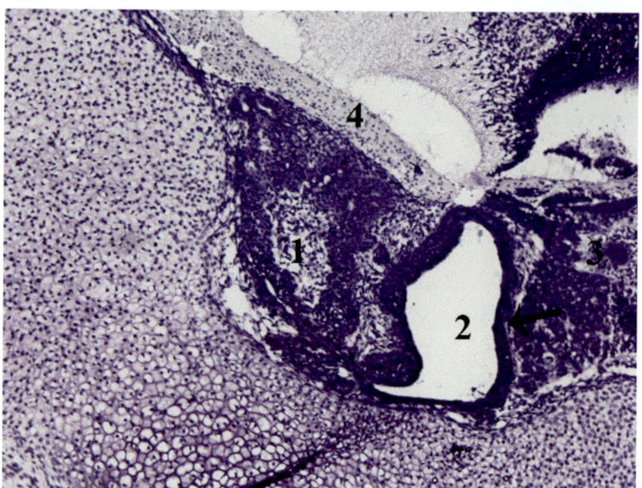

Fig. 1.2 A sagittal tissue section of a 10th week embryo (HE stain, 10 × 20). The mesenchymal cell differentiates to cartilage cell and closes the stomodeum part of Rathke's pouch. The anterior wall of Rathke's pouch continues to grow and forms a cell mass (adenohypophysis primordium). Meanwhile, the posterior Rathke's pouch remains as a tube-like structure with several layers of epithelial cells. An acidophilic stained demarcation can be seen between nervous tissue and Rathke's pouch. (1) Adenohypophysis primordium, (2) Rathke's pouch, (3) neurohypophysis, (4) mesenchymal cell, which is going to develop into the diaphragma sellae. Arrow: Pia mater

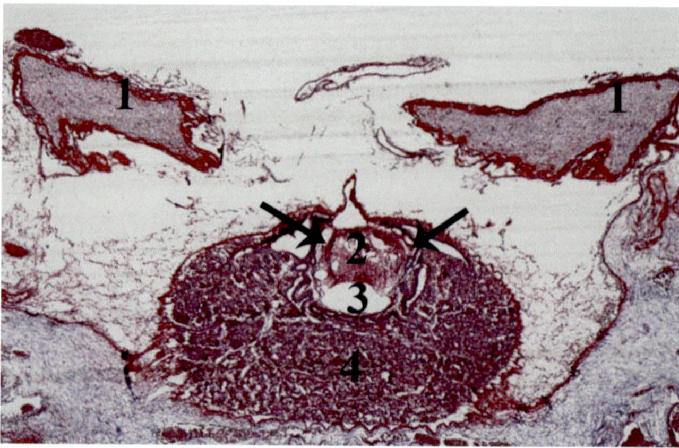

Fig. 1.3 A coronal tissue section of an 18th week fetus (Masson stain, 10 × 20). The collagenous fiber can be demonstrated as red and blue using Masson stain. The arachnoid covered outside of optic nerve can be seen. In the pituitary capsule, the pia mater, stained in red, can be seen. The posterior of Rathke's pouch is atrophied as a single layer of epithelial cells. The intermediate lobe of the pituitary is forming. (1) Optic nerve, (2) neurohypophysis, (3) Rathke's pouch, (4) adenohypophysis. Arrow: Pia mater

1.3 Embryonic Morphogenesis of Membrane Structures in the Sellar Region

The pia mater reportedly appears during early neural tube development from glioblasts. Both the arachnoid and the dura mater are differentiated from ectoderm mesenchymal cells. The arachnoid structure can be observed in the 10th week. As the approach of the anterior pituitary and posterior pituitary occurs during the 5th to 7th week of embryogenetic development, the pia mater and several layers of mesenchymal cells should separate Rathke's pouch and brain tissue (Fig. 1.3). Thus, from the point of view of embryonic development, Rathke's pouch is located in the outside of the pia mater.

1.4 Tumorigenesis of Craniopharyngiomas

The tumorigenesis of craniopharyngiomas remains controversial. However, two hypotheses are widely accepted: the embryonic residual and metaplastic hypotheses.

Adamantinomatous craniopharyngiomas occur predominantly in childhood. Rathke's pouch cells remain along the path of the craniopharyngeal duct during the formation of the adenohypophysis, and the residual cells may start growing to become aCPs after some specific genetic mutations. Mutation of *CTNNB1* exon 3, which will lead to the overactivation of the WNT pathway, is considered to be the key (maybe the only) genetic event during the initiation and growth of aCPs. It was reported that large cystic/solid tumors could be observed in the genetically engineered mouse with deleted exon 3 from the *CTNNB1* locus. The overactivation of the WNT pathway during murine development will lead to the tumor sharing numerous pathological features with aCPs in the sellar region.

Papillary craniopharyngioma mainly occurs in elder patients, and almost all originating points of pCPs are located in the upper part of the pituitary. Squamous metaplasia of the upper part of pituitary cells may be observed with aging. BRAFV600E mutation and overactivation of the MAPK pathway may lead to the formation of squamous cell nests.

Most importantly, both aCP and pCP originate from the adenohypophysis or its progenitor, Rathke's pouch. Combining the successive processes in embryonic development, the pituitary is formed later than the pia mater. Therefore, during the interaction between the adenohypophysis and neurohypophysis, an intact pia mater would separate these two structures (Fig. 1.4). Craniopharyngioma should be treated as an extra-pia mater tumor. The arachnoid around the sellar region may play an important role in the growth pattern of craniopharyngioma (Fig. 1.5).

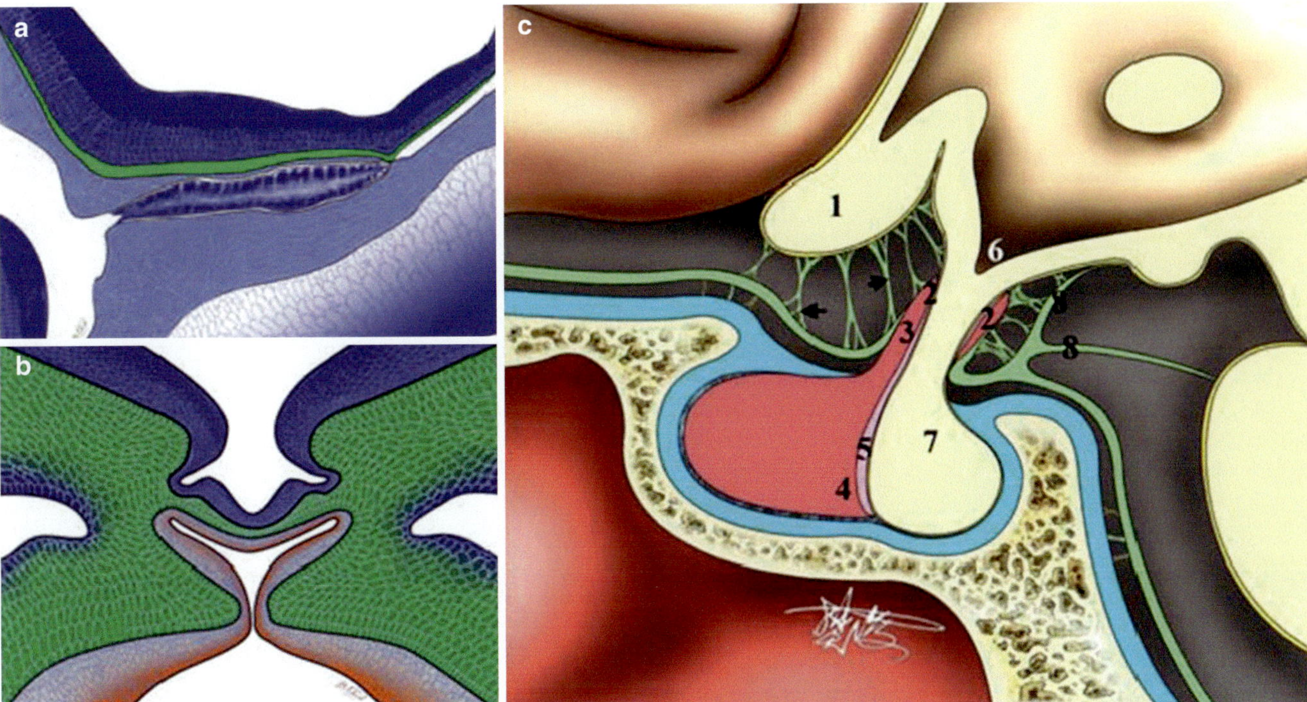

Fig. 1.4 Mode chart of the development of the pituitary. (**a**, **b**) show the sagittal and coronal views, respectively, of a 7th week embryo. (**a**) The green line shows the pia mater separating the nervous tissue from Rathke's pouch. (**b**) Rathke's pouch is shaped as a cup-like structure and is going to contact the incrassated wall of the diencephalon. Green cells represent the mesenchymal cells that are going to differentiate into the membrane structure in the sellar region. (**c**) Sagittal view of the pituitary. The pituitary stalk and neurohypophysis develop from nervous tissue, while pia mater (yellow line) separates them from the adenohypophysis and middle lobe. The inner arachnoid membrane and dura mater are shown as the green line and blue line, respectively. (1) Optic chiasm, (2) pars tuberalis of the pituitary, (3) sleeve segment of the pituitary stalk, (4) pituitary, (5) middle lobe of the pituitary gland, (6) infundibular recess, (7) neurohypophysis, (8) Liliequist membrane. Arrow: Trabecular arachnoid membranes in different diameters

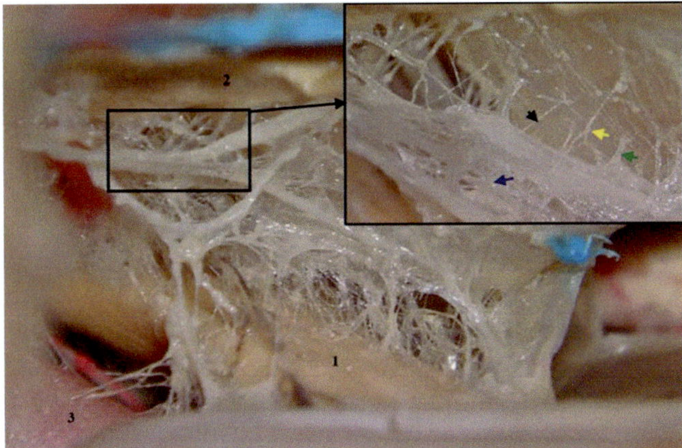

Fig. 1.5 Lateral aspect of the optic nerve (1), olfactory nerve (2), internal carotid (3). From the lateral aspect, the black box shows the arachnoid above the optic nerve. The different diameter arachnoid is displayed in magnification. The black arrow points to the smallest silk-like arachnoid. The cord-like arachnoid is ten times thicker than the silk-like arachnoid, which is shown by the yellow arrow. The green arrow shows the frenum-like arachnoid, which is thicker than the cord-like arachnoid. The blue arrow marks the arachnoid membrane and some naturally formed holes can be seen. These different diameter trabecular arachnoid membranes around the sellar region provide different force of constraint when a tumor grows in the arachnoid space; they will play an important role in the growth pattern of the tumor in the arachnoid space. Besides, the individual variation of the arachnoid trabecular number and diameter and distribution characteristics can be observed frequently in sellar tumor operations or autopsy

2 Surgical Anatomy

Xi'an Zhang, Yun-tao Lu, and Songtao Qi

2.1 Introduction

Craniopharyngioma is a benign tumor in a malignant location. A thorough knowledge of the relevant anatomy is an essential prerequisite for the accurate understanding of a surgical disease, reasonable surgical strategy, and better outcome.

As the anatomy of the sellar region is rich (Fig. 2.1), this chapter will only deal with those membranous structures germane to the issue of how the surrounding structures affect the growth of craniopharyngiomas. Many structures in this region, including the optic nerves, optic chiasma, optic tract, bony pituitary fossa, diaphragma sellae, and internal carotid artery and its branches, offer variable resistance to the progress of sellar region tumors and have been previously addressed. In light of our clinical and anatomical observations, we believe that the membranous structures, due to their considerable tensile strength and intimate relationship with the course of the craniopharyngeal duct, have a major directive effect on the course of craniopharyngiomas. The relationship between tumor and these membranous structures is also the anatomical basis for our novel classification of craniopharyngiomas.

As Atul Goel emphasized the importance of membranes in that: "the anatomical membranes are more primitive embryologically and are physically stronger than many other tissues in the body …… it may appear from an external appearance that the tumour has broken into the anatomical membrane, but on a 'closer' look it can be clear that the membrane may be thinned out or rolled over but never actually torn and transgressed …… it is crucial to understand the 'anatomy' of the tumour growth so that a preoperative impression of the nature of the tumour can be made and accordingly the surgical strategy can be planned" [1].

2.2 The Diaphragma Sellae

The pituitary gland is located within a dural sac, which generally does not easily lend itself to tumor invasion. This dural sac, however, has three potential weak points, at where intrasellar tumor may invade and progress. One is the opening of the diaphragma sellae, and the other two are the lateral walls of the pituitary dural sac. Although the lateral wall is single-layered and much thinner than the other dural walls of the pituitary fossa (Fig. 2.2), it is extremely rare that a newly diagnosed infra-diaphragmatic craniopharyngioma would assume the characteristics of pituitary adenoma in terms of cavernous sinus invasion.

Due to the remarkable variation, the actual dimensions of the opening of the diaphragma sellae determine the least resistant path in an infra-diaphragmatic craniopharyngioma (Figs. 2.3). When the opening of the diaphragma sellae is large and/or the tumor origin is close to the opening, the tumor may extrude through the opening by tracking up alongside the pituitary stalk. In contrast, when the opening of the diaphragma sellae is small and/or the tumor arises deep within the pituitary gland, the tumor's rounded dome is covered by the stretched but intact diaphragma sellae, which withstands more pressure than bone because it cannot be eroded.

X. Zhang (✉) · Y.-t. Lu · S. Qi
Department of Neurosurgery, Nanfang Hospital of Southern Medical University, Guangzhou, Guangdong, China
e-mail: zxa@smu.edu.cn

© Springer Nature Singapore Pte Ltd. 2020
S. Qi (ed.), *Atlas of Craniopharyngioma*, https://doi.org/10.1007/978-981-13-7322-0_2

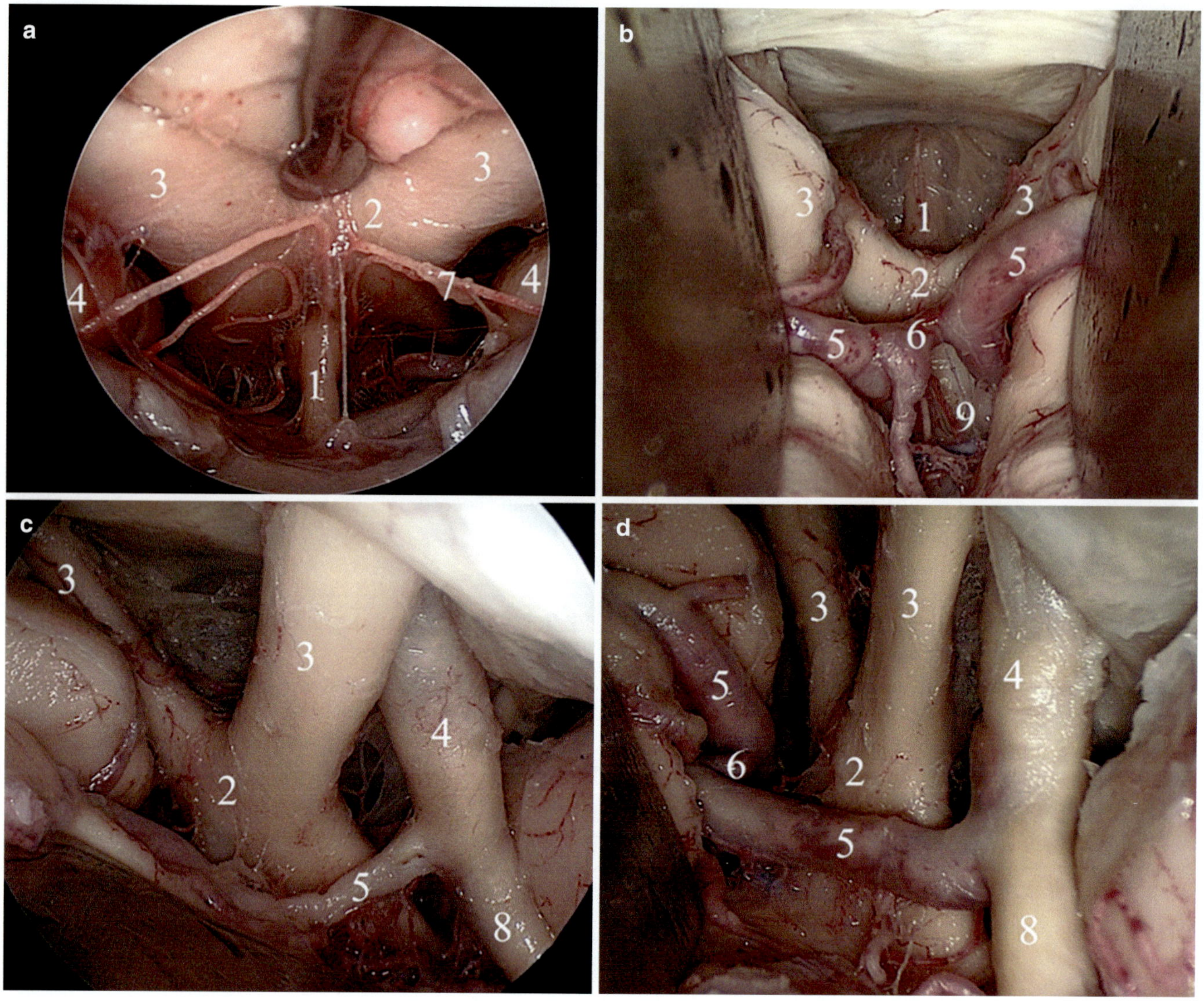

Fig. 2.1 Anatomical view of the sellar region from an endoscopic endonasal (**a**), interhemispheric (**b**), frontolateral (**c**), and pterional (**d**) perspective. (1) Pituitary stalk, (2) optic chiasm, (3) optic nerve, (4) internal carotid artery, (5) anterior cerebral artery, (6) anterior communicating artery, (7) superior hypophyseal artery, (8) middle cerebral artery, and (9) lamina terminalis

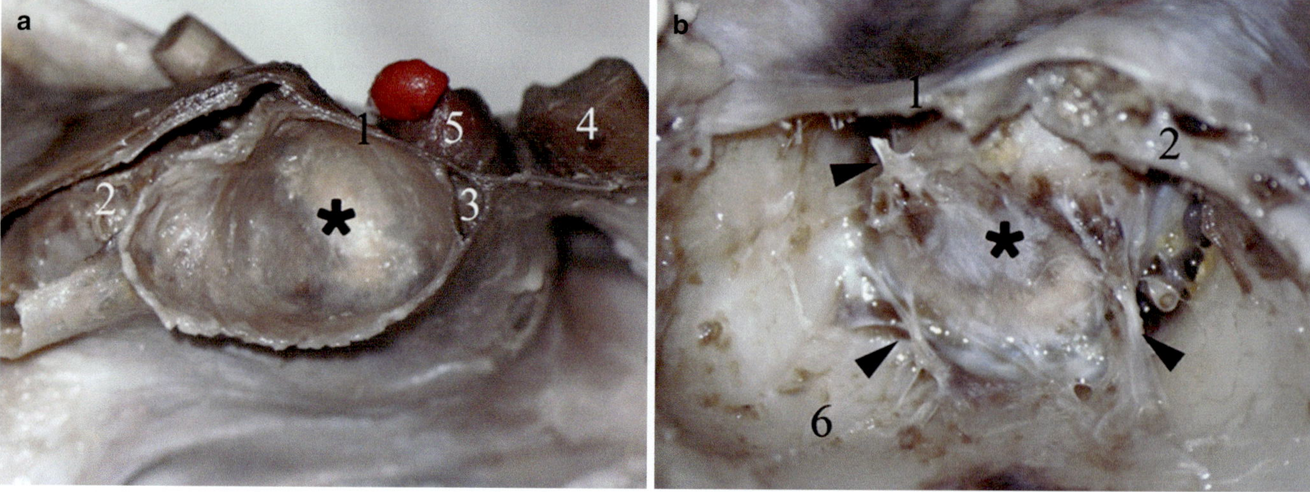

Fig. 2.2 Medial (**a**) and lateral (**b**) views of the pituitary dural sac showing that the meningeal dura-derived lateral wall (asterisks) is intact and anchored to the adjacent endosteal dura by ligaments (arrowheads). (1) Diaphragma sellae, (2) dorsum sellae, (3) inter-cavernous sinus, (4) optic nerve, (5) internal carotid artery, and (6) carotid sulcus

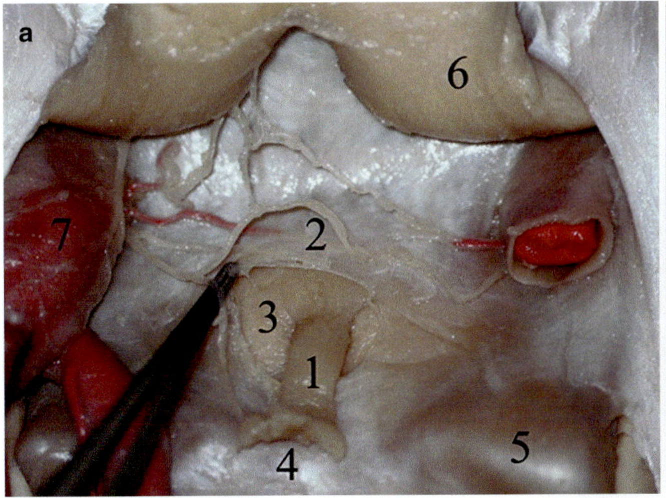

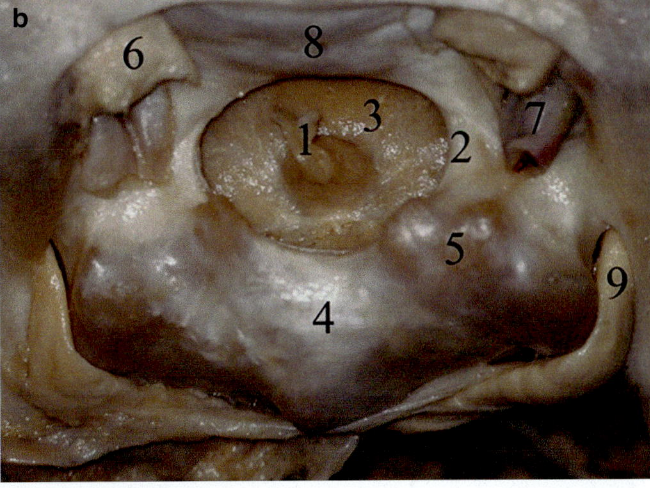

Fig. 2.3 Superior views showing the variable morphology of the opening of the diaphragma sellae among individuals. (**a**) Relatively small opening. (**b**) Large opening. (1) Pituitary stalk, (2) diaphragma sellae, (3) pituitary gland, (4) dorsum sellae, (5) posterior clinoid process, (6) optic nerve, (7) internal carotid artery, (8) tuberculum sellae, and (9) oculomotor nerve

2.3 The Arachnoid Sleeve Enveloping the Pituitary Stalk (ASPS)

The pituitary stalk is enveloped by the arachnoid mater sleeve (ASPS), which is a direct upward extension of the basal arachnoid membrane covering the diaphragma sellae (Figs. 2.4 and 2.5) [3, 4]. At the upper part of the pituitary stalk, the ASPS ends at the top of the pars tuberalis. The arachnoid sleeve is reinforced by the arachnoid trabeculae originating from the adjacent basal and cisternal arachnoid membranes. For a suprasellar craniopharyngioma, the ASPS is, in our opinion, the most important structure in directing the growth of the tumor. The Liliequist membrane and membranes surrounding the internal carotid artery (such as the medial carotid membrane) are also very important and provide an effective barrier for craniopharyngioma to encroach the vascular-rich interpeduncular, carotid, and Sylvian cisterns, when they are dense sheet-like membranes with less and smaller openings.

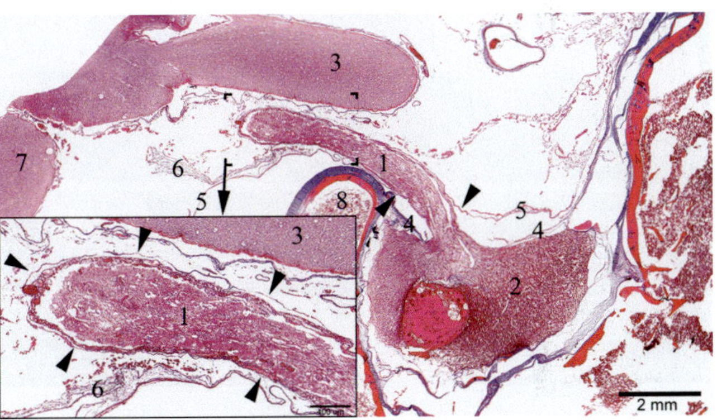

Fig. 2.4 Histological view of the ASPS. Sagittal histologic section through the pituitary stalk (Masson trichrome stain) showing that the ASPS (arrowheads) starts at the lower part of the pituitary stalk near the opening of diaphragma sellae and extends upward to envelop the pituitary stalk (inset). Note that the thickened inner layer of the basal arachnoid membrane covering the dorsum sellae extends superoposteriorly and folds upon itself to form the basal part of the Liliequist membrane (inset) and the latter sends out arachnoid trabeculae to attach to the ASPS [2]. (1) Pituitary stalk, (2) pituitary gland, (3) optic chiasm, (4) diaphragma sellae, (5) basal arachnoid membrane, (6) Liliequist membrane, (7) mammillary body, and (8) dorsum sellae

2.4 The Membrane Separating the Neuro- from the Adenohypophysis

Between the intermediate and posterior lobes, there is a membranous septum, which is direct downwards extension of the pia mater covering the undersurface of the optic chiasma and hypothalamus, courses the full length of the pituitary stalk between pars tuberalis and the neural part of the pituitary stalk. In the pituitary gland, this membranous septum lies between the intermediate and posterior lobes of the pituitary gland (Fig. 2.6) [5]. At the bottom and lateral sides of the interface between the intermediate and posterior lobes of the pituitary gland, this septum appears to fuse with the pituitary capsule. There is no such septum between the intermediate and anterior lobes. We further confirmed that the membranous septum is pia mater (Fig. 2.7).

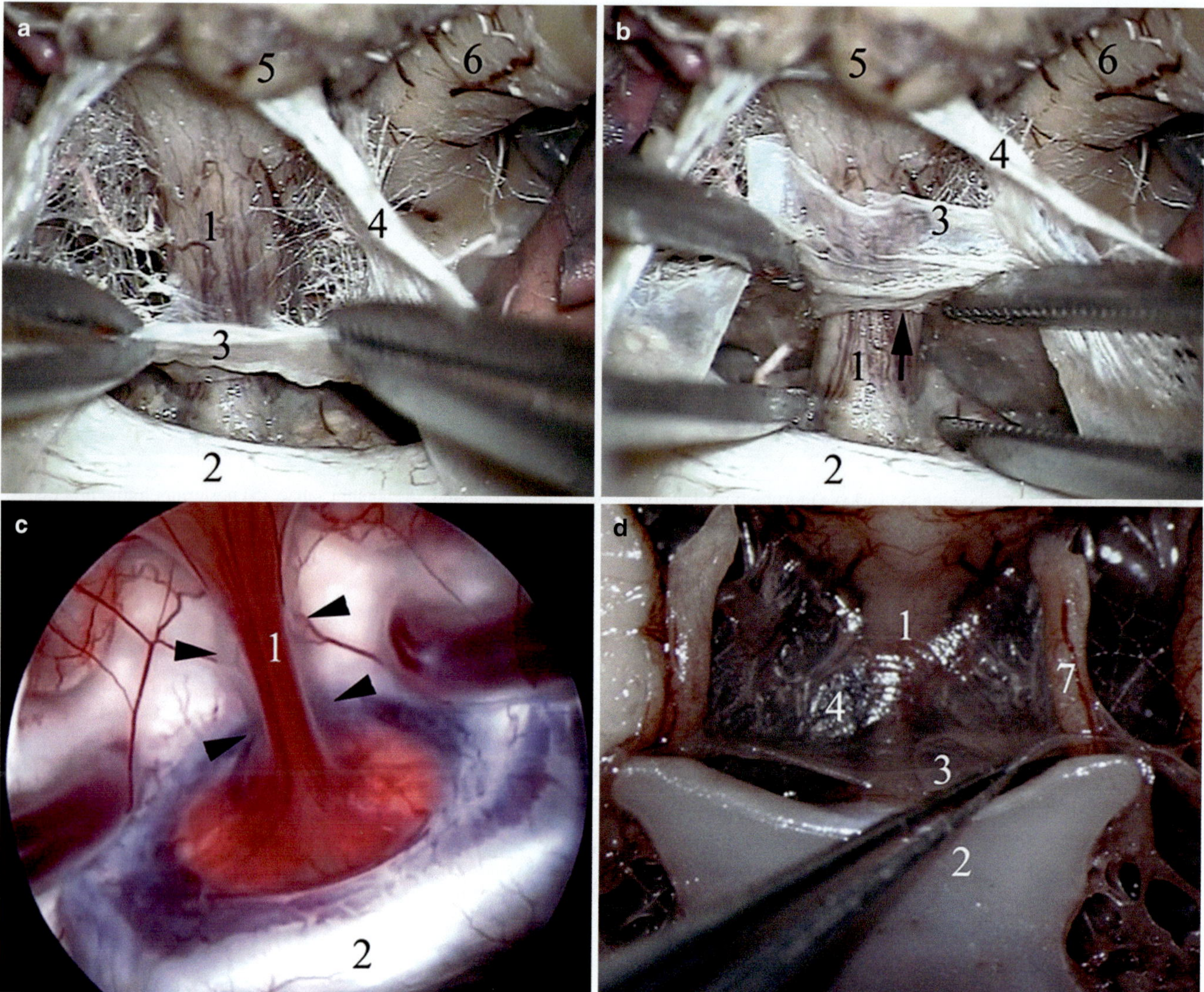

Fig. 2.5 Anatomical and intraoperative views of the ASPS and Liliequist membrane. (**a**, **b**) Posterior views of the ASPS during cadaveric dissection showing that the ASPS (arrow) can be easily stripped upward to the middle part of the pituitary stalk. (**c**) Intraoperative observation of the ASPS in a patient with an interpeduncular cistern arachnoid cyst. Note that after fenestration of the cyst, the irrigation fluid entering the subdural space inflated the ASPS (arrowheads) through tears on the basal arachnoid membrane. (**d**) Posterior views of ASPS during cadaveric dissection showing a totally dense sheet-like Liliequist membrane without opening as compared with the porous trabeculated one shown in figure (**a**). (1) Pituitary stalk, (2) dorsum sellae, (3) basal arachnoid membrane optic chiasm, (4) Liliequist membrane, (5) mammillary body, (6) optic tract, and (7) oculomotor nerve

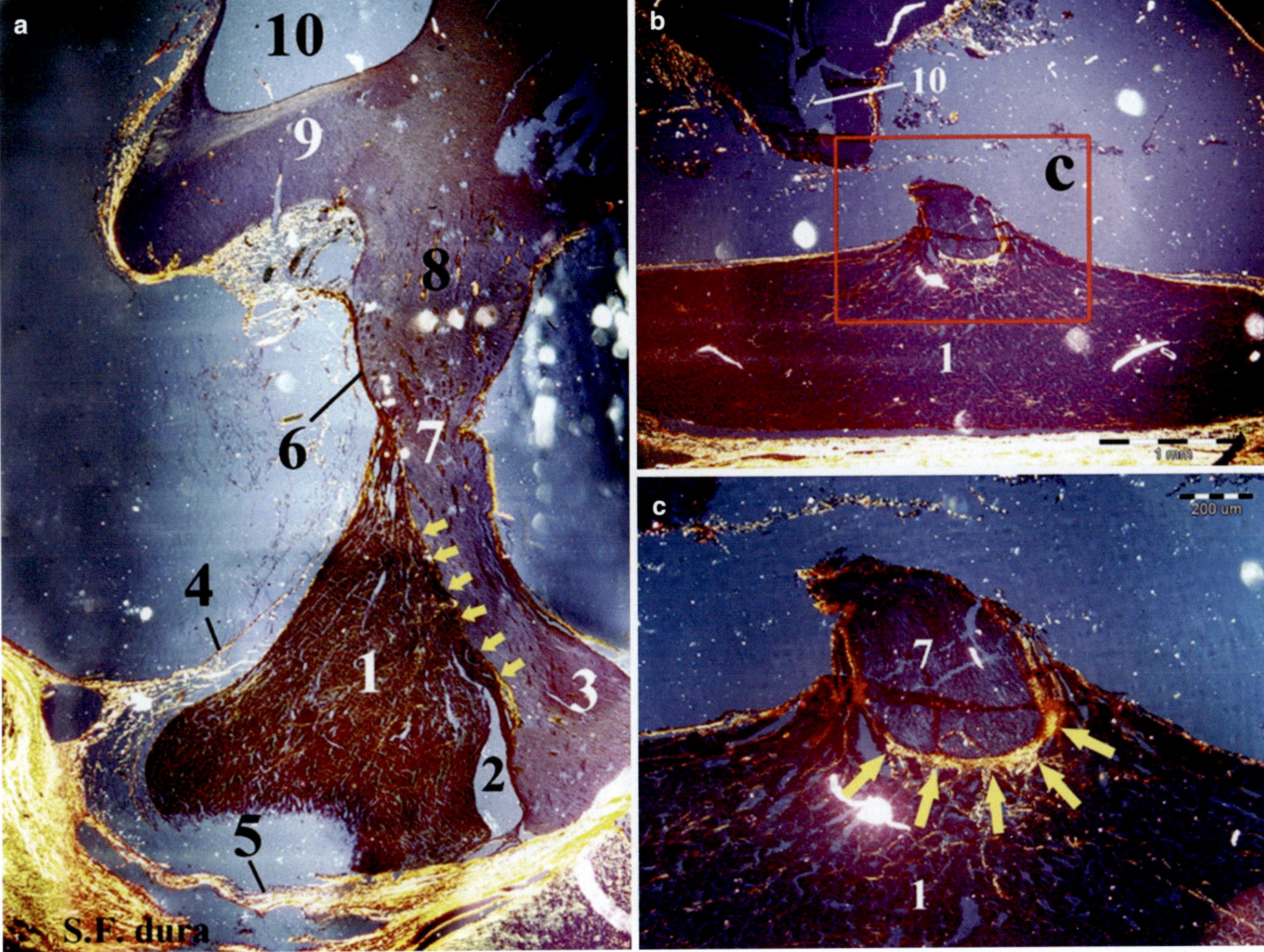

Fig. 2.6 Sagittal (**a**) and coronal (**b**, **c**) sections of the pituitary gland showing the membranous septum (yellow arrows) between the adeno- and the neurohypophysis (picrosirius red staining in combination with polarization microscopy). (1) Adenohypophysis, (2) intermediate lobe of the gland, (3) posterior lobe, (4) diaphragma sellae, (5) pituitary capsule, (6) pars tuberalis, (7) pituitary stalk, (8) infundibular tuberculum, (9) optic chiasm, and (10) third ventricle

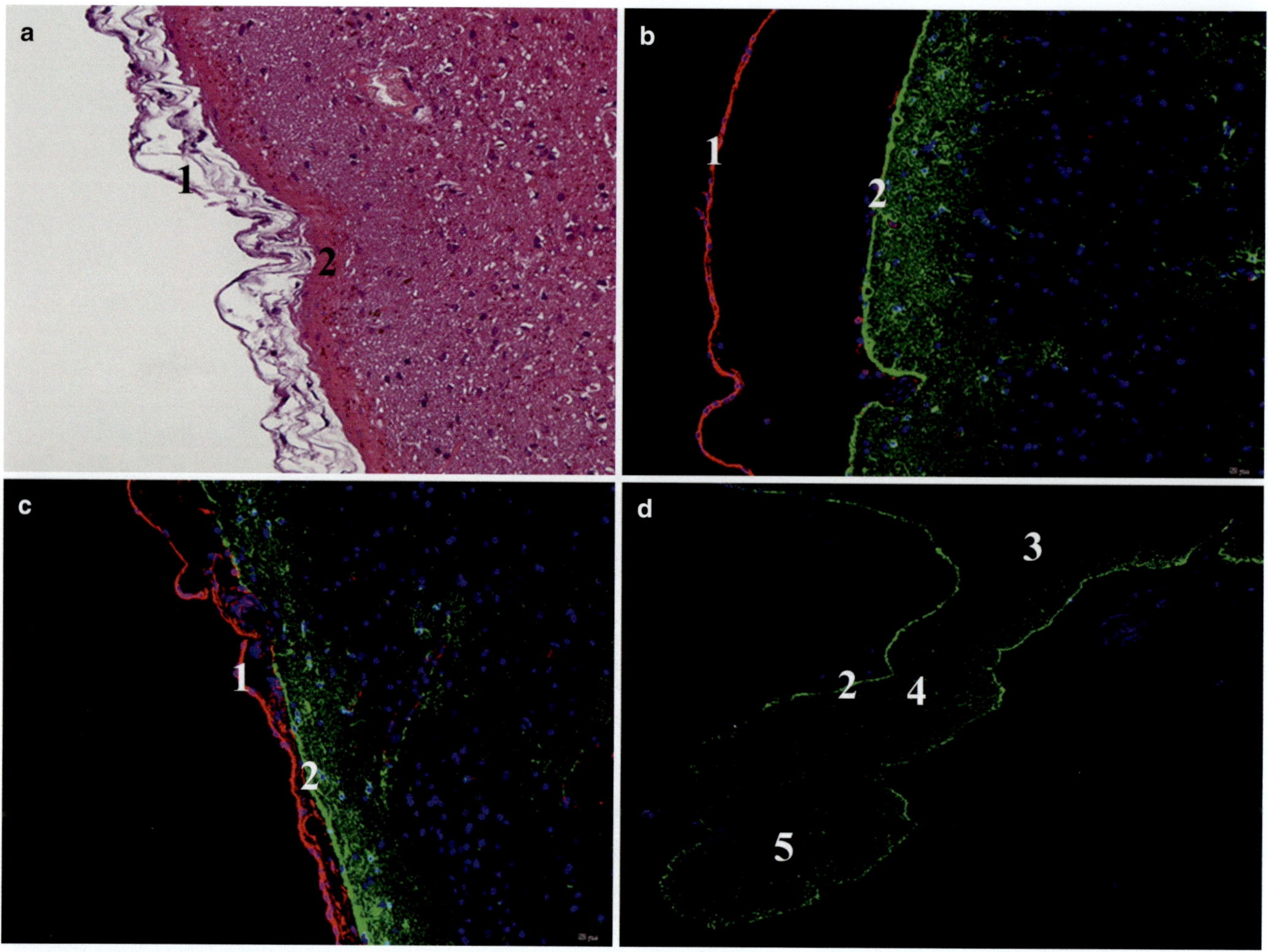

Fig. 2.7 (**a–c**) Immunofluorescence staining of arachnoid and pia mater of brain, the red is for arachnoid and green for pia mater. (**d**) Immunofluorescence staining of the pituitary stalk, which confirmed the membranous septum is pia mater. (1) Arachnoid, (2) pia mater, (3) third ventricle floor, (4) pituitary stalk, and (5) neurohypophysis

References

1. Goel A. Expert's comments. On: Ohata K, Tsuyuguchi N, Morino M, Takami T, Goto T, Hakuba A, Hara M. A hypothesis of epiarachnoidal growth of vestibular schwannoma at the cerebello-pontine angle: surgical importance. J Postgrad Med. 2002;48(4):253–9.
2. Zhang XA, Qi ST, Huang GL, Long H, Fan J, Peng JX. Anatomical and histological study of Liliequist's membrane: with emphasis on its nature and lateral attachments. Childs Nerv Syst. 2012;28(1):65–72.
3. Song-tao Q, Xi-an Z, Hao L, Jun F, Jun P, Yun-tao L. The arachnoid sleeve enveloping the pituitary stalk: anatomical and histologic study. Neurosurgery. 2010;66(3):585–9.
4. Qi S, Lu Y, Pan J, Zhang X, Long H, Fan J. Anatomic relations of the arachnoidea around the pituitary stalk: relevance for surgical removal of craniopharyngiomas. Acta Neurochir. 2011;153(4):785–96.
5. Lu YT, Qi ST, Xu JM, Pan J, Shi J. A membranous structure separating the adenohypophysis and neurohypophysis: an anatomical study and its clinical application for craniopharyngioma. J Neurosurg Pediatr. 2015;15(6):630–7.

3 QST Classification for Craniopharyngioma and Histopathological Aspect

Yi Liu, Chao-hu Wang, and Songtao Qi

3.1 Introduction

The pathological diagnosis of craniopharyngioma is not complicated; however, it is very important to understand the relationship between tumors and the adjacent structures and to clarify the true origin and growth pattern of craniopharyngioma from the histological level. Therefore, the main contents of this chapter is to show the pathological manifestations of craniopharyngioma itself, as well as the relationship between tumor and pituitary stalk, the third ventricle floor, and the pituitary gland. The purpose of this chapter is not only to prove that the tumor was epi-pia mater originated. At the site of tumor origin, the pia mater between tumor and third ventricle floor and pituitary stalk could be disappeared, and the tumor could directly contact with third ventricle floor and pituitary stalk. All of this is the basis of QST classification and is important for protection of the surrounding structure.

Craniopharyngioma is divided into two pathological types, namely, adamantinomatous craniopharyngioma (aCP) and papillary craniopharyngioma (pCP), in the 2017 version of the WHO central nervous system pathological classification. This chapter describes the typical pathological features of the two types of craniopharyngioma, as well as the pathological relationship between the tumor and surrounding structures.

3.2 Adamantinomatous Craniopharyngioma (aCP)

Typical pathological features of aCP include whorl-like cells, stellate reticulum, and palisade-like epithelial cells. Within the tumor parenchyma, wet keratin and varying degrees of calcification are observed. In some cystic tumors, cysts of different sizes can be seen. The cystic cavity is mainly composed of cholesterol crystals and necrotic tumor cells (Fig. 3.1).

3.3 Papillary Craniopharyngioma (pCP)

The typical pathological feature of pCP is the stratified papillary squamous epithelium. At the center of the squamous epithelium, the fibrous vascular core is visible. The cells around the fiber core are called the basal cells. In the tumor parenchyma, new blood vessels of different sizes and densities can be seen. In pCP, calcification and wet keratin are rare, and cystic cavities are still visible in some tumor parenchyma (Fig. 3.2).

Y. Liu (✉) · C.-h. Wang · S. Qi
Department of Neurosurgery, Nanfang Hospital of Southern Medical University, Guangzhou, Guangdong, China

© Springer Nature Singapore Pte Ltd. 2020
S. Qi (ed.), *Atlas of Craniopharyngioma*, https://doi.org/10.1007/978-981-13-7322-0_3

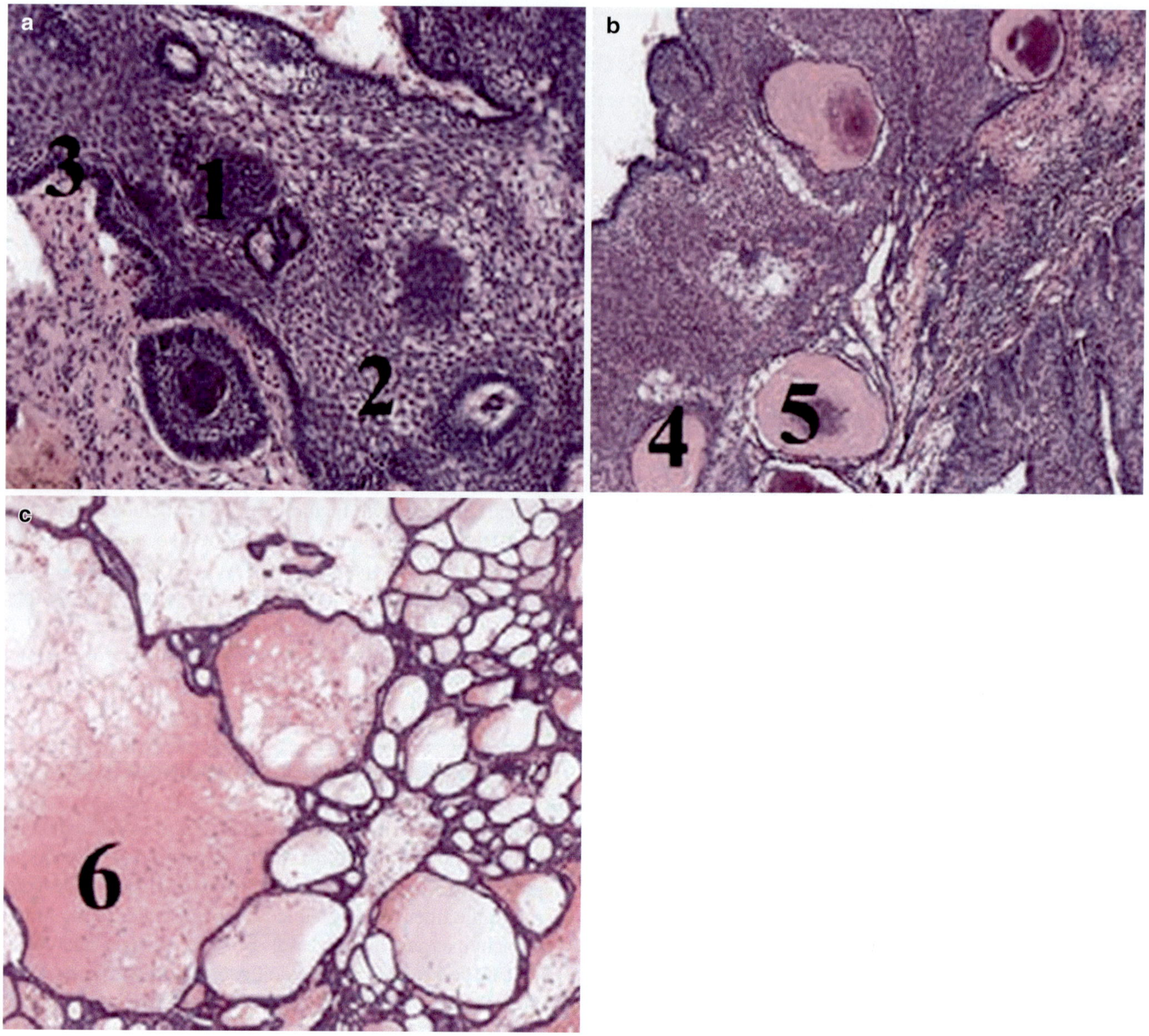

Fig. 3.1 Pathological manifestation of aCP (**a**–**c**). (1) Whorl-like cells, (2) stellate reticulum, (3) palisade-like cells, (4) wet keratin, (5) calcification, (6) cysts

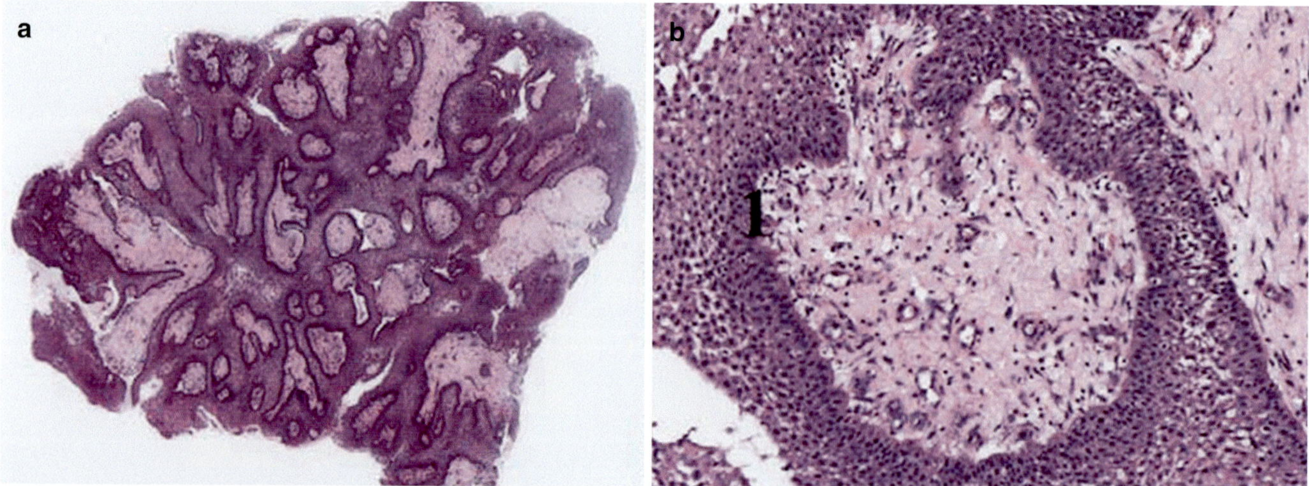

Fig. 3.2 Typical pathological performance of pCP (**a**, **b**). (1) Basal cells

3.4 The Four Segments of Pituitary Stalk

Previously, we found that the suprasellar arachnoid arising from the basement membrane of the arachnoid envelops the pituitary stalk to form an arachnoidal sleeve (ASPS). The pituitary stalk was divided into four segments in accordance with the folds of the ASPS, namely, the infradiaphragmatic, extra-arachnoidal, intra-arachnoidal, and subarachnoidal segments (Fig. 3.3).

3.5 QST Typing System for Craniopharyngioma

On the basis of the tumor origin and on the presence of an arachnoid envelope around the pituitary stalk (ASPS), we established a QST typing system for craniopharyngioma (Fig. 3.4). Type Q tumors originate below the diaphragma, and the pituitary gland is therefore most likely to be involved. Type S tumors originate from pars tuberalis adherent to the

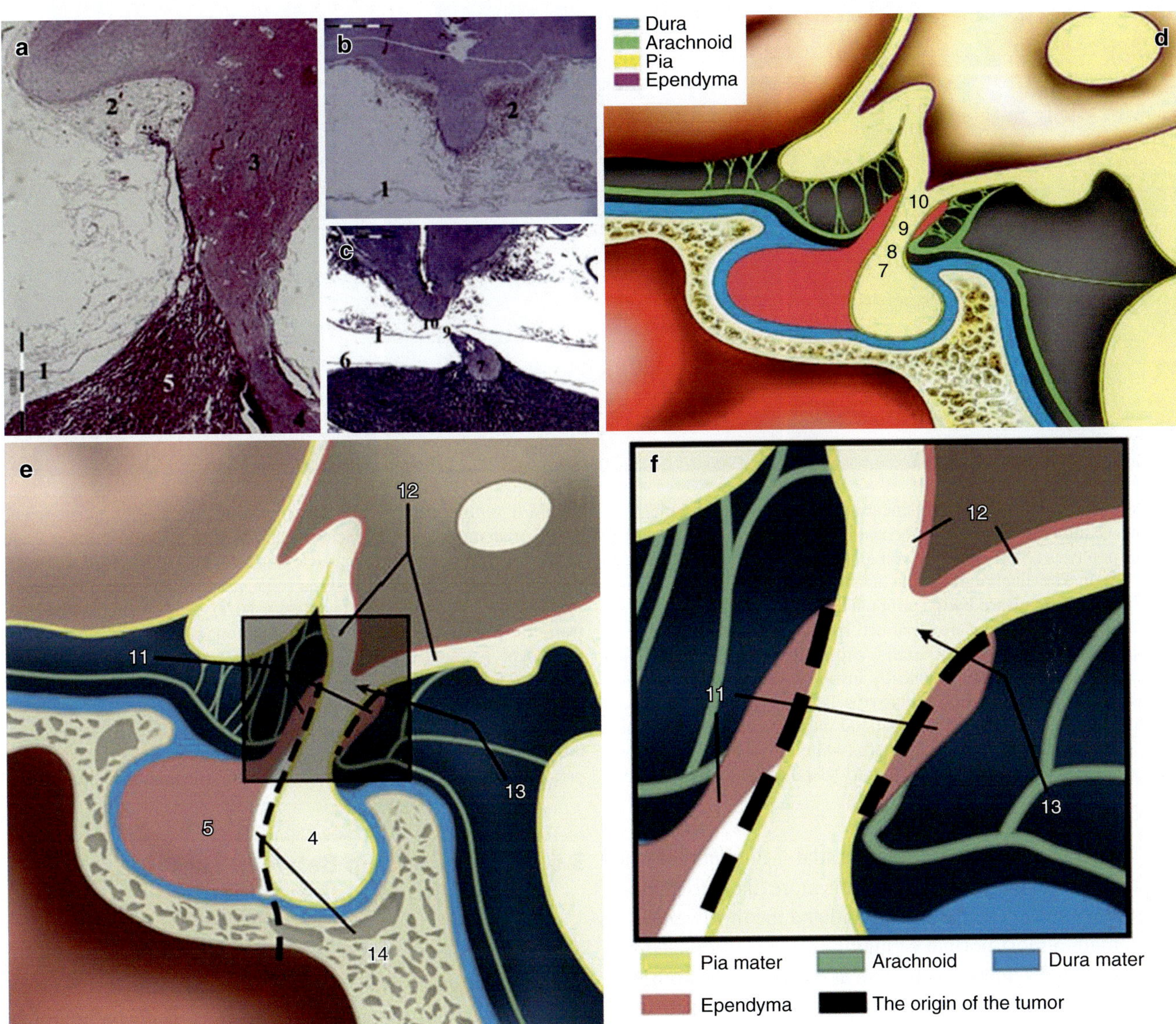

Fig. 3.3 The four segments of pituitary stalk and membrane structures in sellar area (**a–f**). (1) Basal arachnoid membrane (BAM), (2) arachnoid trabecula, (3) pituitary stalk, (4) neurohypophysis, (5) pars distalis, (6) diaphragma sellae, (7) infradiaphragmatic segment, (8) extra-arachnoidal segment, (9) intra-arachnoidal segment, (10) subarachnoidal segment, (11) pars tuberalis, (12) median eminence, (13) infundibular, (14) intermediate lobe

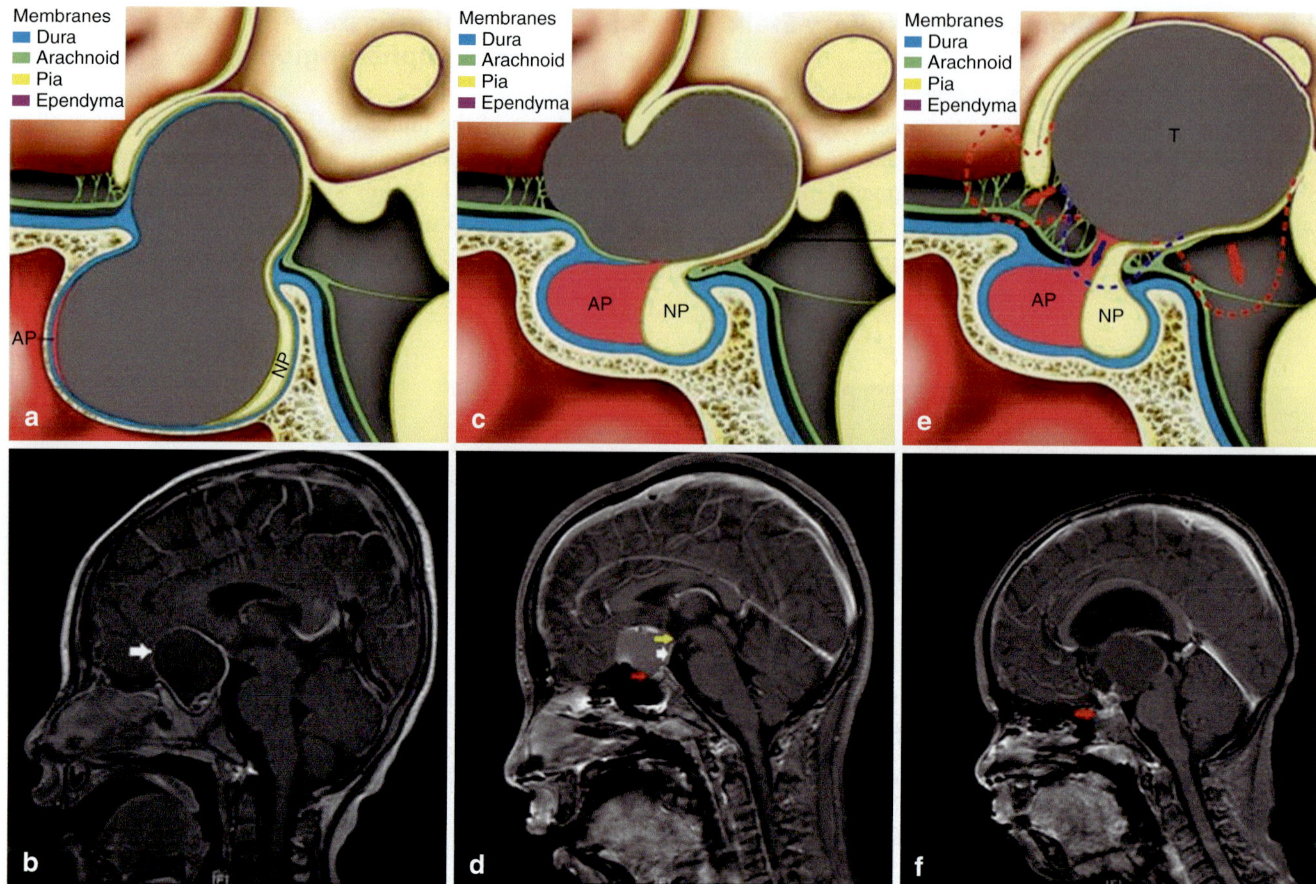

Fig. 3.4 Schematic of QST classification for craniopharyngioma. (**a**, **b**) Type Q tumors (T) originate beneath the diaphragma sellae. The adenohypophysis (AP) and the neurohypophysis (NP) were compressed by the tumor. The diaphragm (while arrow head) covers the tumor and was often pushed upward by the tumor. The tumor and the nerve layer of the third ventricle floor are separated by a multilayered membrane structure. Even when the tumor extends suprasellarly, the nerve layer of the third ventricle floor is not typically involved. (**c**, **d**) Type S tumors originate from Rathke's pouch precursor cells that remain in pars tuberalis adherent to the extra-arachnoidal and intra-arachnoidal segments of the pituitary stalk. The pituitary stalk (white arrow head) was most likely involved by the tumor. The pituitary gland (red arrow head) and the third ventricle floor (yellow arrow head) were often normal. The ASPS or an inner layer of arachnoid can be seen between the tumor and the nerve layer of the third ventricle floor, which makes surgical separation fairly simple. The diaphragma sellae prevent the tumor from growing downward into the pituitary fossa. (**e**, **f**) Type T tumors originate from Rathke's pouch precursor cells that remain in the top of pars tuberalis. Type T tumors are located beneath the basal arachnoid membrane and outside the pia mater. The lower part of the pituitary stalk (PS) and the pituitary gland (red arrow) was often normal. The third ventricle floor could be not appeared in MRI. Some type T tumors can grow through the ASPS or break through the inner arachnoid layer near the pars tuberalis, subsequently growing into the subarachnoid space

extra-arachnoidal and intra-arachnoidal segments of the pituitary stalk, and this type of tumor is more likely to involve the pituitary stalk. The pituitary gland and the third ventricle floor remain almost normal or may be slightly displaced by the tumor. Type T tumors originate at the top of pars tuberalis. These tumors are located in the subarachnoid space, outside the pia mater, and usually occupy the third ventricle cavity, involving the third ventricle floor and the proximal pituitary stalk; the distal pituitary stalk and pituitary gland are usually normal.

3.6 Relationship Between Tumor and Surrounding Structure

According to the QST classification, Q-type tumors are all almost belongs to aCP, and the tumor mainly involves the pituitary gland (Figs. 3.5, 3.6, and 3.7). Both pathological types can be found in S-type and T-type tumors. S-type tumors mainly involve the pituitary stalks (Fig. 3.8), while T-type tumors mainly involve both the third ventricle floor (hypothalamus) and pituitary stalk (Figs. 3.9–3.12).

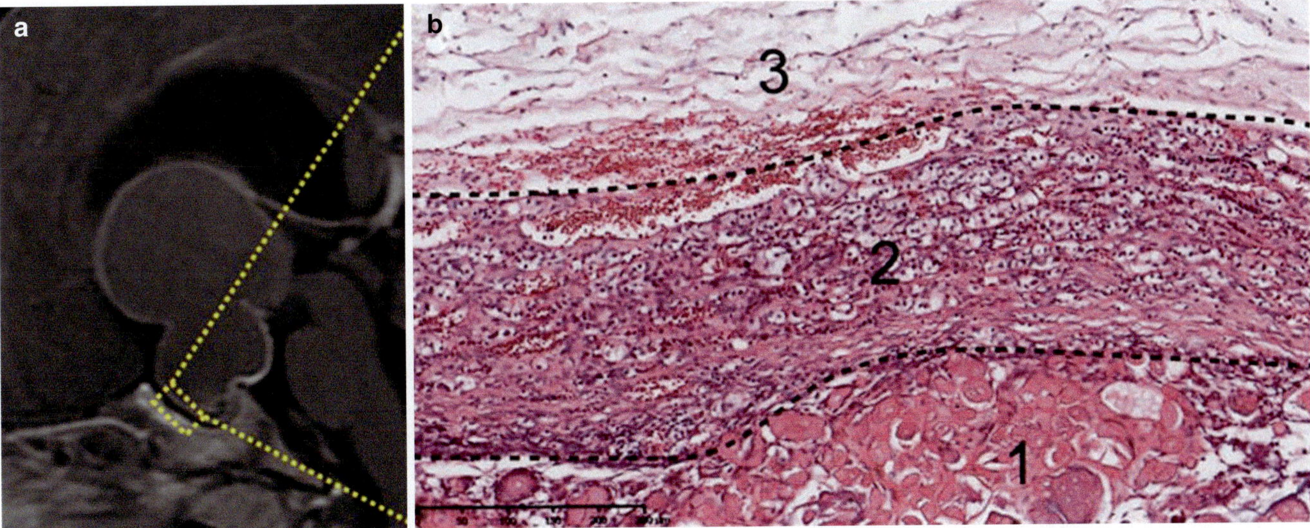

Fig. 3.5 Relationship between Q-type tumor and adenohypophysis (**a**, **b**). The boundary between the tumor and adenohypophysis is clear. (1) Tumor, (2) adenohypophysis, (3) pituitary capsule

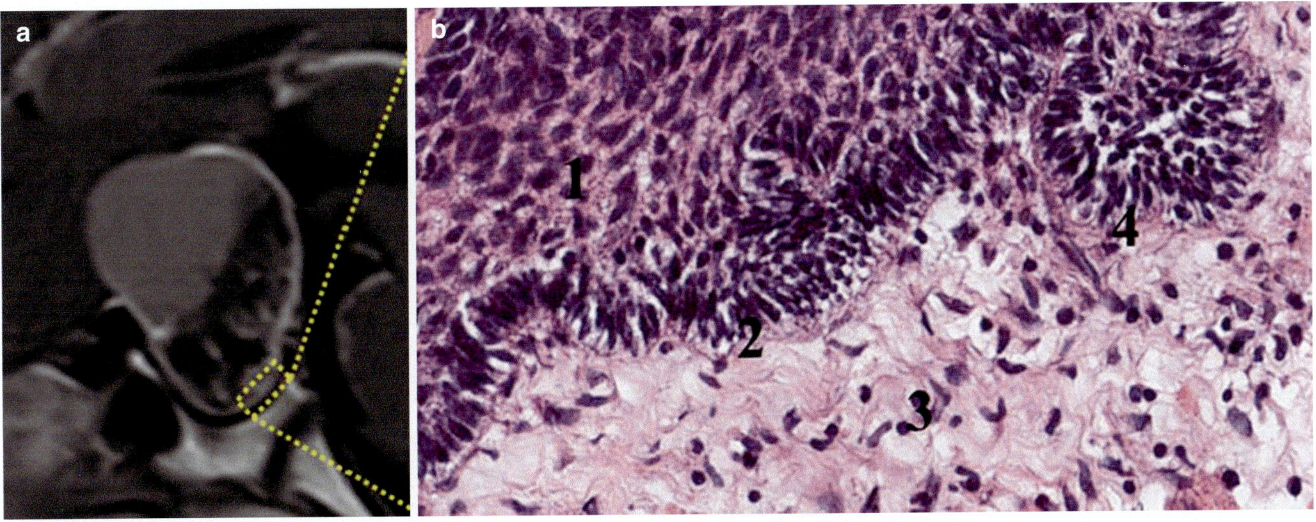

Fig. 3.6 Relationship between Q-type tumor and neurohypophysis (**a**, **b**). Sometimes the mortise-like structure can be seen between tumor and neurohypophysis, and the pia mater could be disrupted. (1) Tumor, (2) pia mater, (3) neurohypophysis, (4) mortise-like structure

3.6.1 Relationship Between Q-Type Tumor and Peripheral Structure

3.6.2 Relationship Between S-Type Tumor and Peripheral Structure

Both pathological types can occur in S-type tumors, and S-type tumors mainly involve pituitary stalks (Fig. 3.8).

3.6.3 Relationship Between T-Type Tumor and Peripheral Structure

From HE staining, we defined the relationship between ACP and the third ventricle floor as three types, including mortise and tenon(m-t)-like (Fig. 3.9), moat-like and marsh-like types (Fig. 3.10). M-t-like type is more common at the origin site of the tumor, and the latter two are more common at the

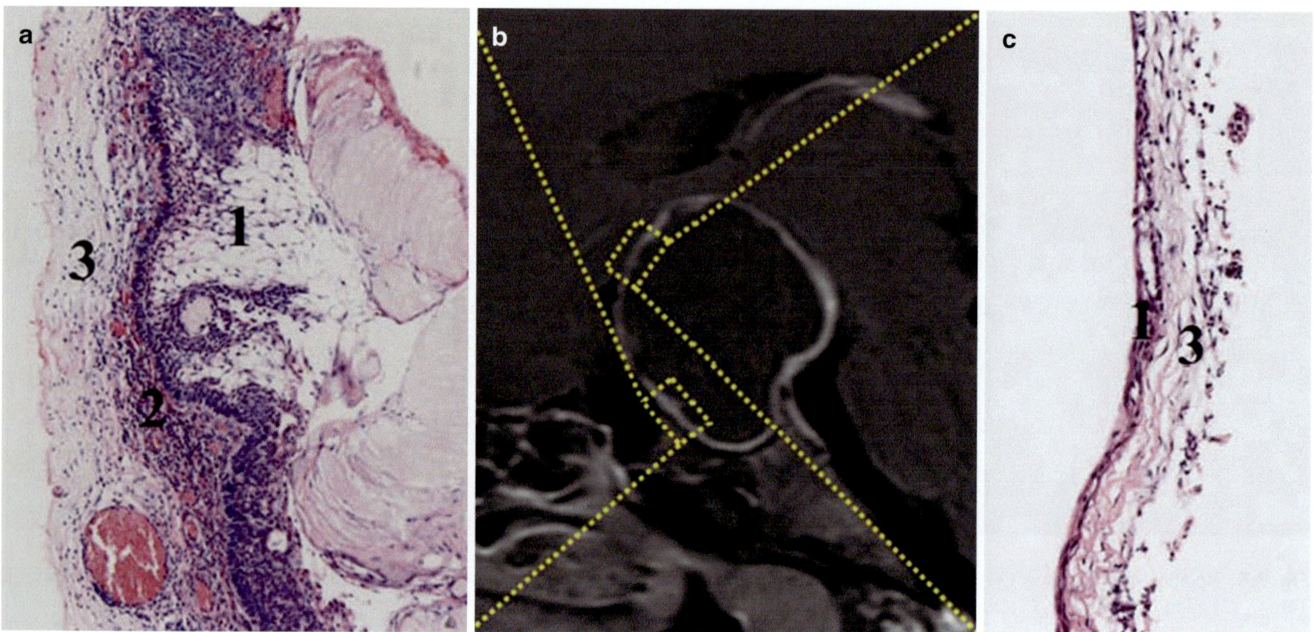

Fig. 3.7 The relationship between type Q tumor and diaphragma sella (**a**–**c**). The boundary between the tumor and diaphragma sella is clear. Sometimes adenohypophysis was compressed by the tumor and was attached to the diaphragma sella. (1) Tumor, (2) adenohypophysis, (3) diaphragma sella

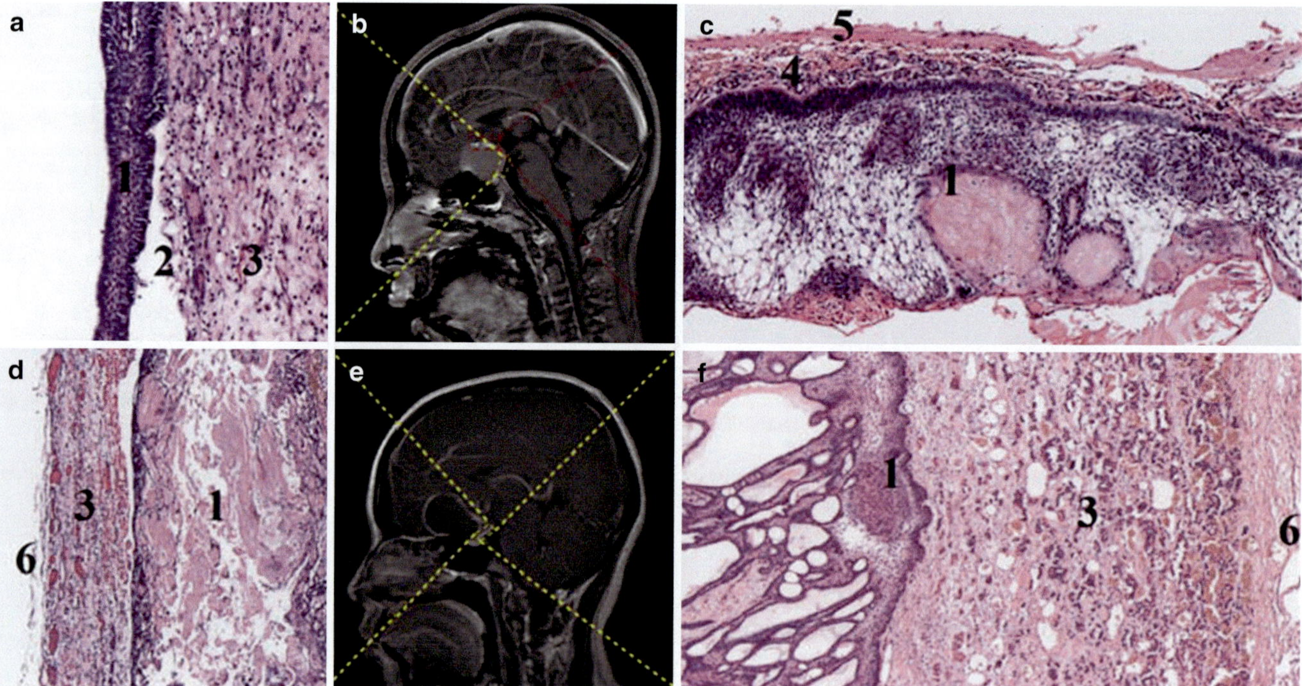

Fig. 3.8 The relationship between type S tumor and the pituitary stalk and third ventricle floor. In upper case, the boundary between the S-type aCP and the pituitary stalk is clear, and there is still pia mater between tumor and pituitary stalk (**a**, **b**). The third ventricle floor is involved by the tumor; however, there is still arachnoid trabecula separating the tumor and the third ventricle floor (**c**). At the lower case, the tumor grows within the ASPS and only compresses the stalk at the non-origin site (**d**, **e**). At the origin site of the tumor, the pia mater between the tumor and the pituitary stalk can be destroyed, resulting in the pituitary stalk being involved (**f**). (1) Tumor, (2) pia mater, (3) pituitary stalk, (4) arachnoid trabecula, (5) third ventricle floor, (6) ASPS

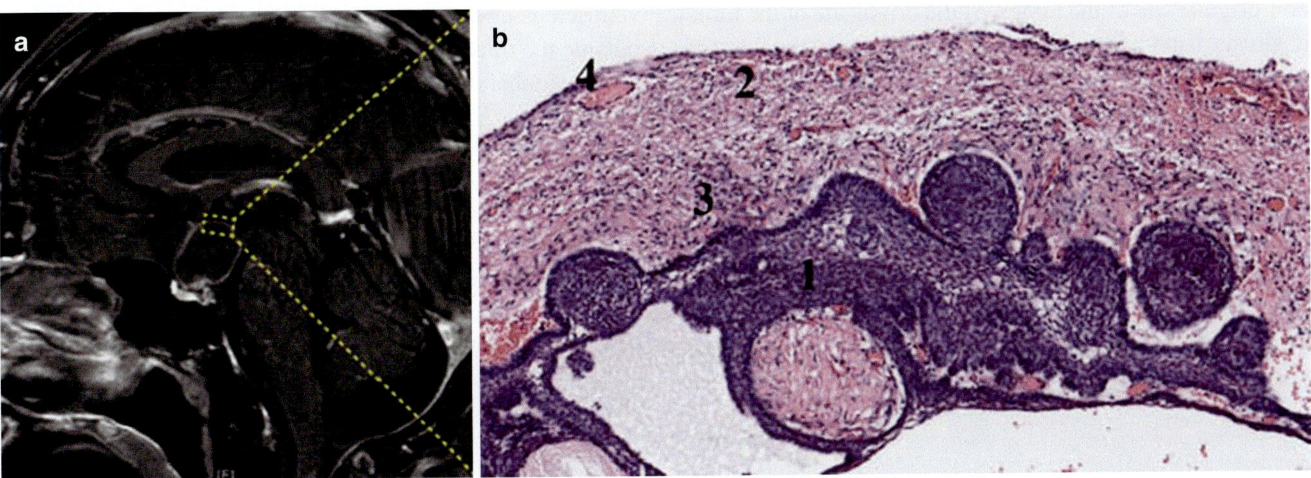

Fig. 3.9 T-type aCP forms m-t-like type with the third ventricle floor (**a**, **b**). There is always the gliosis band between tumor and the nervous layer of the third ventricle floor. (1) Tumor (m-t-like structure), (2) nerve tissue of third ventricle floor, (3) gliosis band, (4) ependymal cells

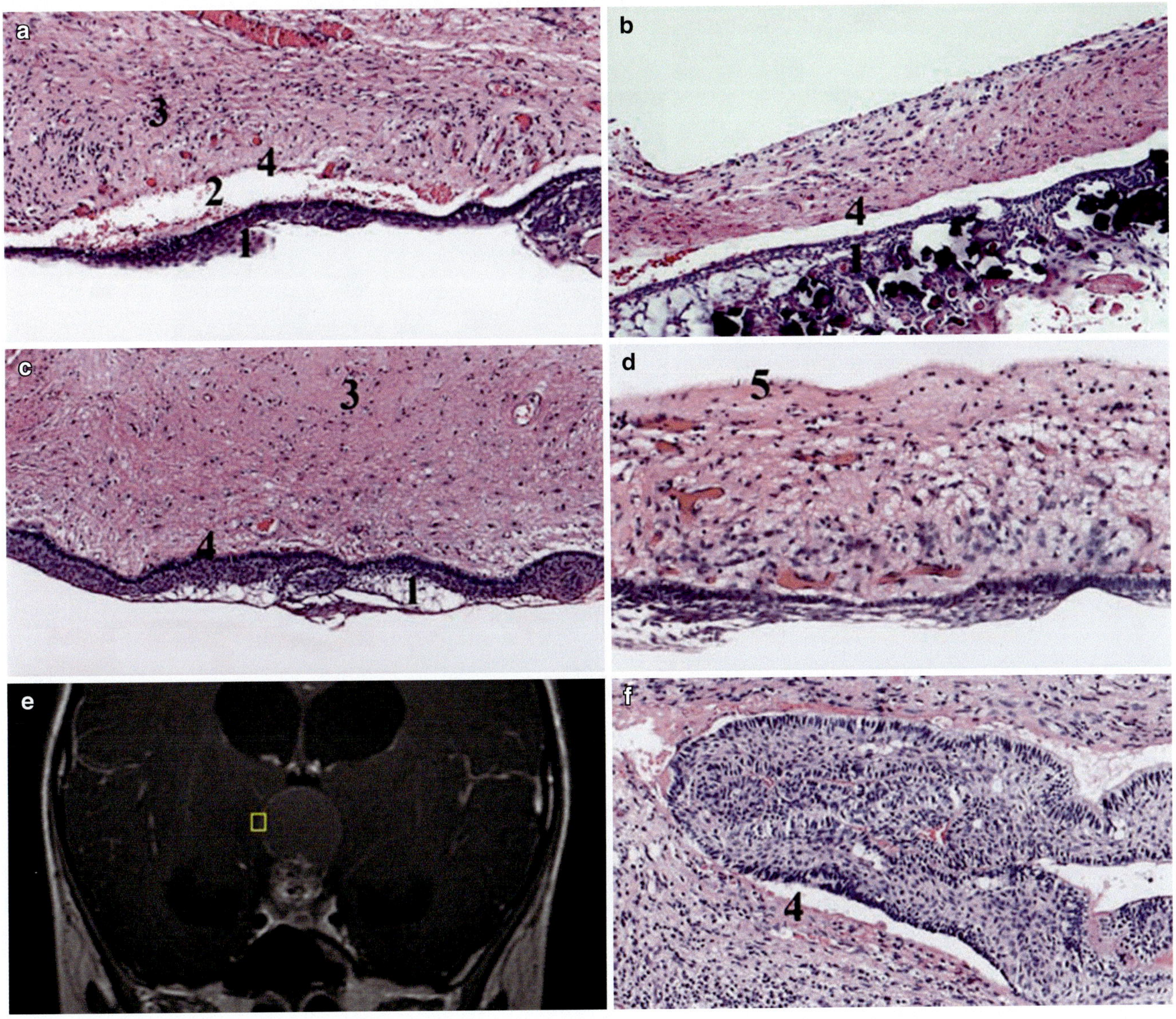

Fig. 3.10 T-type ACP form marsh-like (**a**, **b**) and moat-like (**c**, **d**) type structures with the third ventricle floor at non-origin site (**e**). The pia mater between tumor and the third ventricle could be seen which indicate that tumor could not invade the third ventricle floor at non-origin site (**f**). (1) Tumor, (2) moat-like structure, (3) nerve tissue of third ventricle floor, (4) pia mater, (5) ependymal cells

non-original site of the tumor. At the origin site of the tumor, a gliosis band (Fig. 3.11) was always appeared between tumor and the nervous layer of the third ventricle floor, which provide a dissect plane during operation.

Although T-type aCP forms a variety of relationships with the third ventricle floor, the ependymal layer of the third ventricle is always intact, which means the tumor is located outside the third ventricle. Therefore, the term "third ventricle craniopharyngioma" is inaccurate (Fig. 3.12)

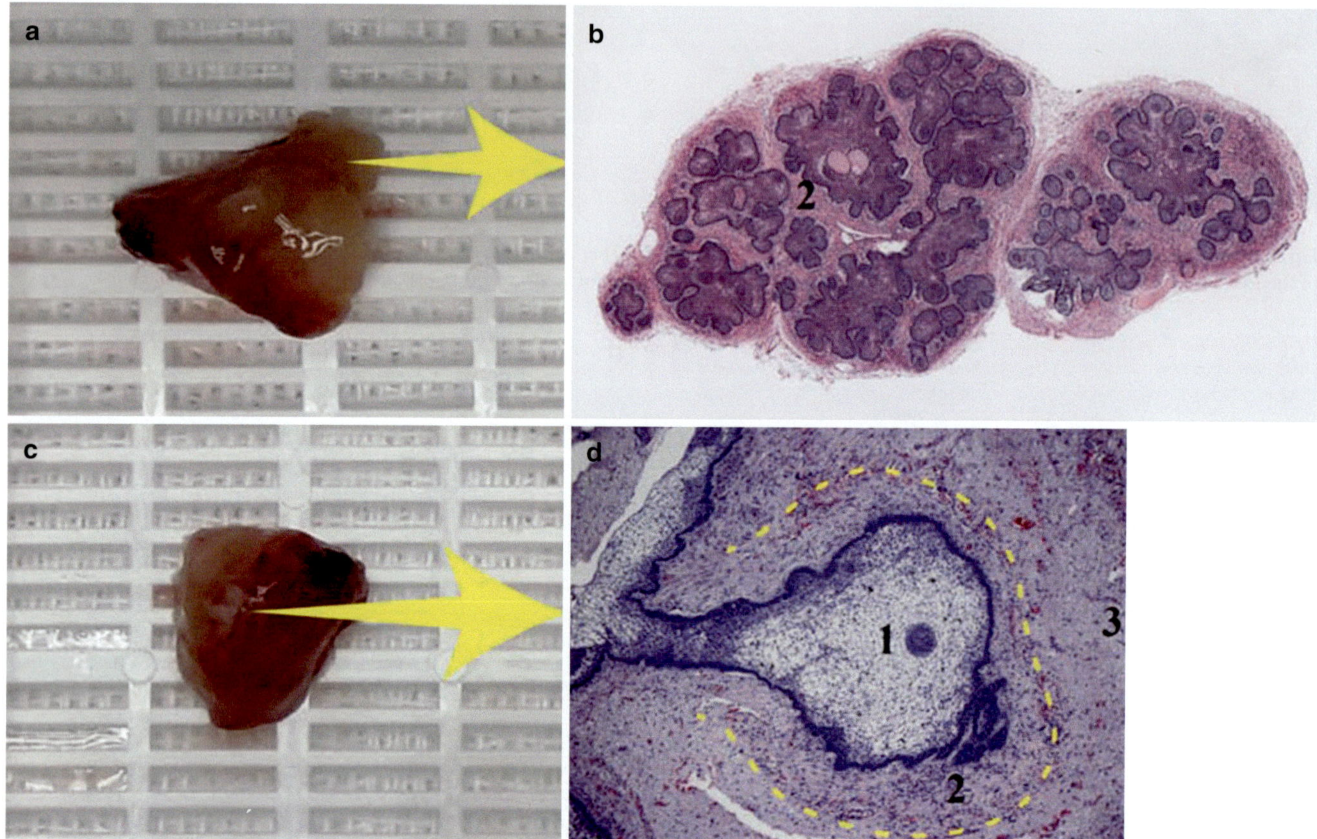

Fig. 3.11 A gliosis band could be seen between tumor and third ventricle floor (**a**–**d**). The tumor could be totally removed when separated along the gliosis band. (1) Tumor, (2) gliosis band, (3) third ventricle floor

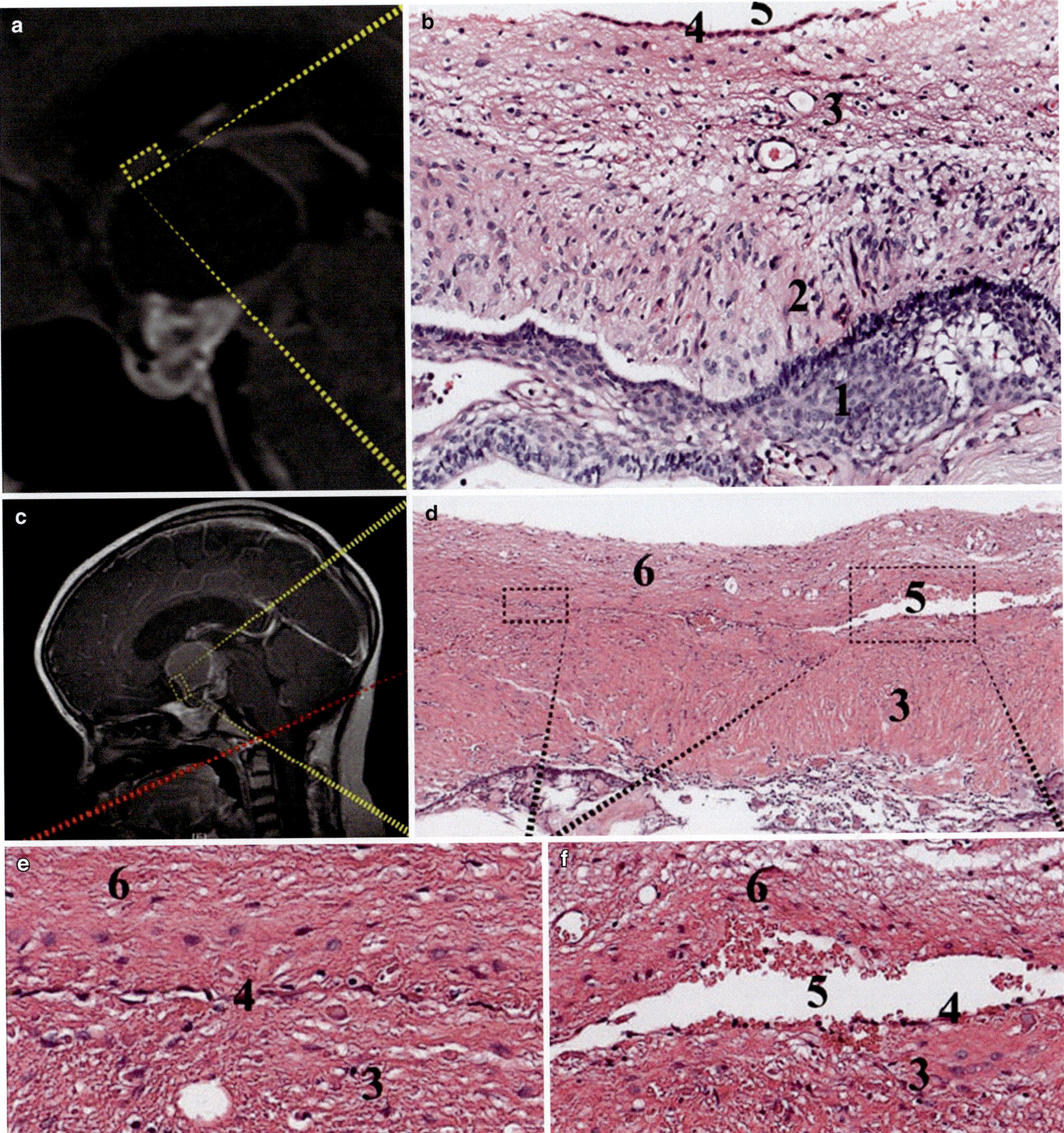

Fig. 3.12 The relationship between type T tumor and the third ventricle. At the origin site of the tumor (**a**, **b**), the m-t-like structure was formed, and the gliosis band could be seen. Although the tumor located in the third ventricle in MRI (**a**, **c**), the pathology demonstrate that the tumor is still outside the third ventricle (**b**). When tumor was resected through anterior interhemispheric fissure approach (**c**), the lamina terminalis should be incised. The pathology of (**b**–**f**) further demonstrated that the tumor originated outside the third ventricle floor and the third ventricle was pushed into a fractured shape. (1) Tumor, (2) gliosis band, (3) nerve tissue of third ventricle floor, (4) ependymal cells, (5) third ventricle, (6) lamina terminalis

Comparison Between the QST Scheme and Other Schemes for Craniopharyngiomas

4

Yun Bao and Songtao Qi

4.1 Introduction

The classification of craniopharyngioma should have the following characteristics: it should be consistent with embryonic origin and with clinical symptoms and the development of diseases, it should be conducive to the choice of treatment methods and surgery, it should be accurate in determining the difficulty of treatment and the prognosis, and it should involve sufficient histopathology evidence.

The QST classification introduced in this chapter is based on the origin, combined with the influence of the peripheral membrane structure on the tumor growth mode, and is fully in line with the surgical requirements for tumor classification.

Over the past 30 years, numerous important neurosurgical experts have markedly contributed to the idea that craniopharyngioma can be cured by surgery. There have been multiple important craniopharyngioma classifications, which can be roughly summarized as the author's experience, the intraoperative findings, the relative relationship with important structures, and even the classifications made for inductive analysis. These classifications require improvement:

1. The tumor originates from the residual Rathke's pouch cells, not the embryonic origin of nervous tissue. Because of this, purely intraventricular tumors do not exist.
2. The tumor is huge, the growth mode is complex, and the tumor is difficult or impossible to classify, for example, *pre-chiasmatic*, *retro-chiasmatic*, *preinfundibular*, *transinfundibular*, and *retroinfundibular* types.
3. Classification is inconsistent with clinical symptoms and prognosis, such as the classification according to the degree of pushing of the third ventricle and hypothalamus and the classification by tumor size without consideration to tumor origin. This type of defect can lead to the wrong choice of surgical approach and methods, extension of the learning curve, and even failure of treatment. It is also the reason why treatment methods used for malignant tumors such as radiotherapy, stereotactic radiotherapy, cystic fluid aspiration, and internal irradiation and chemotherapy are also used for the benign tumor of craniopharyngioma. The reason is that these classification methods lack embryological views and pathological histological evidence.

The main assertion of this chapter is that craniopharyngioma originates from outside the nerve tissue and is impossible to grow in the third ventricle. Craniopharyngioma is difficult to cure and must be treated by experienced neurosurgeons with increased perioperative management and precise endocrine support and in a center of vital functional remodeling capabilities. In order to change the status of craniopharyngioma, it is very important to select and apply the correct surgical classification. Learning, understanding, and using QST classification correctly are critical steps toward changing the status of craniopharyngioma, from incurable to curable. Therefore, the content of this chapter constitutes the core of the book and an importance showcase of the author's work.

Craniopharyngiomas can arise anywhere along the craniopharyngeal canal. Various classification systems have been proposed to aid in the planning of surgical routes based either on preoperative MRI or on intraoperative views of the anatomical structures involved with or surrounding the tumor (Table 4.1). In Pascual's classification scheme, the distinction among the pseudo-intraventricular, infundibulo-tuberal, and true intraventricular types is precisely based on the original site of development of the lesion. In addition, both Kassam's and Pascual's schemes take into consideration the position and status of the pituitary-hypothalamic structures adjacent to the lesion.

However, most classification systems do not emphasize the Rathke's pouch cell origin and the peripheral structures, especially the membrane structure on the growth pattern of the tumor, which leads to the following two situations. First,

Y. Bao (✉) · S. Qi
Department of Neurosurgery, Nanfang Hospital of Southern Medical University, Guangzhou, Guangdong, China

© Springer Nature Singapore Pte Ltd. 2020
S. Qi (ed.), *Atlas of Craniopharyngioma*, https://doi.org/10.1007/978-981-13-7322-0_4

Table 4.1 Summary of schemes for craniopharyngiomas

Authors	Classification system	Comment
Yasargil	(a) Purely intrasellar-infradiaphragmatic (b) Intra- and suprasellar, infra- and supradiaphragmatic (c) Supradiaphragmatic parachiasmatic, extraventricular (d) Intra- and extraventricular (e) Paraventricular in respect to the third ventricle (f) Purely intraventricular	Purely intraventricular type may lead to the misunderstanding that the tumor originated from nervous tissues
Hoffman	Intrasellar Pre-chiasmatic Retro-chiasmatic Giant	Many tumors are classified into "giant" type which is not suitable for guiding the surgical approach
Samii	(I) Intrasellar or infradiaphragmatic (II) Occupying the cistern with/without an intrasellarcomponent (III) Lower half of the third ventricle (IV) Upper half of the third ventricle (V) Reaching the septum pellucidum or lateral ventricles	Tumors classified as IV and V may have a good prognosis, which is not in line with common sense as the complicated surrounding structure
KC Wang	*Grade 0*, a tumor of subdiaphragmatic origin with competent diaphragma sellae growing in the pre-chiasmatic direction *Grade 1*, a tumor of subdiaphragmatic origin with incompetent diaphragma sellae growing through the diaphragmatic aperture in the retro-chiasmatic direction *Grade 2*, a tumor of supradiaphragmatic origin growing retrochiasmatically in the direction of the third ventricular floor or into adjacent cerebrospinal fluid spaces	Plenty of tumors growing pre-chiasmatically
Kassam	Preinfundibular Transinfundibular Retroinfundibular Isolated intraventricular	This classification may lead to the misunderstanding that the tumor originated from nervous tissues
Songtao Qi	Q, originating beneath the diaphragma S, originating from the extra-arachnoidal and intra-arachnoidal segments of the pituitary stalk T, originating at the tubero-infundibulum	Based on embryology and originating sites Based on surrounding membranous structures

some classification systems violate the embryology perspective, for example, *intraventricular craniopharyngioma*. Second, some classification systems are only based on the relative position of the tumor and anatomical structure, which does not allow for the classification of some large tumors, thus losing the guiding meaning of treatment.

The QST scheme supports Erdheim's embryological theory regarding the origin of these lesions from remnants of incompletely involuted hypophyseal duct/Rathke's pouch remnants along the pituitary-hypothalamic axis. In particular, Erdheim found the presence of squamous cells, the presumed remnants of Rathke's pouch migratory pathway, at two specific sites, that is, the dorsal surface of the pituitary gland (which may well correspond to the development of type Q) and the distal end swelling of the pars tuberalis just beneath the chiasm-infundibulum junction. This second location matches the high rate of T-type lesions found in this study. Curiously, Erdheim found small nests of squamous cells along the middle extension of the pars tuberalis wrapping the pituitary stalk, between the pituitary gland and the infundibulum, and the S type developing around the middle area of the pituitary stalk was the least often found (when CPs are erroneously categorized as "suprasellar" lesions in most textbooks and monographs).

The QST scheme incorporates analysis of the meningeal relationships at the tumor boundaries, that is, the arachnoid and pia mater, which can affect the growth patterns of tumors. Morphological heterogeneity among CPs may well correspond to the pattern of meningeal covering proposed in the QST scheme. Multiloculated lesions could develop when ASPS allows the expansion of the tumor throughout the intra-arachnoidal spaces of the chiasmatic cistern for the S and T types.

In the QST system, the tumor origin determines the tumor type, but the surrounding membrane structure can affect the tumor growth pattern. Understanding the pathological relationship between tumors and peripheral structures is of great significance for identifying and protecting important structures during surgery.

4.2 Some Case of Craniopharyngiomas Difficult to Be Classificated

This is a case of giant type Q craniopharyngioma. In other classification systems, it is not possible to classify this tumor because the tumor is so large that it is difficult to discern the relationship between the tumor and surrounding structures. At the same time, the tumor occupied the space of the third ventricle. In previous classification systems, there was no suitable type for the tumor. In the QST system, we classified this tumor as type Q because the tumor originated in the

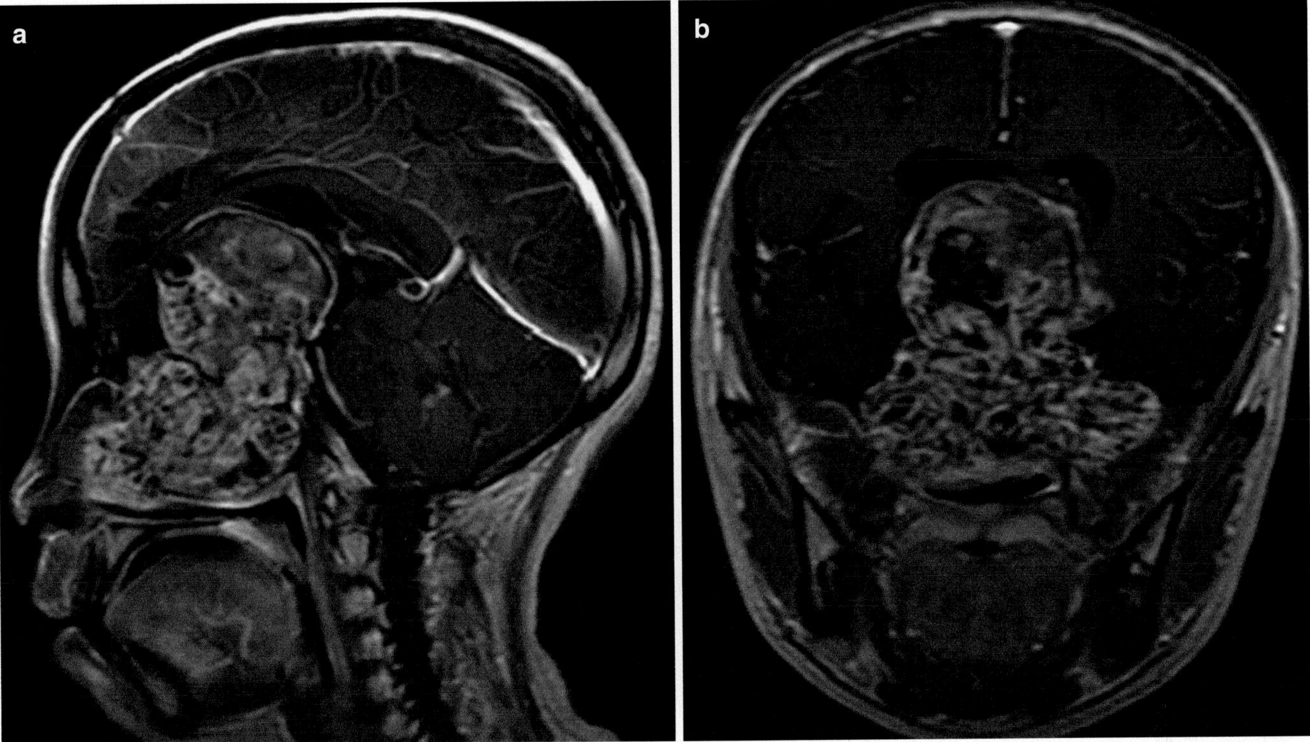

Fig. 4.1 MRI enhancement images in sagittal and coronal images of type Q craniopharyngioma

pituitary fossa and grew upward; although it occupied the space of the third ventricle, there was a multilayer membrane structure between the tumor and the third ventricle floor. Previous typing methods couldn't classify this huge tumor. This case will be classified as level 4 if applying the previous typing method, which implicated the worst prognosis according to their statement. But as we know that this is a tumor of type S and will result optimistic outcome regularly (Fig. 4.1).

This is a type S tumor. This shape of tumor is irregular and cannot be classified in other systems. On MRI, we can see that the pituitary fossa is not enlarged and the pituitary gland is visible, indicating that the tumor does not have a subsellar origin. This tumor originates from the remnants of the Rathke's' pouch precursor cells around the pituitary stalk. For some part of the ASPS and Liliequist membrane is not strong enough, the tumor could expand around the pituitary stalk, even into the space of the cervical spinal cord. The third ventricle floor is pushed upward by the tumor, but there remains membrane structure separating the tumor and the third ventricle floor (Fig. 4.2).

This is also a type S tumor. The tumor shape is irregular and lobulated, which is difficult to classify in other systems. This tumor originates from the remnants of Rathke's pouch precursor cells around the pituitary stalk. The pituitary gland and pituitary stalk are visible on MRI, and the tumors expand around the pituitary stalk. Although the tumor occupied the space of the third ventricle, there remains a multilayered membrane structure separating the third ventricle floor, and the tumor just pushes the third ventricles floor upward instead of invading. Figures 4.2 and 4.3 showed that both are type S craniopharyngioma, but the growth pattern is not the same because of the differences of peripheral membranous structure (Fig. 4.3).

This is a case of type T tumors. Although the morphology of this tumor is similar to Q-type tumor, they have a completely different origin and growth pattern. This tumor originates from the remnants of Rathke's pouch precursor cells near tuberalis. The cystic part occupies the space of the third ventricle, and some of the tumor break through the inner arachnoid and expanded into the subarachnoid space. Some other tumors break through the pia mater of the pituitary stalk, and grow into the stalk, and then expand into the pituitary fossa. Therefore, the pituitary stalk and pituitary gland are often not visible on the MRI. Previous typing methods couldn't classify this huge tumor. This case will be classified as level 4 if applying the previous typing method, which implicated the worst prognosis according to their statement. But as we know that this is a tumor of type Q and will result optimistic outcome regularly (Fig. 4.4).

This is a classic type T tumor. The tumor originates from the pars tuberalis, which often occupies the space of the third ventricle. The third ventricle floor and the upper end of the pituitary stalk may not appear on MRI, but the lower segment of the pituitary stalk and the pituitary gland are often visible. Figures 4.4 and 4.5 showed that both are type T craniopharyngioma, but the

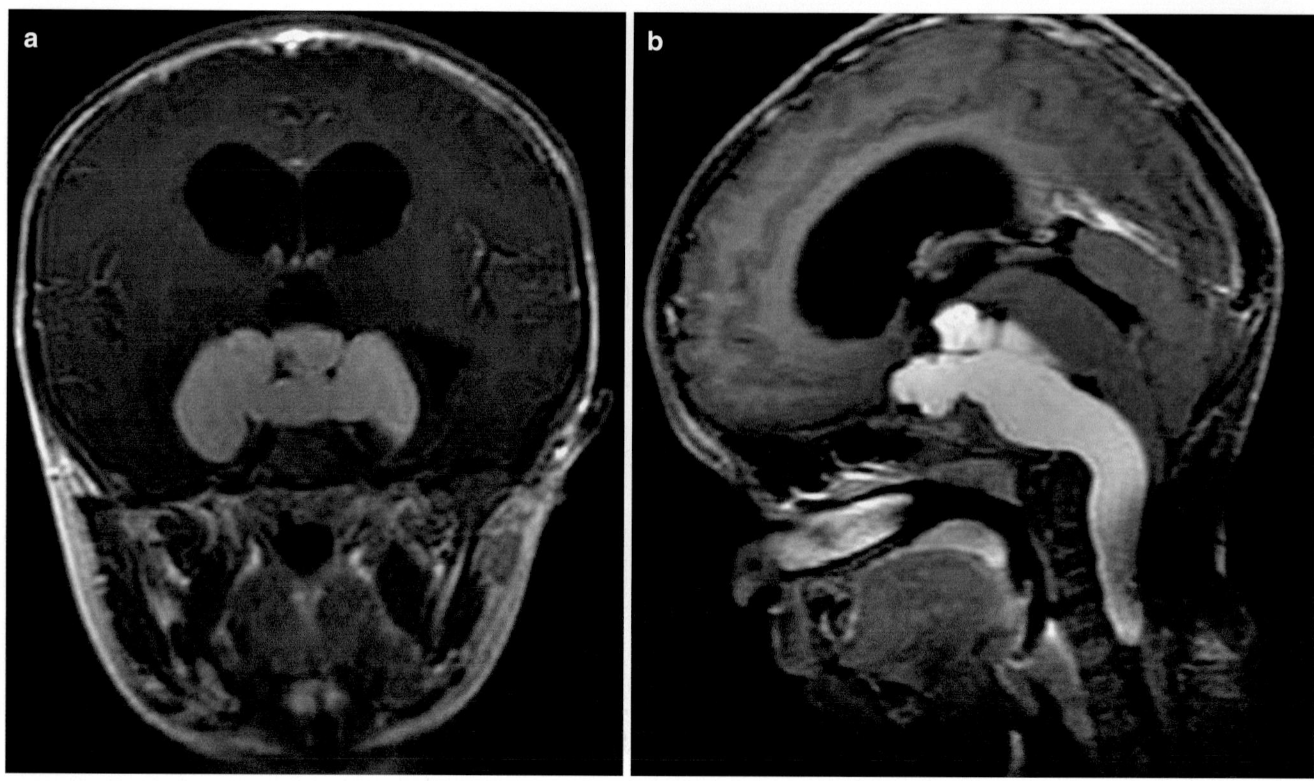

Fig. 4.2 MRI enhancement images in sagittal and coronal images of type S craniopharyngioma

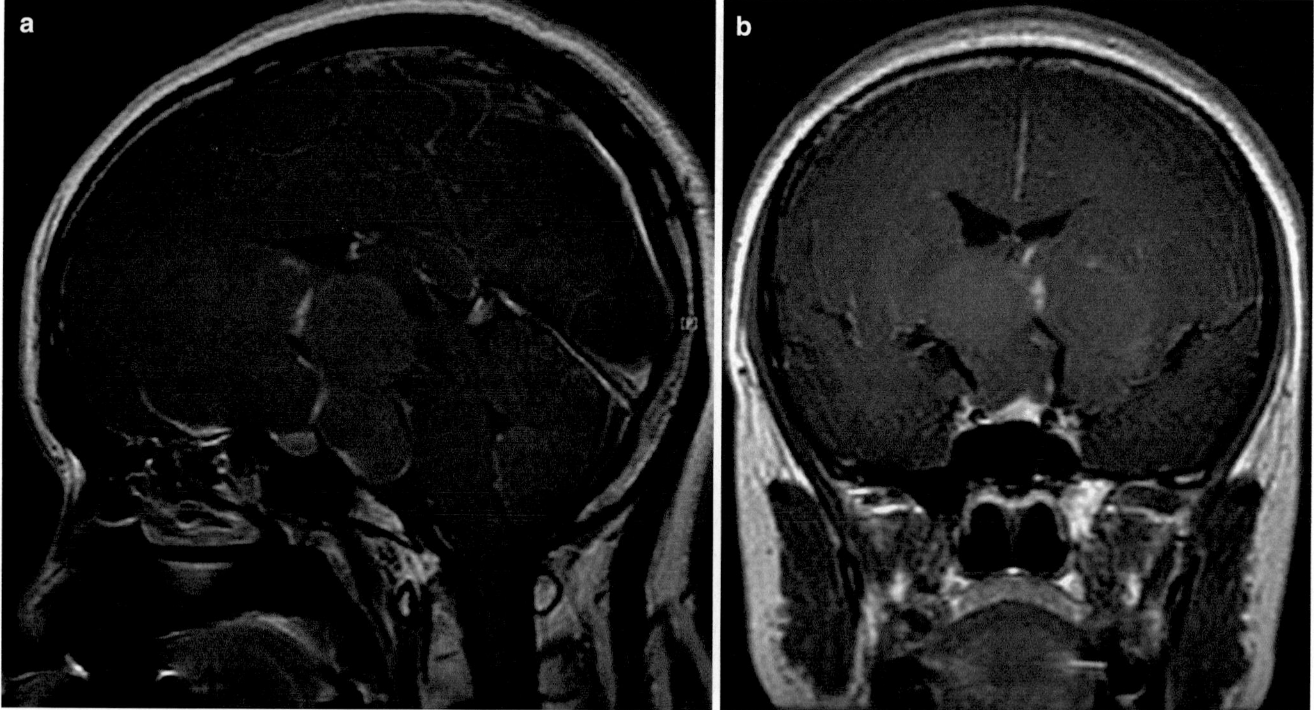

Fig. 4.3 MRI enhancement images in sagittal and coronal images of type S craniopharyngioma

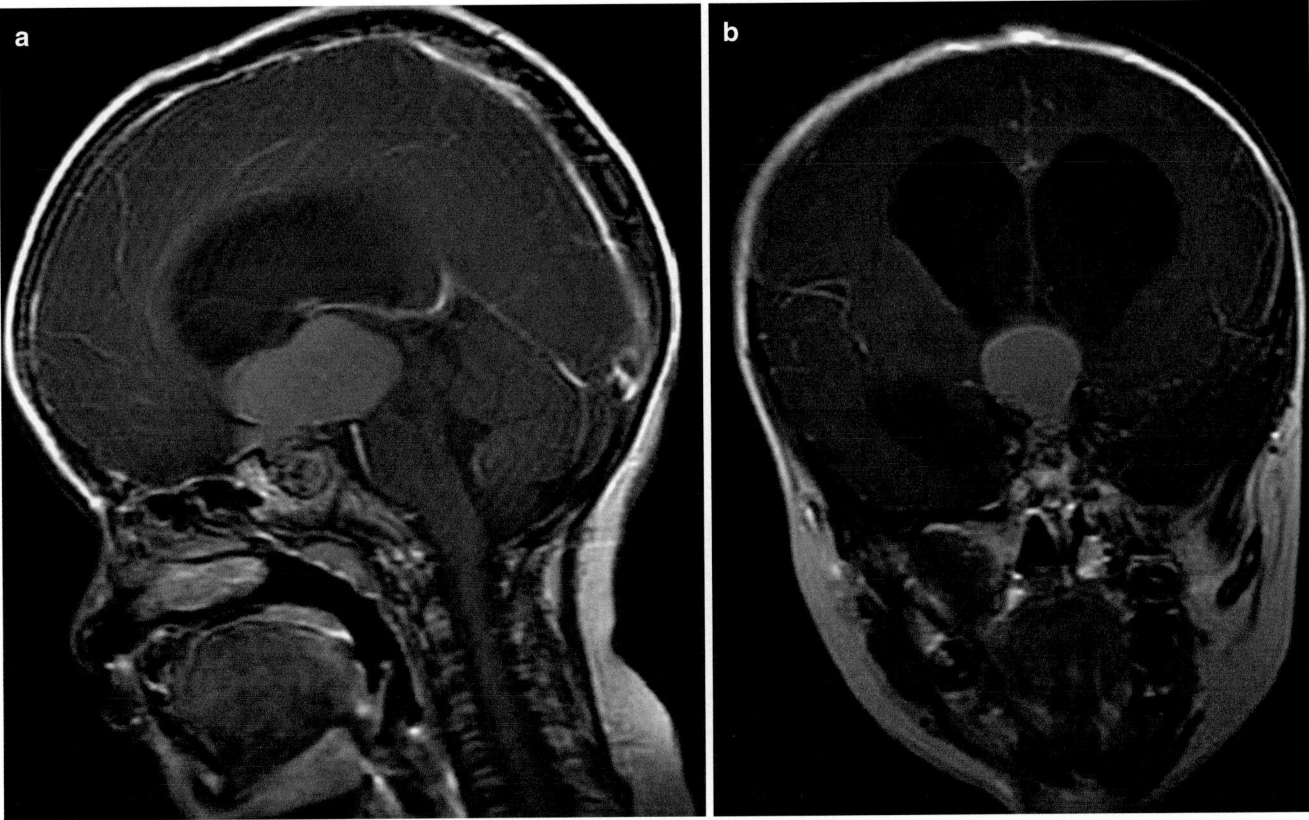

Fig. 4.4 MRI enhancement images in sagittal and coronal images of type T craniopharyngioma

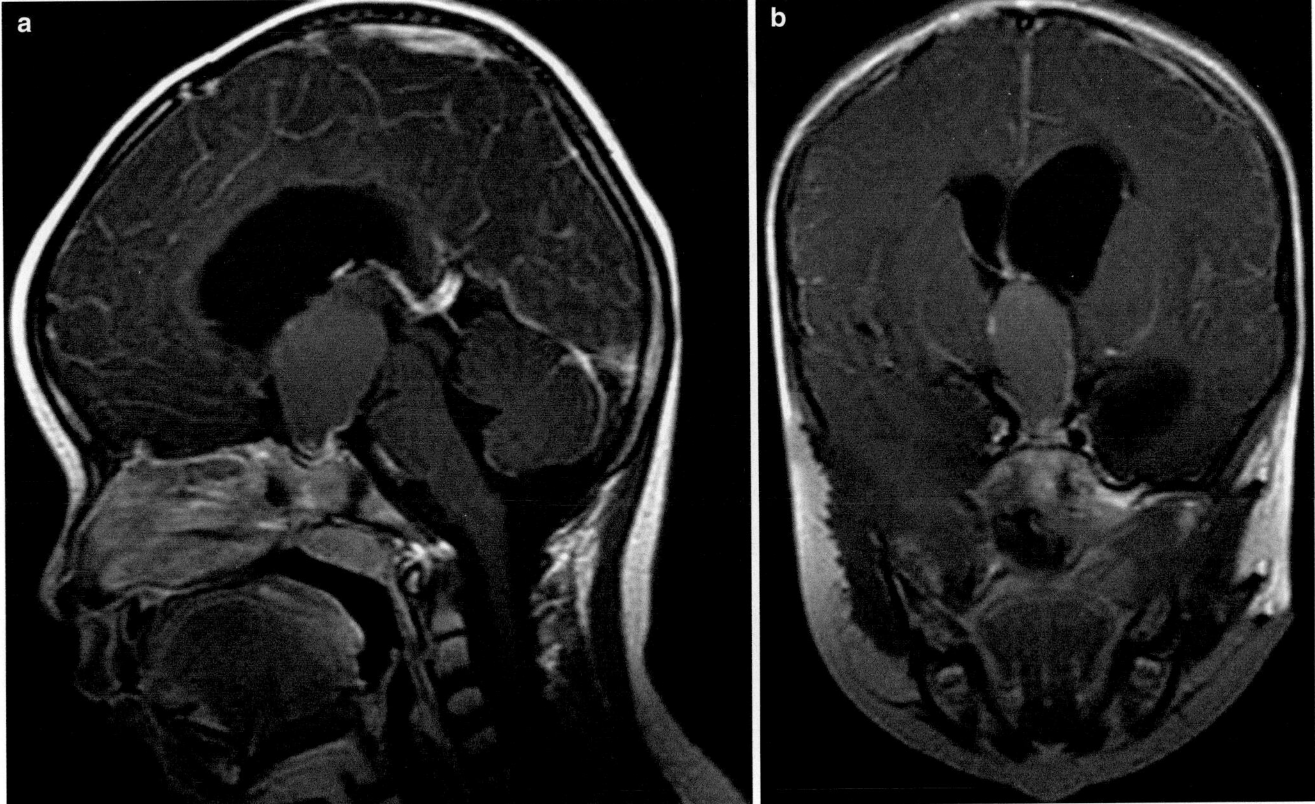

Fig. 4.5 MRI enhancement images in sagittal and coronal images of type T craniopharyngioma

growth pattern is not the same because of the difference in peripheral membranous structure (Fig. 4.5).

4.3 The Goal of Surgical Treatment of Craniopharyngioma, Which Is Difficult to Be Classified

The neurosurgeon should remove craniopharyngioma as much as possible safely. En bloc complete resection can be performed, and important peripheral structures can be preserved, even in patients with large tumor (Fig. 4.6), with severely calcified craniopharyngioma (Fig. 4.7), or after radiotherapy (Fig. 4.8). As shown in first case of type Q tumors in Chap. 6, the vision of this patient in preoperative period was poor and significantly improved after surgery (the visual acuity of the right eye was 0.08, and it became 0.8 after operation, and the left eye was 1.2 both before and after surgery). The endocrine status of some patients was poor in preoperative period, which significantly improved after surgery. Soma patients had their own children after surgery. For example, a male patients (in Fig. 4.9) and female patients (Fig. 4.10) had their own children 2 and 3 years after surgery, respectively. The goal of surgical treatment of craniopharyngioma is to completely remove tumor, improve the endocrine status, and improve the vision. Finally, patients with craniopharyngioma can be cured.

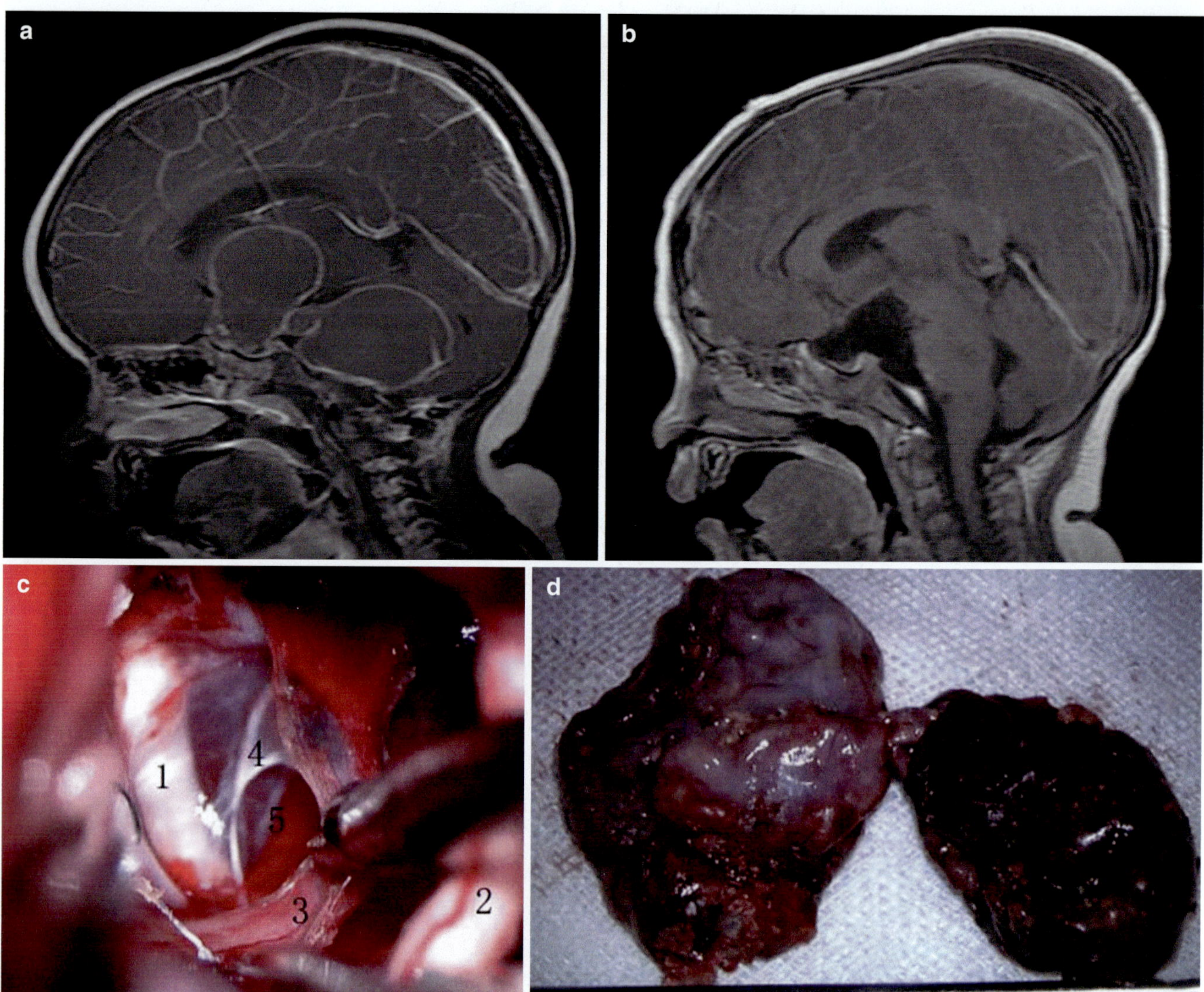

Fig. 4.6 This was a case of a 2-year-old girl with type S tumor. The tumor expands to posterior fossa. The posterior fossa tumor can be fully exposed through the cerebellar hiatus. The tumor is so huge calcification, which can be en bloc total resected. (**a**, **b**) Pre- and postoperative MR sagittal images, (**c**) important peripheral structures be preserved, (**d**) tumor specimen after en bloc resection. (1) Right side optic nerve, (2) left side optic nerve, (3) pituitary stalk, (4) ASPS (arachnoid sleeve of pituitary stalk), (5) arachnoid hole (tumor protruding to posterior fossa from this arachnoid hole)

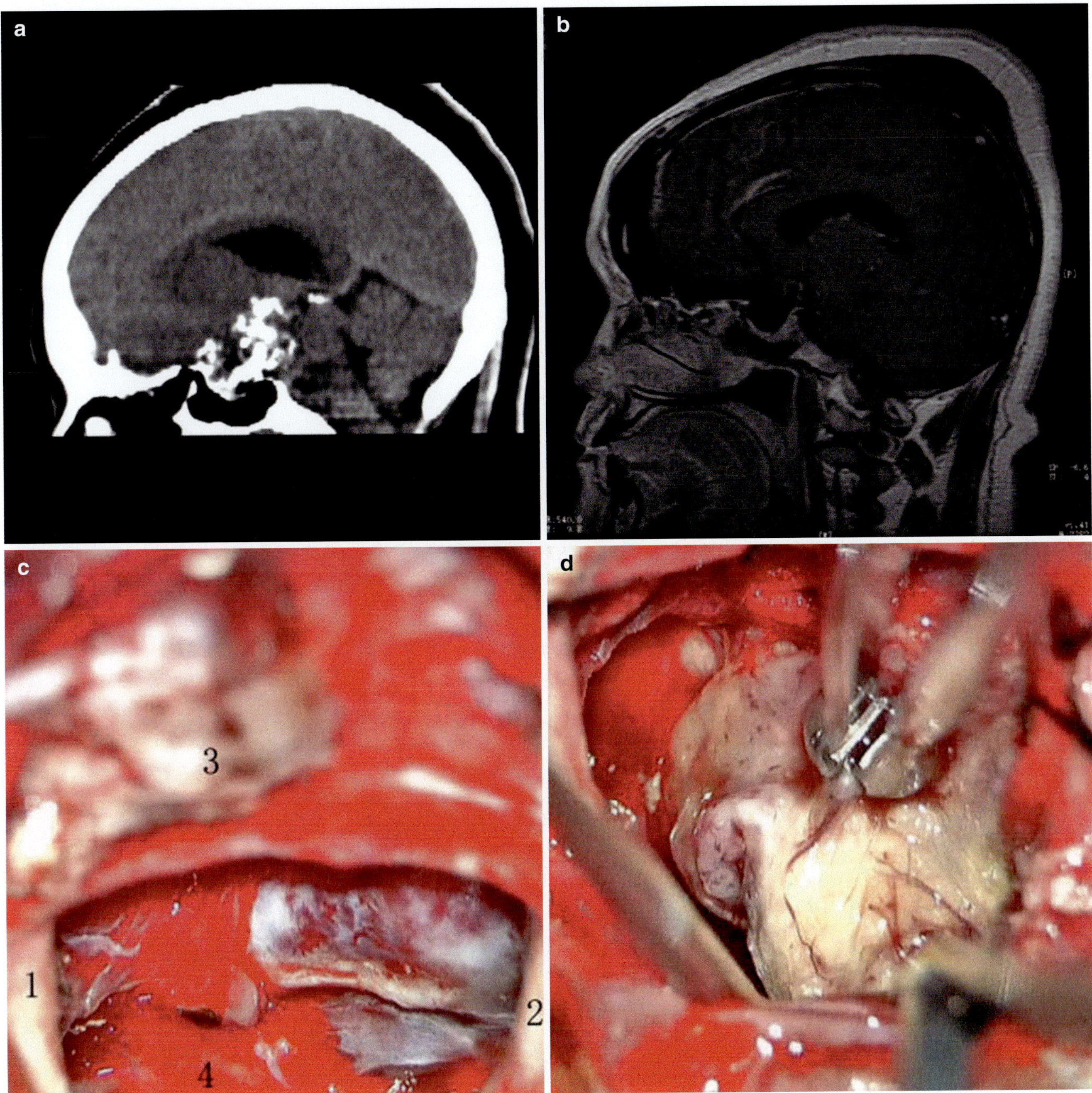

Fig. 4.7 This was a case of a 42-year-old female patient with type S tumor. The tumor had huge calcification, which can be en bloc total resected even if the difficulties of resection of this kind of tumor. (**a**, **b**) Pre- and postoperative MR sagittal images, (**c**) important peripheral structures be preserved, (**d**) tumor specimen after en bloc resection. (1) Left side optic nerve, (2) right side optic nerve, (3) dorsum sellae, (4) pressed pituitary stalk (the origin point of tumor)

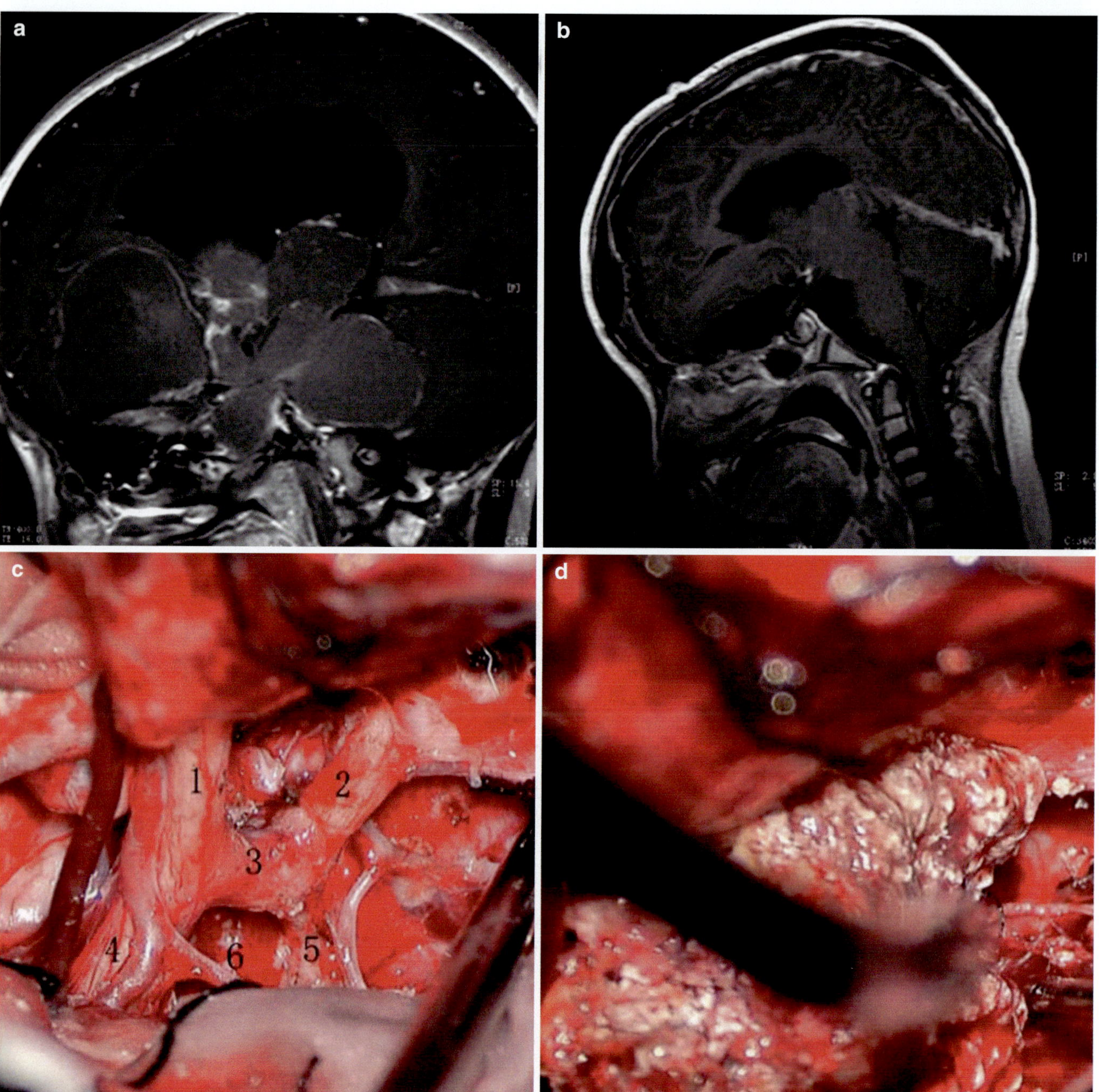

Fig. 4.8 This was a case of an 8-year-old girl with type S tumor, who only received radiotherapy before surgery. The tumor expands to the anterior, middle, and posterior cranial fossa. The patient's right eye was completely blinded for 2 years. The tumors adhered very tightly to right optic tract, for total resected tumors, some part of right optic tract was be removed. (**a**, **b**) Pre- and postoperative MR sagittal images, (**c**) important peripheral structures be preserved, (**d**) tumor specimen after en bloc resection. (1) Left side optic nerve, (2) right side optic nerve, (3) optic chiasma, (4) left optic tract, (5) right optic tract, (6) the third ventricle floor

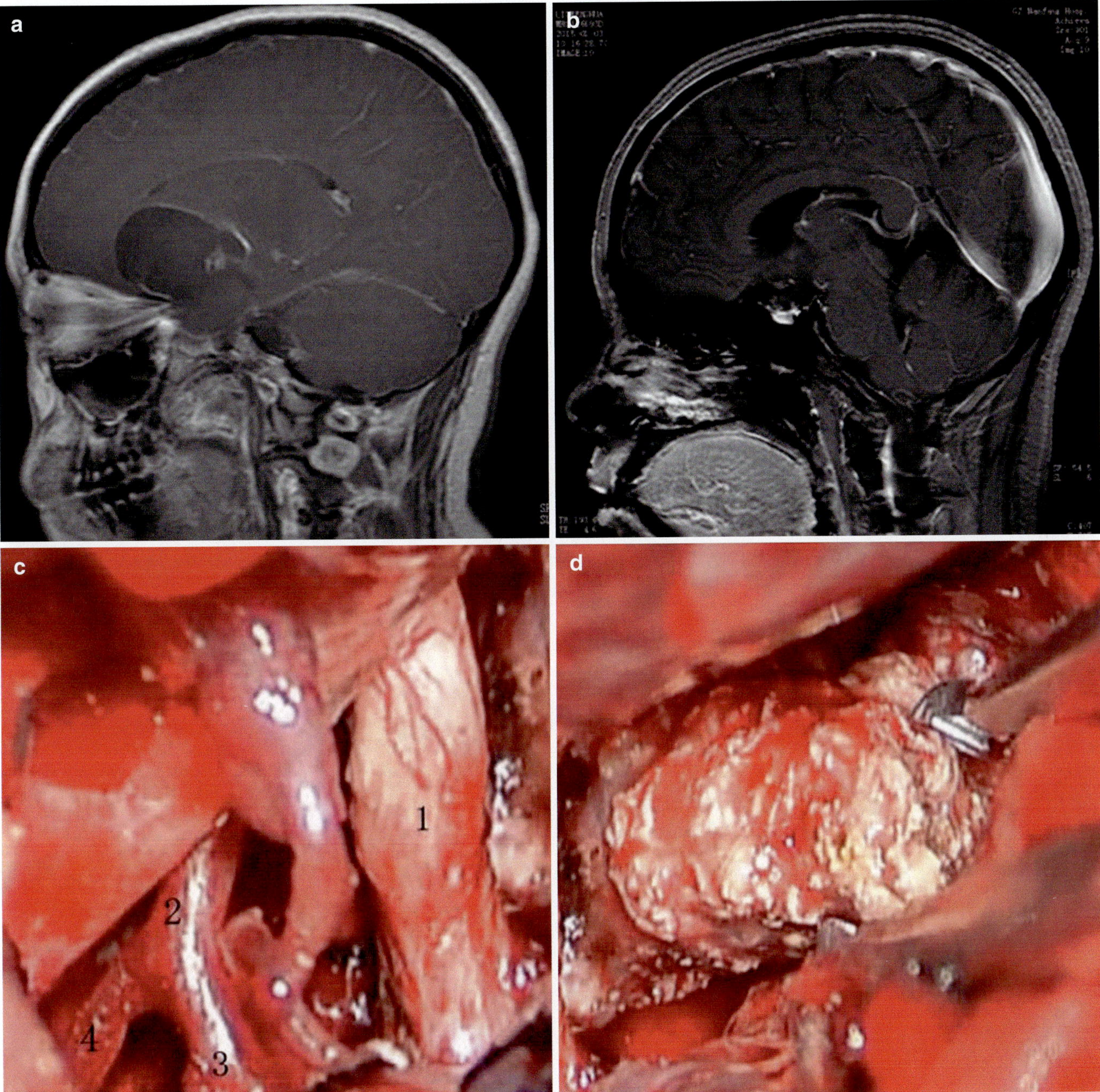

Fig. 4.9 This was a case of a 24-year-old female patient with type S tumor. The tumor had a giant calcification. It is difficult to remove this kind of tumor piece by piece for the giant calcification. En bloc resection is very difficult for the narrow surgical space. The good news is that the patient can also have her own children 3 years after surgery. (**a**, **b**) Pre- and postoperative MR sagittal images, (**c**) important peripheral structures be preserved, (**d**) tumor specimen after en bloc resection. (1) Left optic nerve, (2) right side ICA, (3) right anterior cerebral artery, (4) left middle cerebral artery

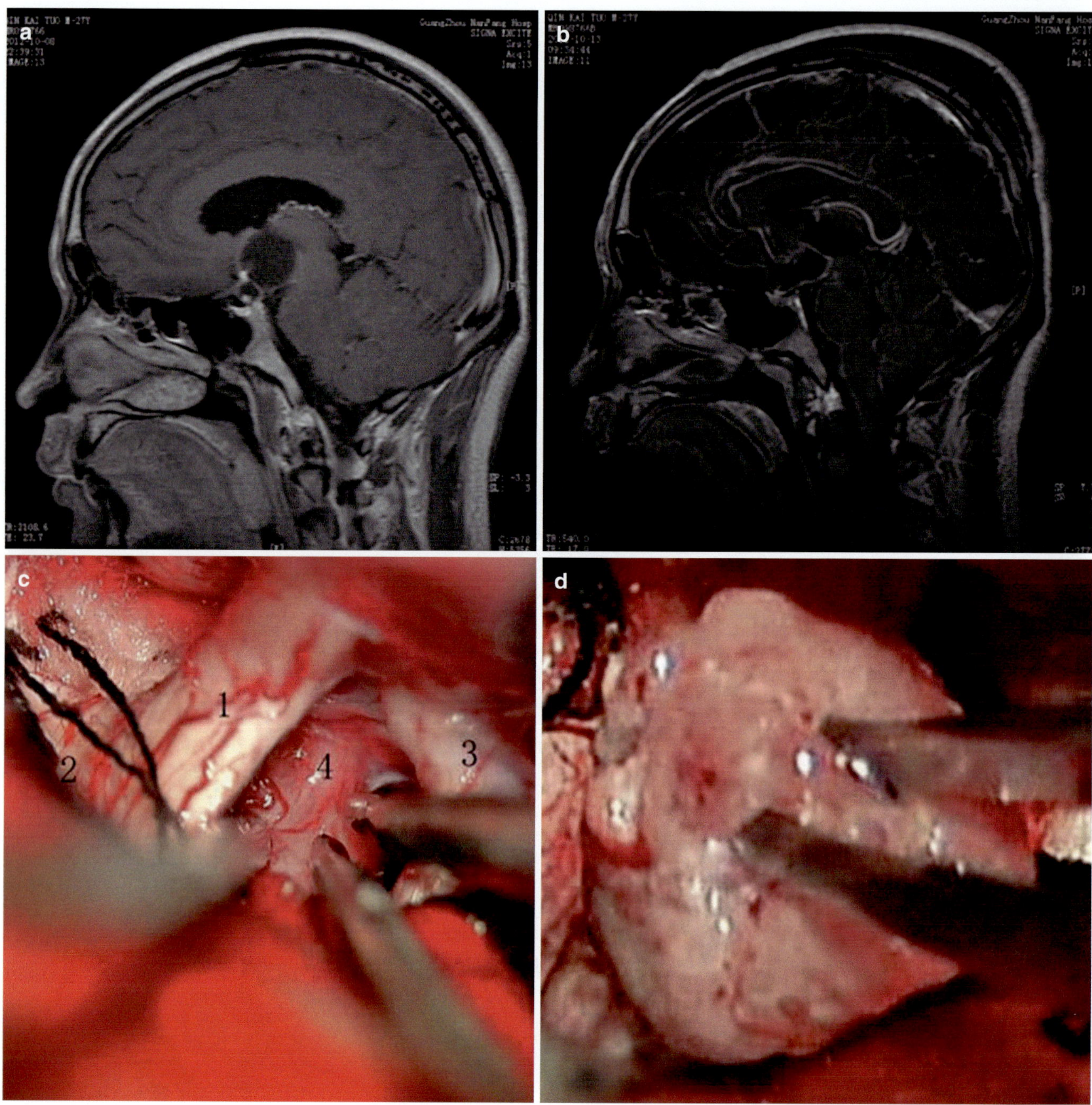

Fig. 4.10 This was a case of a 27-year-old male patient with type T papillary craniopharyngioma. Some part of tumor expands into the sleeve of pituitary stalk. Most part of tumor is smooth, except the origin point. The patient can have his own children 2 years after surgery. (1) Right side optic nerve, (2) optic chiasm, (3) right side ICA, (4) pituitary stalk. (**a**, **b**) Pre- and postoperative MR sagittal images, (**c**) important peripheral structures be preserved, (**d**) tumor specimen after en bloc resection

4.4 Mainly Schemes of Craniopharyngiomas

Table 4.1 is summary of mainly schemes of craniopharyngiomas.

Tables 4.2, 4.3, and 4.4 are summaries of endocrine disorder in various types of craniopharyngioma of 116 patients with primary craniopharyngioma who underwent surgical treatment at our hospital from August 2013 to July 2016. These included 64 male patients and 52 female patients ranging in age from 4 to 68 years. Dates showed that QST classification is highly correlated with preoperative endocrine status, and other types are not very highly correlated with to preoperative endocrine status. Patients with type Q were more likely to have hypopituitarism. Because the Q type originated under the saddle, it directly oppressed and affected the pituitary. The endocrine dysfunction rate of type S is low, because this type of tumor pituitary and hypothalamus is less affected by tumors.

Table 4.2 Endocrine disorder in various types of craniopharyngioma

	QST classification				Yasargil classification						
Endocrine disorder	Q type $n = 32$	S type $n = 23$	T type $n = 61$	*P* value	a $n = 5$	b $n = 3$	c $n = 20$	d $n = 30$	b + c $n = 23$	b + d $n = 35$	*P* value
ACTH deficiency	14 43.8%	4 17.4%	13 21.3%	0.039*	1 20.0%	3 100%	2 10%	9 30%	7 30.4%	9 25.7%	0.057
FSH/LH deficiency	14 43.8%	3 13.0%	17 27.9%	0.047*	2 40%	2 66.7%	5 25%	8 26.7%	13 56.5%	20 57.1%	0.035*
GH deficiency	26 81.3%	7 30.4%	18 29.5%	0.001*	3 60%	2 66.7%	12 60%	26 86.7%	18 78.3%	24 68.6%	0.239
TSH deficiency	15 46.9%	2 8.7%	11 18.0%	0.001*	1 20%	2 66.7%	2 10%	1 3.3%	4 17.4%	12 34.3%	0.005*

$^*P < 0.05$

Table 4.3 Endocrine disorder in various types of craniopharyngioma

	Samii classification					
Endocrine disorder	I $n = 5$	II $n = 45$	III $n = 27$	IV $n = 37$	V $n = 2$	*P* value
ACTH deficiency	1 20%	12 26.7%	7 26.0%	10 27.0%	1 50%	0.954
FSH/LH deficiency	2 40%	19 42.2%	11 40.7%	16 43.2%	2 100%	0.603
GH deficiency	3 60%	31 68.9%	20 74.1%	30 81.1%	1 50%	0.626
TSH deficiency	1 20%	8 17.8%	2 7.4%	11 29.7%	0 0%	0.227

Table 4.4 Endocrine disorder in various types of craniopharyngioma

	Hoffman classification					KC Wang classification			
Endocrine disorder	1 $n = 8$	2 $n = 23$	3 $n = 83$	4 $n = 2$	*P* value	0 $n = 24$	1 $n = 26$	2 $n = 66$	*P* value
ACTH deficiency	3 37.5%	8 34.8%	20 24.1%	0 0%	0.520	8 33.3%	9 34.6%	14 21.2%	0.303
FSH/LH deficiency	3 37.5%	15 65.2%	32 38.6%	0 0%	0.075	11 45.8%	12 46.2%	27 40.9%	0.860
GH deficiency	5 62.5%	15 65.2%	63 75.9%	2 100%	0.520	15 62.5%	18 69.2%	52 78.8%	0.264
TSH deficiency	2 25%	7 30.4%	13 15.7%	0 0%	0.360	6 25%	7 26.9%	9 13.6%	0.243

Part II

Surgical Treatment of Craniopharyngioma

5 Endoscopic Transsphenoidal Surgery for Craniopharyngioma

Jun Fan, Yi Liu, and Songtao Qi

5.1 Introduction

The advantages of craniopharyngioma endoscopic resection are summarized as follows. First, the original site of the tumor can be well exposed under the endoscopic transsphenoidal approach, and the relationship between the tumor and peripheral structures could be well identified. Second, for type Q tumors, it is very important to protect pituitary function by identifying the tumor and remaining pituitary tissue under the endoscope. Third, the optic nerve and chiasm are less disturbed, which is one of the reasons why the postoperative vision of patients is better. With the development of neuro-endoscopic devices and the improvement of instruments, the endoscopic transsphenoidal approach may attain a broader application spectrum.

The main perspective of this book on endoscopic resection of craniopharyngioma is based on total tumor resection as the ultimate goal. In endoscopic operations, there are several points to be noted, with the first being patient safety. Whenever surgeons encounter difficulties or risks during endoscopic surgery, they need to stop and switch to craniotomy surgery. Second, in clinical practice, the physician's physical condition should be taken into account because it is difficult to ensure the quality of surgery if the surgeon is overexerted. Third, both neurosurgical microscopy and neuro-endoscopy are important tools for the resection of craniopharyngioma, and the proper application of these two tools ensures that each patient is properly treated.

The endoscopic transsphenoidal approach has recently emerged and is widely used in the treatment of craniopharyngioma. Compared with traditional microscopic craniotomy, endoscopic surgery has the following advantages:

1. Almost no brain retraction.
2. It can fully expose the tumor located on the ventral side of the optic chiasm. Endoscopic observation can better identify the relationship between the tumor and the surrounding structures and increase the protection of the surrounding structures.
3. Transsphenoidal surgery does not leave visible surgical scars, which can meet the patients' cosmetic needs.

However, endoscopic surgery also has the following disadvantages:

1. The learning curve is longer. This approach requires the tacit cooperation between the main surgeon and the assistant.
2. Endoscopic operation is sometimes limited by space and high requirements for surgical equipment.
3. Patients are prone to developing cerebrospinal fluid leakage postoperatively, and some patients have severe nasal complications after the operation.
4. Vascular rupture during surgery, often leading to catastrophic consequences.
5. For some tumors involving the pituitary stalk, it is often necessary to remove the pituitary stalk to ensure complete tumor resection, while separation under the microscope can sometimes maintain the continuity of the pituitary stalk.

J. Fan (✉) · Y. Liu · S. Qi
Department of Neurosurgery, Nanfang Hospital of Southern Medical University, Guangzhou, Guangdong, China

© Springer Nature Singapore Pte Ltd. 2020
S. Qi (ed.), *Atlas of Craniopharyngioma*, https://doi.org/10.1007/978-981-13-7322-0_5

Therefore, we should select the most suitable approach according to the patient's preoperative images and tumor classification. We believe that transsphenoidal surgery is not suitable in the following situations based on our more than 20 years of experience:

1. The operation of craniopharyngioma should be based on the concept of total resection. Therefore, if transsphenoidal surgery does not achieve the goal of total resection, it should not be used.
2. Tumors involving multiple skull base fossae, such as S-type tumors extending to the anterior skull base or even the posterior skull base or laterally expanding tumors, are not suitable for this approach.
3. Tumors involving the main blood vessels, including the ACA, internal carotid artery, and PCA, may cause blood vessel rupture during resection, which is not suitable for the approach.
4. Recurrent tumors, especially those that have undergone internal and external radiation, which results in severe adhesion to the surrounding structure, are not suitable for this approach.
5. Previous studies have reported that the sphenoid sinus with poor gasification or no gasification is a relative contraindication to transsphenoidal surgery. According to our experience, the size of the nasal cavity and the degree of sphenoid sinus gasification should not be the reason for limiting the approach.

We will illustrate the application of this approach in the treatment of craniopharyngioma, both in pediatric and in adult patients.

5.2 Application of the Endoscopic Transsphenoidal Approach in Pediatric Patients with Craniopharyngioma

5.2.1 Case 1: A Case of Q-Type Craniopharyngioma in a Child (Figs. 5.1, 5.2, 5.3, 5.4, 5.5, 5.6, 5.7, 5.8, 5.9, and 5.10)

5.2.2 Comment

This is a case of Q-type craniopharyngioma in a child, and the origin was located beneath the diaphragma sellae. Therefore, the transsphenoidal approach could well treat the

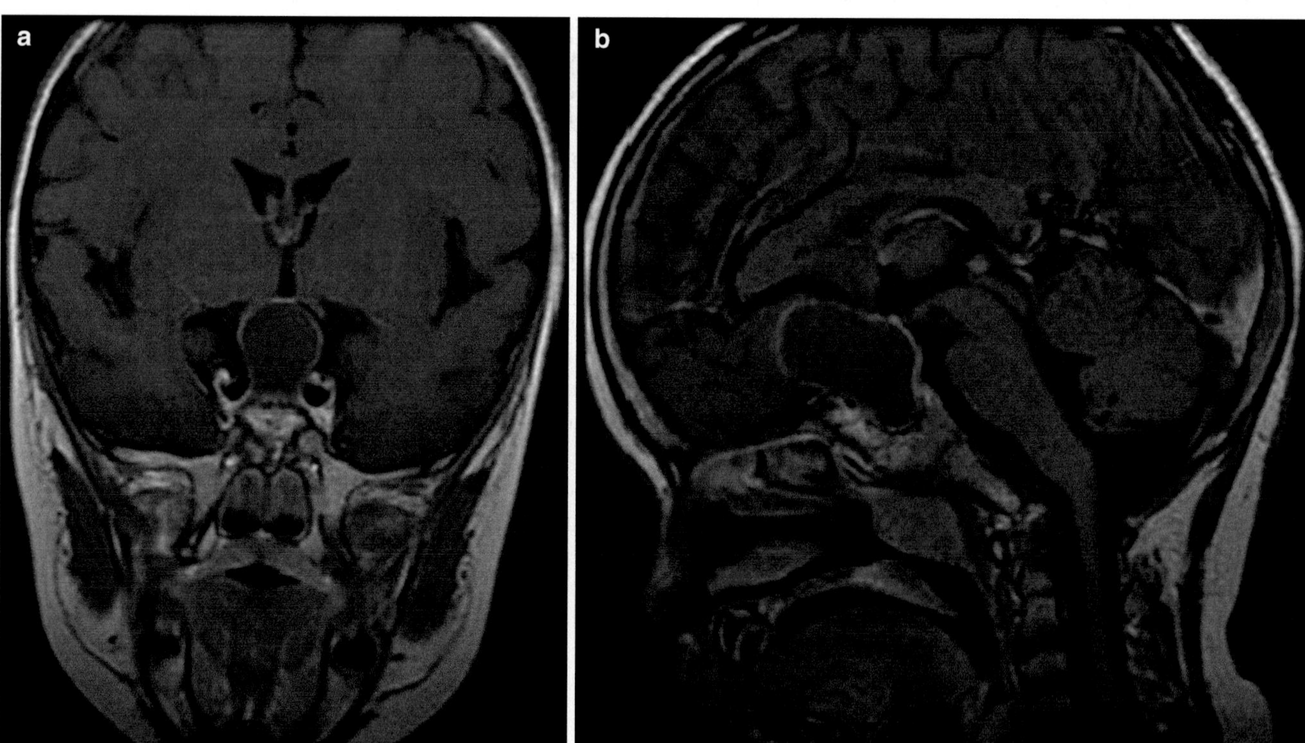

Fig. 5.1 Preoperative MRI of type Q craniopharyngioma in a child. (**a**) Coronal view showing that the tumor is located beneath the diaphragma sellae and the optic chiasm is pushed upward; the bilateral cavernous sinuses are not involved. (**b**) Sagittal view showing that the pituitary fossa is enlarged; the pituitary gland and pituitary stalk are unrecognizable. The tumor protrudes into the anterior skull base, and the bottom of the third ventricle is pushed by the tumor

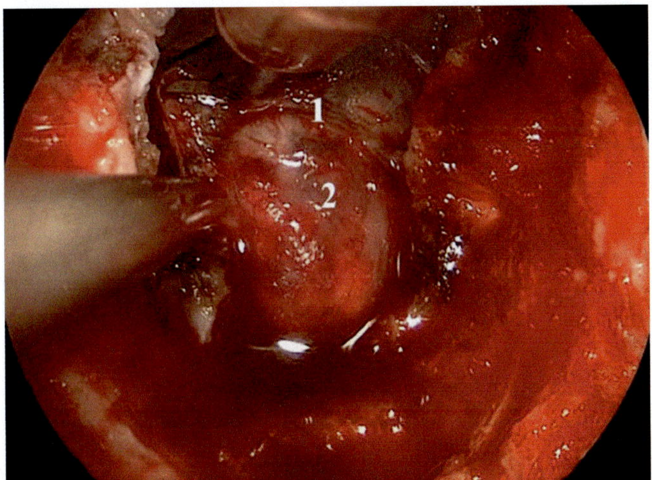

Fig. 5.2 Double nostril expanded transsphenoidal approach. The dura and pituitary sac are opened, and the tumor is visible. The tumor originates beneath the diaphragma sellae and is a Q-type tumor. (1) Pituitary sac, (2) tumor

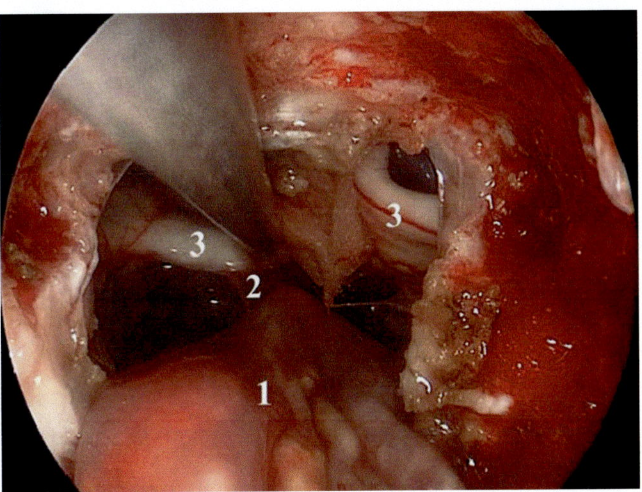

Fig. 5.4 Separating the tumor from the suprasellar structures. Diaphragma sellae and arachnoid remain between the tumor and suprasellar structures. (1) Diaphragma sellae on the surface of the tumor, (2) arachnoid between the tumor and optic chiasm, (3) optic nerve and optic chiasm

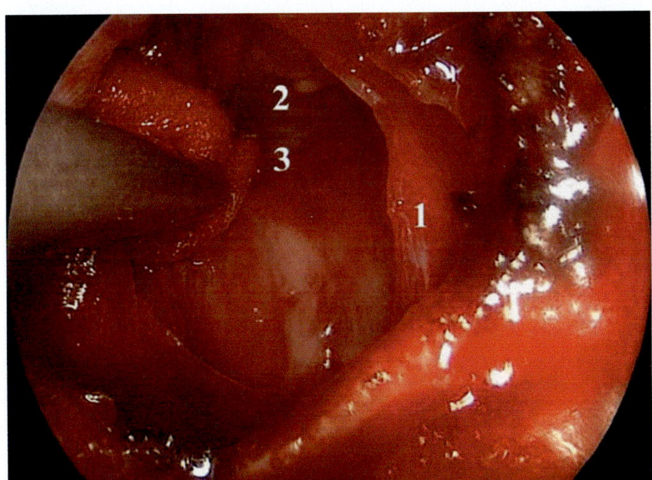

Fig. 5.3 Separating the intra-sellar tumor from the normal pituitary; the boundary between the tumor and the pituitary gland is clear. (1) Pituitary gland, (2) tumor, (3) boundary

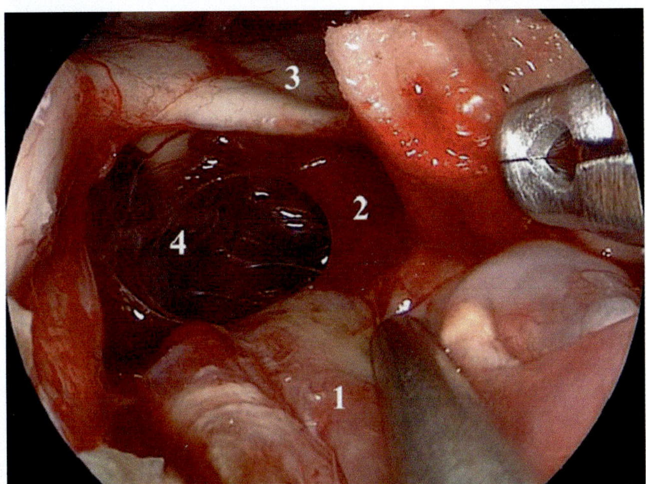

Fig. 5.5 The pituitary stalk is revealed. (1) Tumor, (2) pituitary stalk, (3) optic chiasm, (4) Liliequist membrane

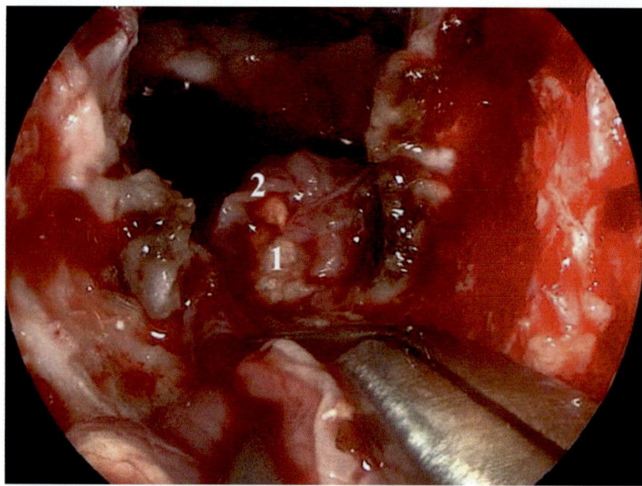

Fig. 5.6 Detachment of the diaphragma sellae for better separation. (1) Tumor, (2) diaphragma sellae

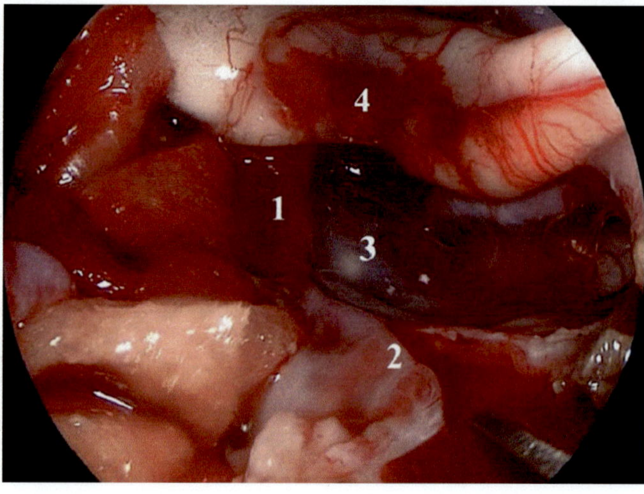

Fig. 5.8 Detachment of the diaphragma sellae to free the pituitary stalk. (1) Pituitary stalk, (2) diaphragma sellae, (3) Liliequist membrane, (4) optic chiasm

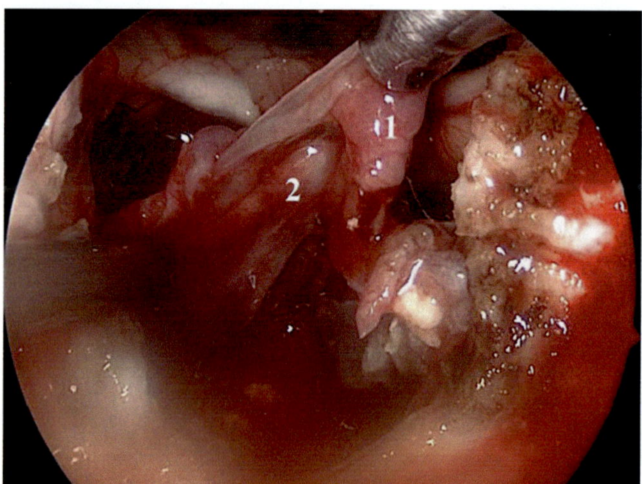

Fig. 5.7 Separation of the tumor and the diaphragma sellae; a clear boundary is observed between the tumor and diaphragma sellae. (1) Tumor, (2) diaphragma sellae

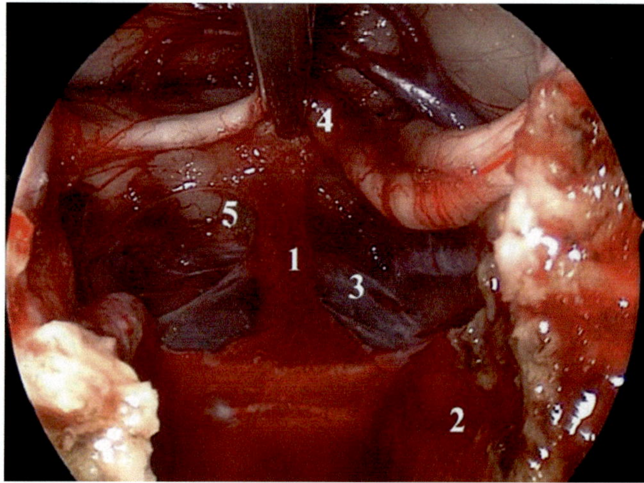

Fig. 5.9 Structures were well protected after the tumor resection. (1) Pituitary stalk, (2) pituitary gland, (3) Liliequist membrane, (4) optic chiasm, (5) third ventricle floor

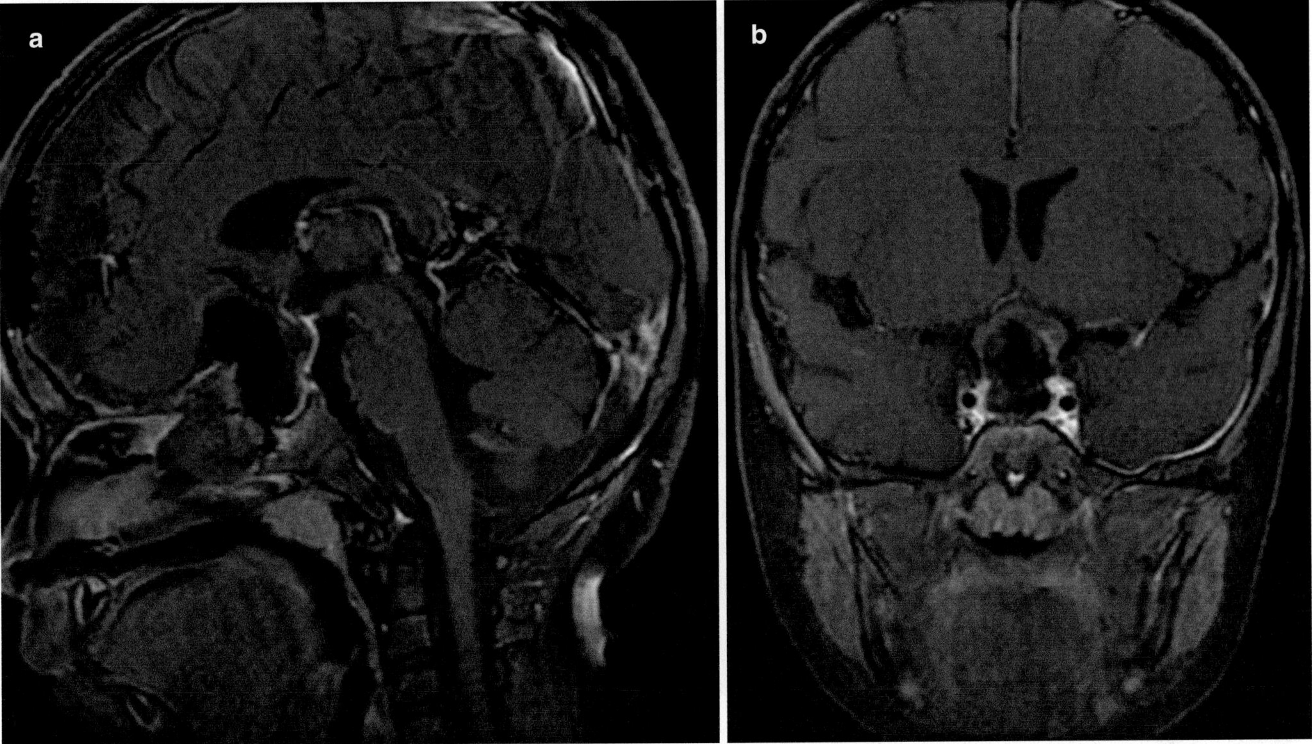

Fig. 5.10 Postoperative MRI (**a**, **b**) showing that the tumor was completely resected and that the third ventricle floor and pituitary stalk were intact

origin of the tumor. Although the tumor had reached the level of the third ventricle floor, diaphragma sellae and arachnoid remained between the tumor and important structures, providing a natural interface for separation.

The tumor protruded into the anterior skull base through the anterior chiasm space, and transcranial surgery could also achieve satisfactory resection through the anterior chiasm space. However, the patient's pituitary fossa was deepened, and the transcranial approach was blocked by tuberculum sellae, which rendered it difficult to expose the tumor's origin. Tuberculum sellae had to be removed to achieve satisfactory exposure.

5.2.3 Case 2: A Case of Q-Type Craniopharyngioma Extending to the Floor of the Third Ventricle in a Child (Figs. 5.11, 5.12, 5.13, 5.14, 5.15, 5.16, 5.17, 5.18, 5.19, 5.20, and 5.21)

5.2.4 Comment

This is also a Q-type tumor. Compared with Case 1, the tumor in this case expanded more toward the third ventricle. Although some tumors protrude into the space of the third ventricle, there remain multiple layers of tumor and the third ventricle

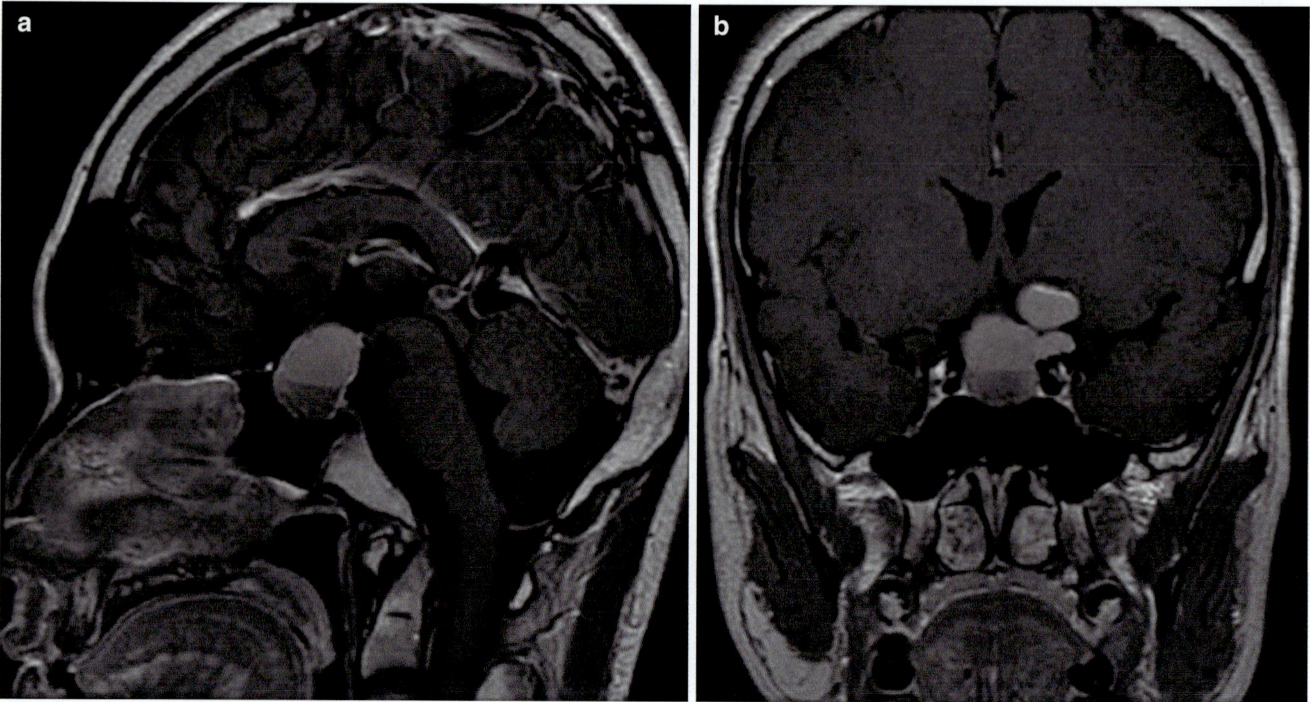

Fig. 5.11 A case of Q-type craniopharyngioma involving the third ventricle floor. (**a**) Sagittal view showing that the pituitary fossa is enlarged and the tumor mainly extends upward to the level of the third ventricle floor. (**b**) Coronal view showing that part of the tumor grows into the para-sellar space

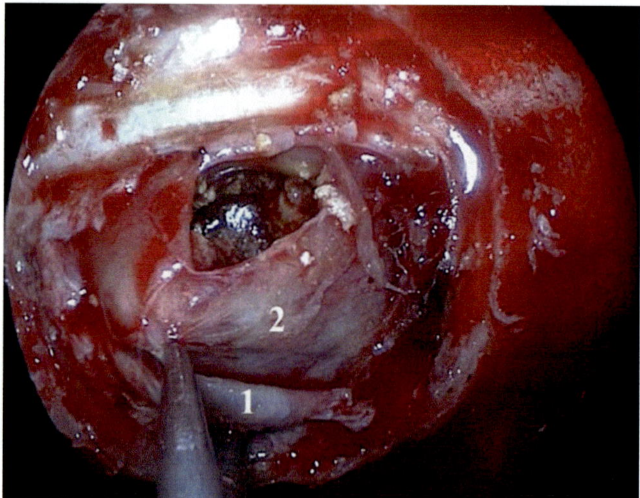

Fig. 5.12 Opening of the dura and exposure of the tumor. (1) Pituitary sac, (2) tumor

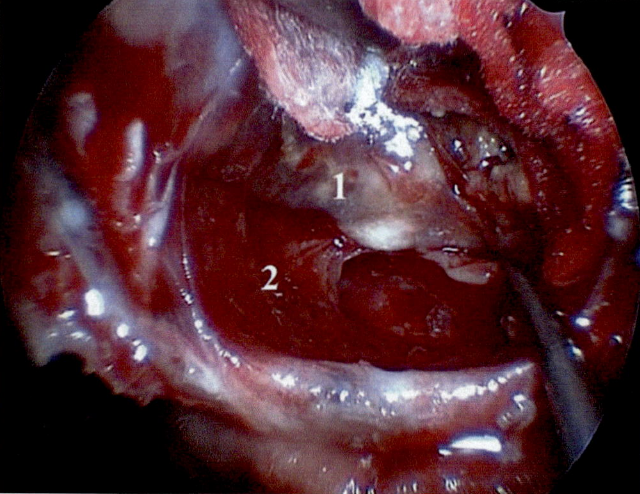

Fig. 5.13 Separation of the tumor from the pituitary gland; a clear boundary between the tumor and the pituitary gland is visible. (1) Tumor, (2) normal pituitary

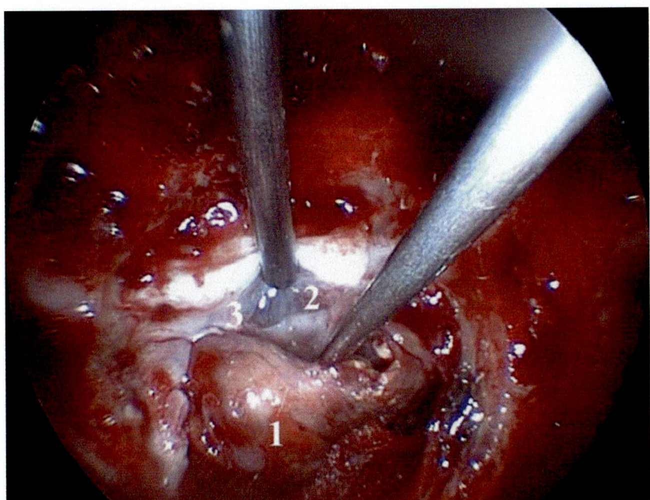

Fig. 5.14 Diaphragma sellae and arachnoid cover the tumor. (1) Tumor, (2) arachnoid, (3) diaphragma sellae

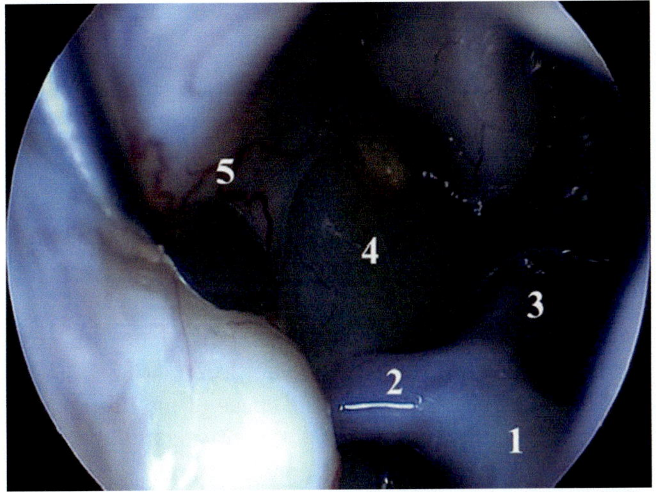

Fig. 5.15 Exploration of the tumor in the para-sellar space. (1) Internal carotid artery, (2) anterior cerebral artery, (3) middle cerebral artery, (4) tumor, (5) optic chiasm

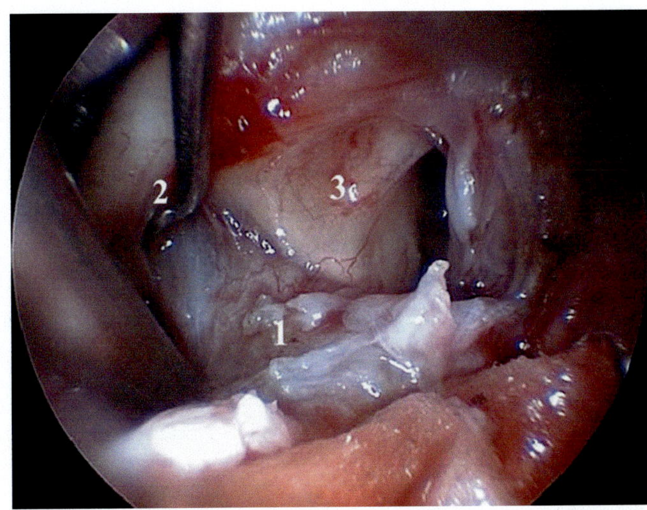

Fig. 5.16 Separation of the tumor from the third ventricle floor; the boundary between the tumor and the third ventricle floor is clear. (1) Tumor, (2) optic chiasm, (3) third ventricle floor

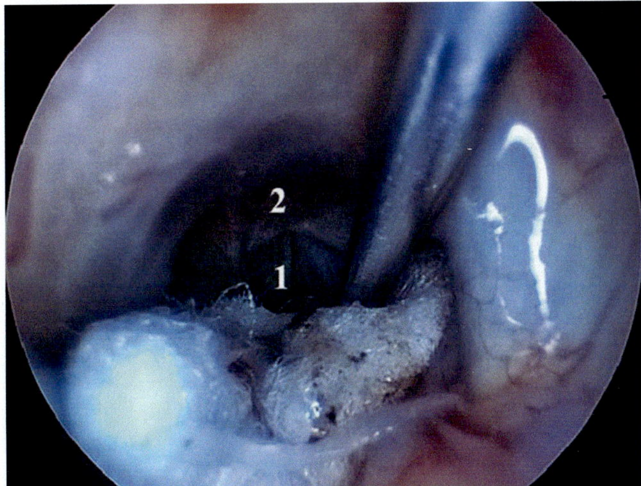

Fig. 5.17 Although the tumor occupies the space of the third ventricle, it is easy to separate the tumor from third ventricle floor because of the presence of a multimembrane structure. (1) Tumor, (2) third ventricle floor

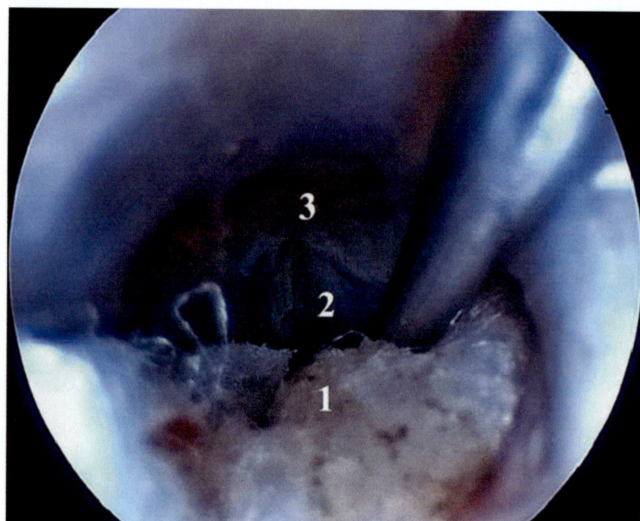

Fig. 5.18 Using brain cotton as a separation tool, the tumor wall is completely pulled out from the third ventricle floor. Attention should be given to protecting the intact tumor wall and avoiding missing tumors. (1) Brain cotton, (2) tumor wall, (3) third ventricle

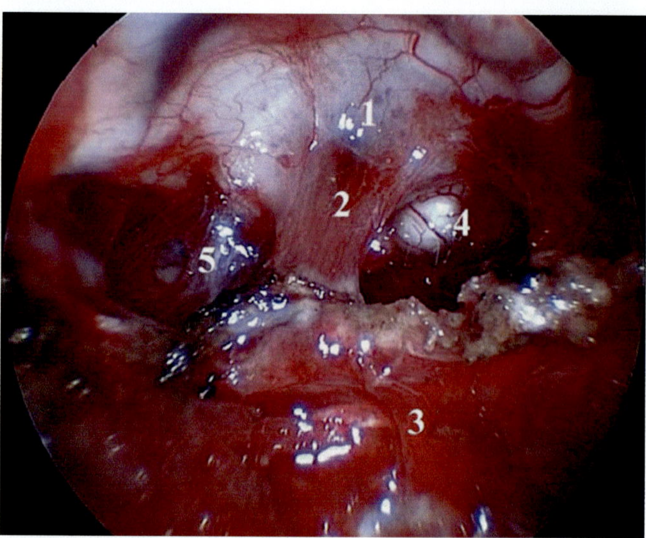

Fig. 5.20 After the tumor is totally resected, it can be seen that the structures are well protected and that the third ventricle floor is intact. (1) Third ventricle floor, (2) pituitary stalk, (3) pituitary gland, (4) mammillary body, (5) Liliequist membrane

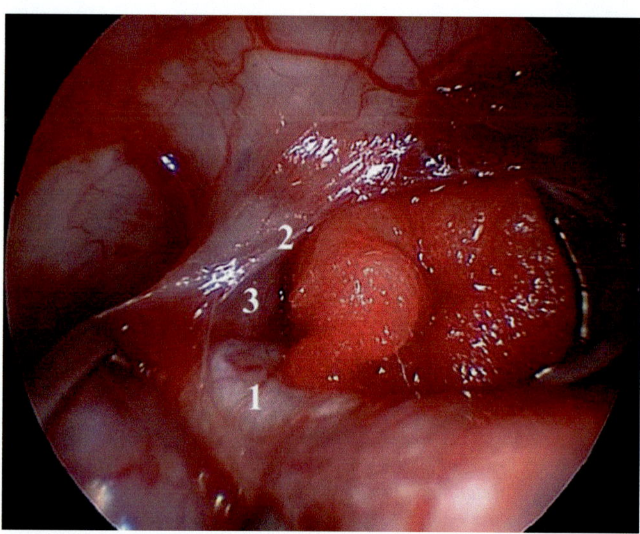

Fig. 5.19 After the tumor involving the third ventricle floor is pulled out, we can see that there remains pia mater between the tumor and the third ventricle floor. (1) Tumor, (2) pia mater, (3) third ventricle floor

floor. Membrane structure was the anatomical basis for the complete preservation of the third ventricle floor in this patient. Some of the tumors are mainly cystic. When removing the tumor, it should not be separated piece by piece but in an en bloc pattern, otherwise tumor tissue will be easily missed.

5.2.5 Case 3: A Large T-Type Craniopharyngioma Occupying the Space of the Third Ventricle (Figs. 5.22, 5.23, 5.24, 5.25, 5.26, 5.27, 5.28, 5.29, 5.30, 5.31, and 5.32)

5.2.6 Comment

It can be seen from the intraoperative picture that the tumor in this case is a T-type tumor, originating from the pars tuberalis and occupying the space of the third ventricle, and the pituitary gland is not involved. At the point of origin, there was no obvious separation interface between the tumor and the third ventricle floor, which required sharp separation. This is why this type of tumor can cause hypothalamic injury. However, at the non-origin point of the tumor, there is usually pia mater or inner arachnoid membrane to separate the tumor and the third ventricle floor. However, if the tumor is of large volume and the pia mater at the non-origin point of the third ventricle is pushed and becomes thin, it may be unable to provide a separation interface. There is often a gliosis band between the tumor and the third ventricle floor, which can be used as a boundary for separation.

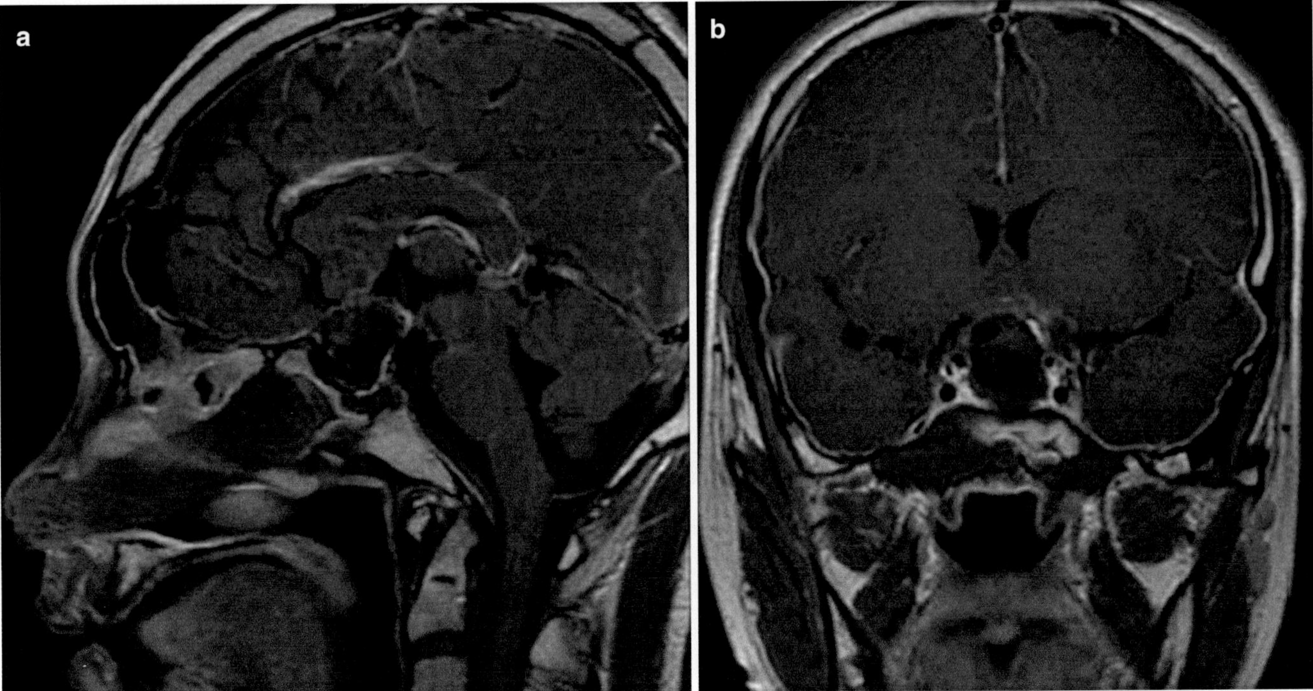

Fig. 5.21 Postoperative MRI (**a**, **b**) showing that total resection was achieved

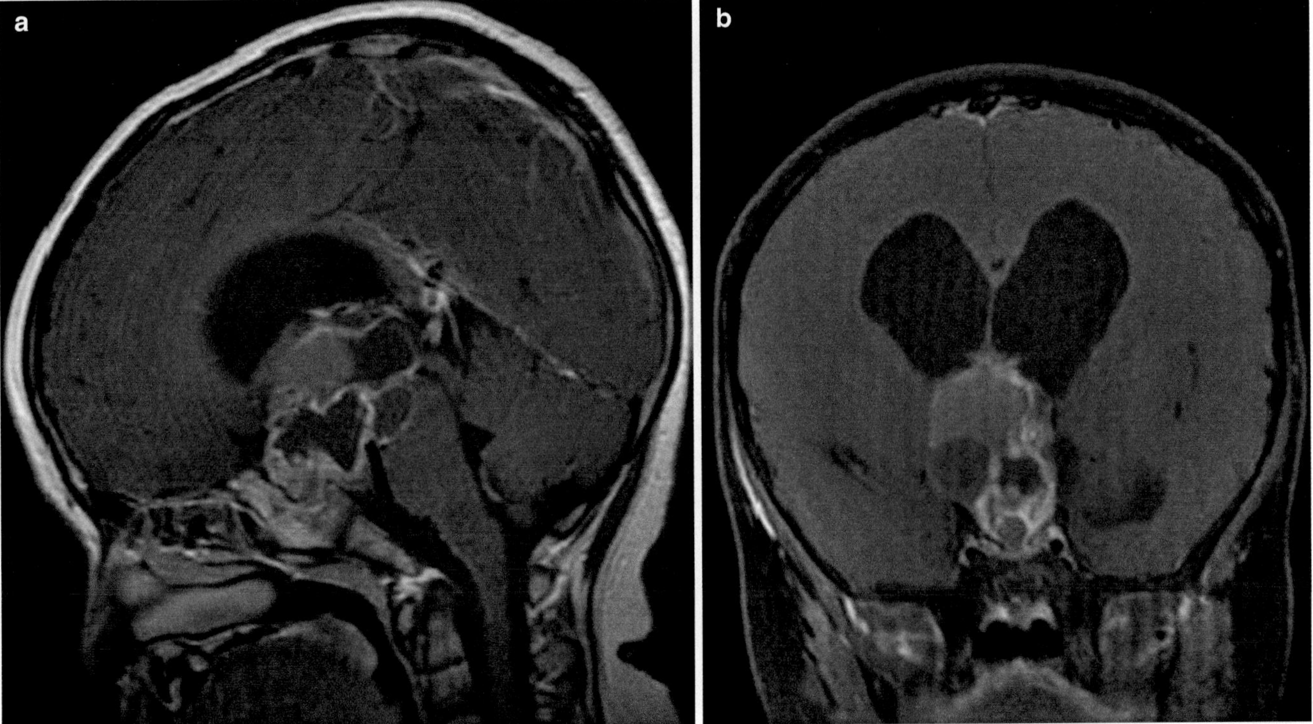

Fig. 5.22 Preoperative MRI (**a**, **b**) image showing that the tumor originates from the pars tuberalis and occupies the space of the third ventricle. It blocks the foramen of Monro and causes hydrocephalus. The pituitary gland is visible

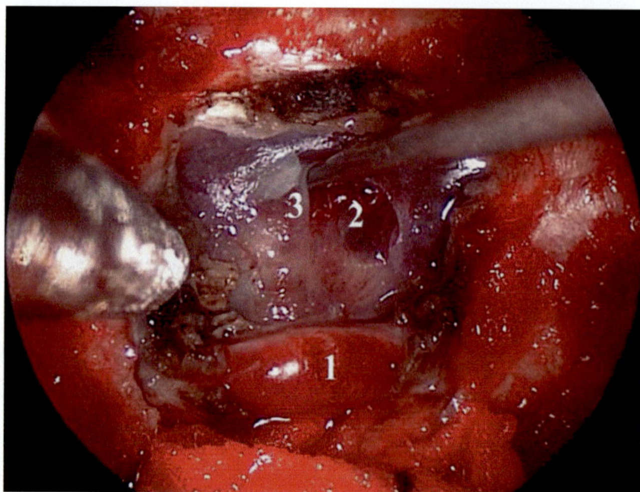

Fig. 5.23 After the dura is opened, the tumor is found located in the subarachnoid space, and the pituitary gland below is not involved. (1) Pituitary gland, (2) tumor, (3) arachnoid

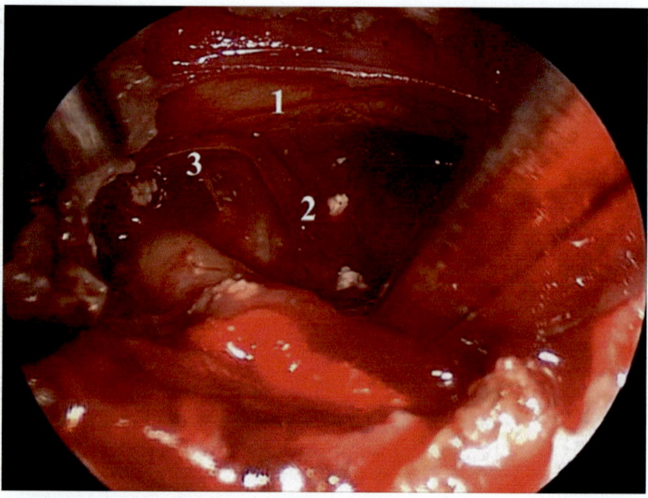

Fig. 5.25 Exploring the upper pole of the tumor. The tumor protrudes into the third ventricle floor. (1) Optometry, (2) tumor, (3) third ventricle floor

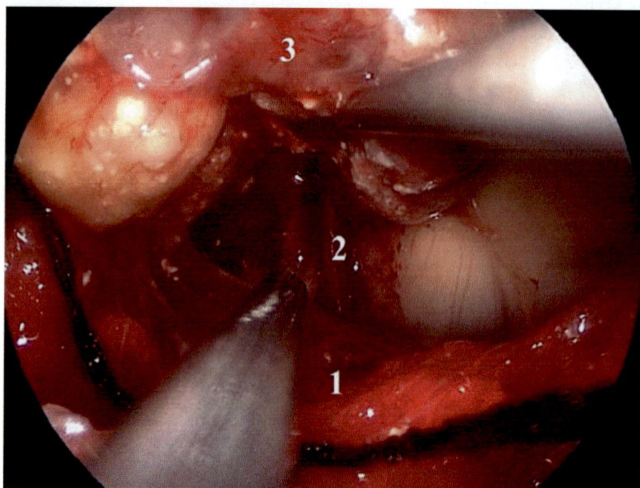

Fig. 5.24 Exploration of the lower pole of the tumor. The tumor is located inside the basal arachnoid, and the lower part of the pituitary stalk is visible. (1) Basal arachnoid, (2) pituitary stalk, (3) tumor

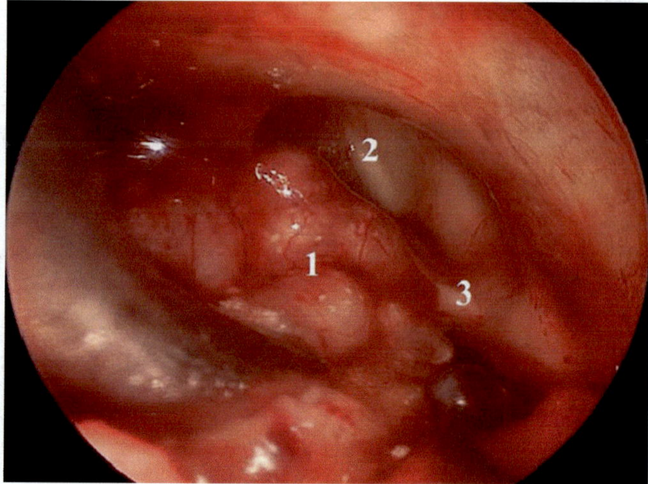

Fig. 5.26 Separation of the tumor from the third ventricle floor. The tumor at the point of origin has obvious adhesion to the third ventricle wall. At the non-origin point, the tumor is easily separated from the third ventricle wall. (1) Tumor, (2) the non-origin point of third ventricle, (3) tumor origin site

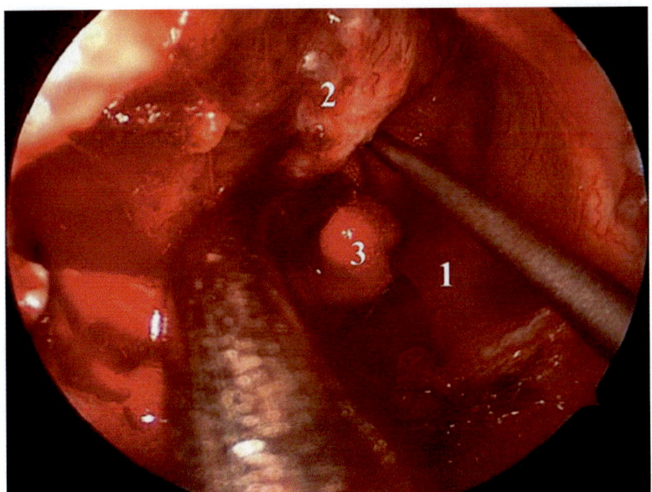

Fig. 5.27 Using brain cotton as a tool to separate tumors. The boundary between the tumor and the third ventricle is clear at the non-origin site. (1) Origin point, (2) tumor, (3) brain cotton

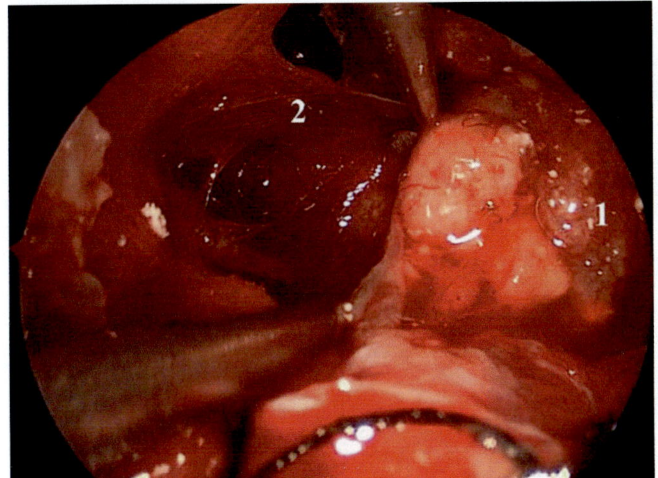

Fig. 5.28 Separation of the right border of the tumor, showing inner arachnoid separation between the tumor and the right third ventricle. (1) Tumor, (2) inner arachnoid

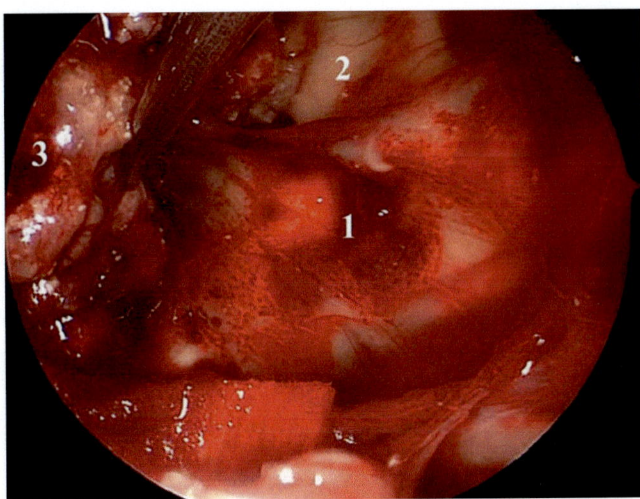

Fig. 5.29 There is no obvious boundary tumor at the point of tumor origin, which requires sharp separation. (1) Origin point, (2) non-origin point, (3) tumor

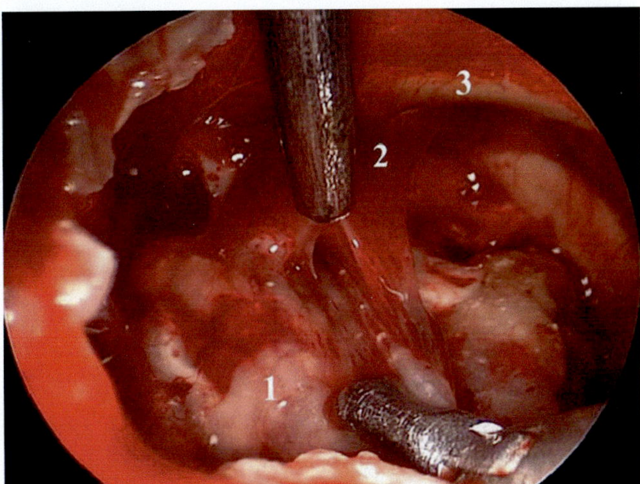

Fig. 5.30 There is a gliosis band between the tumor and the third ventricle floor. (1) Tumor, (2) gliosis band, (3) third ventricle floor

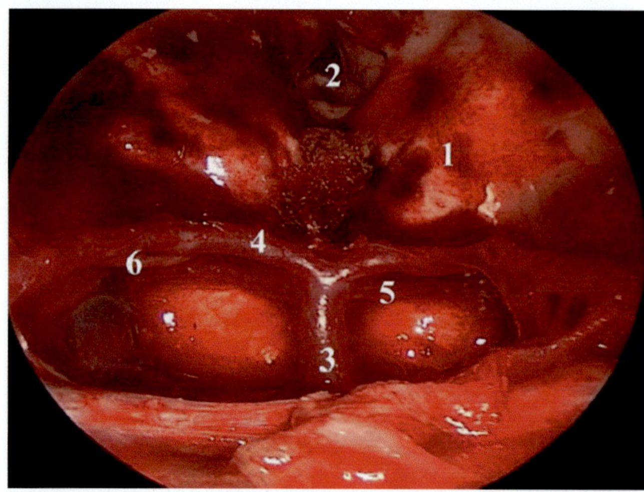

Fig. 5.31 The structure is well protected, and the third ventricle floor is partially opened after tumor total resection. (1) Third ventricle floor (tumor origin), (2) third ventricle, (3) basilar artery, (4) posterior cerebral artery, (5) superior cerebellar artery, (6) oculomotor nerve

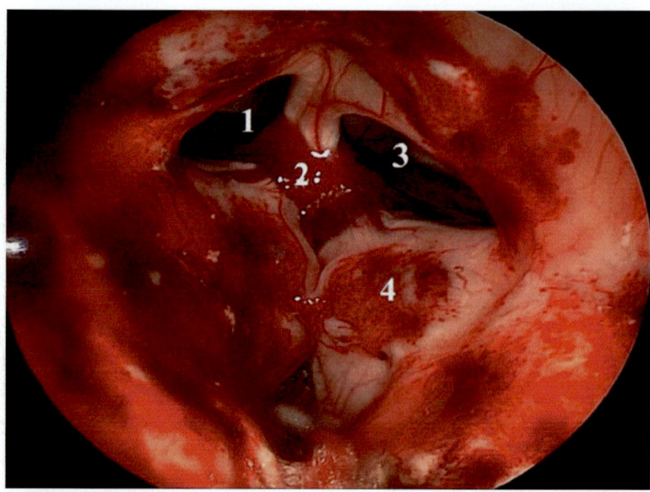

Fig. 5.32 View of the third ventricle floor. (1) Right foramen of Monro, (2) choroid plexus, (3) left foramen of Monro, (4) thalamus

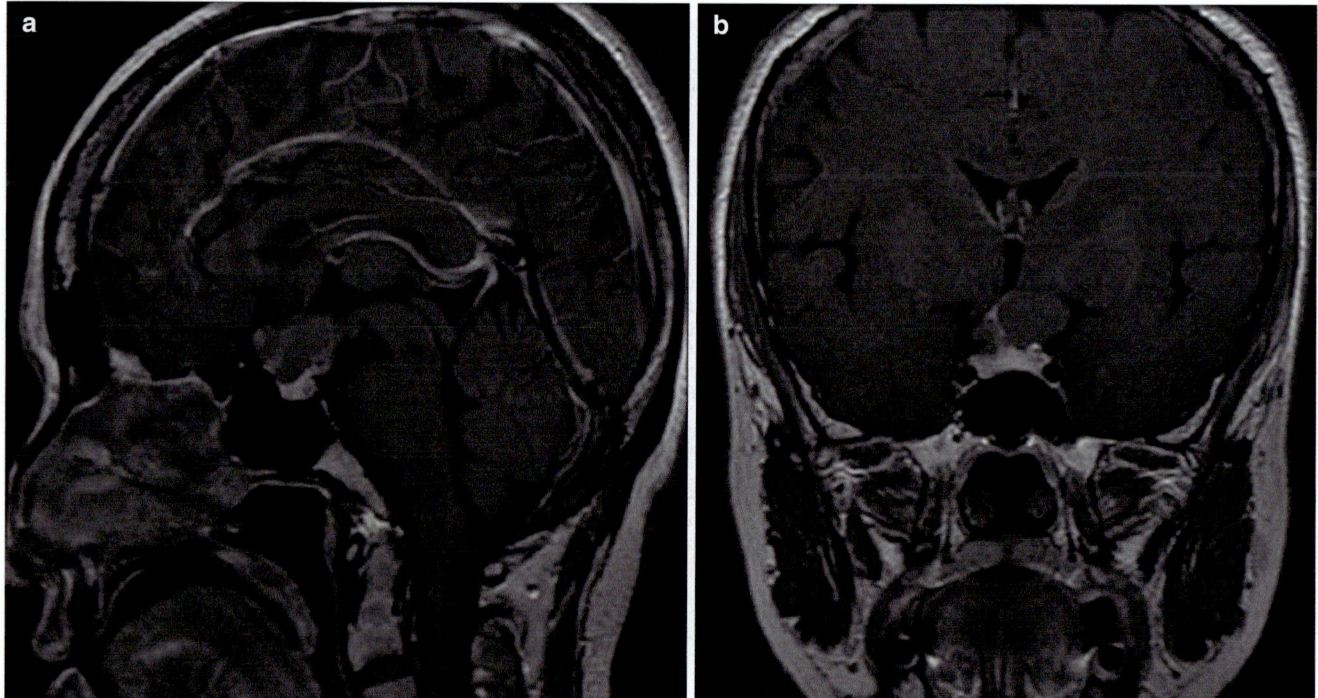

Fig. 5.33 The S-type craniopharyngioma originates from the pituitary stalk. The pituitary stalk is generally visible in MRI (**a**, **b**) but often interrupted or pushed by the tumor. The pituitary gland below is relatively normal, and the third ventricle above may be pushed

5.3 Application of the Endoscopic Transsphenoidal Approach in Adult Craniopharyngioma

5.3.1 Case 1: A Case of S-Type Craniopharyngioma in an Adult

(Figs. 5.33, 5.34, 5.35, 5.36, 5.37, 5.38, 5.39, 5.40, and 5.41)

5.3.2 Comment

S-type tumors originate from Rathke's pouch precursor cells that remain in the pituitary stalk. Therefore, the origin of the tumor is located in the pituitary stalk. There are membrane structures (including the arachnoid sleeve of pituitary stalk, inner arachnoid, and pia mater) between the tumor and the third ventricle floor. The pituitary gland

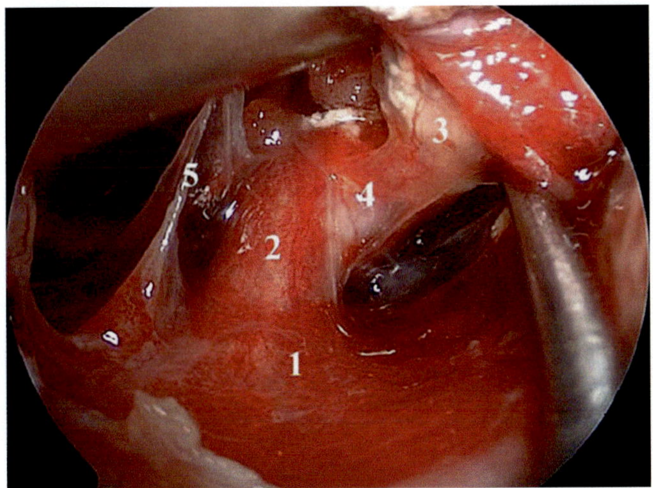

Fig. 5.34 After opening the dura mater at the tuberculum sellae, the tumor is exposed. It can be seen that the tumor originates from the pituitary stalk and is located inside the arachnoid sleeve of the pituitary stalk. The pituitary is not involved. (1) Pituitary gland, (2) pituitary stalk, (3) tumor, (4) tumor origin point, (5) pituitary stalk arachnoid sleeve

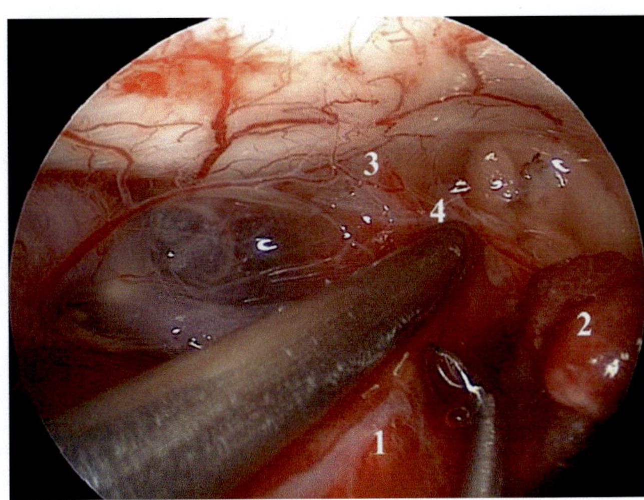

Fig. 5.36 Separation of the tumor origin from the pituitary stalk. (1) Pituitary stalk, (2) tumor, (3) third ventricle floor, (4) arachnoid

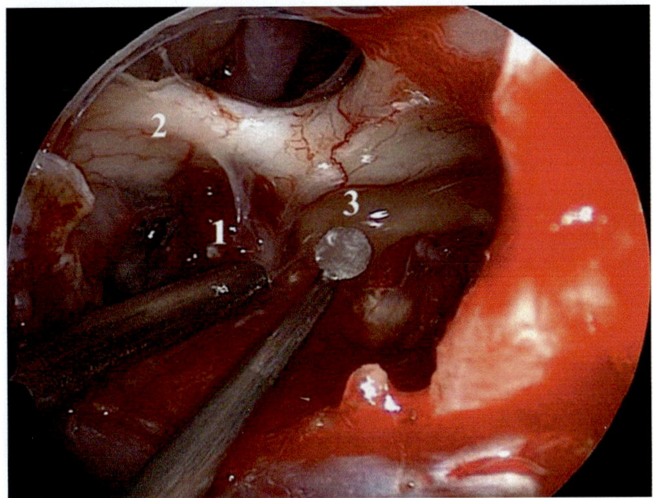

Fig. 5.35 Arachnoid remains between the tumor and the third ventricle floor. (1) Tumor, (2) optic nerve, (3) third ventricle floor

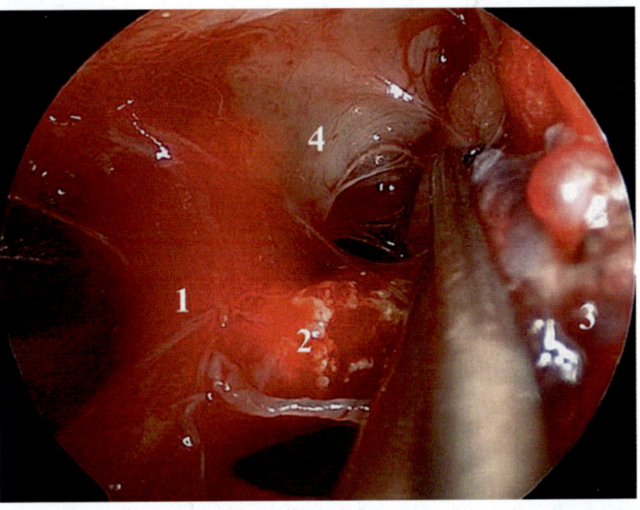

Fig. 5.37 The tumor origin in the pituitary stalk can be clearly seen, and the third ventricle is intact. (1) Pituitary stalk, (2) origin point, (3) tumor, (4) third ventricle floor

is protected from the tumor involving the diaphragma sellae. The tumor can involve the pituitary stalk and expand in all directions. The stalk involvement pattern is related to the height and tightness of the ASPS. When the ASPS is loosely attached to the pituitary stalk, the tumor tends to grow into the subarachnoid space because the arachnoid offers no restriction. In these cases, the pituitary stalk is almost normal or is only pushed by the tumor. Invasion can be seen in the tumor origin site of the pituitary stalk, similar to the brain invasion displayed by type T tumors. In extreme cases, these tumors can even involve three cranial fossae by extending into the subarachnoid space. When the ASPS is tightly attached to the pituitary stalk, the tumor tends to grow through the pituitary stalk due to the mechanical restriction offered by the ASPS. Some tumors even penetrate through the pituitary stalk and pass through the diaphragma sellae, thus involving the hypophyseal fossa.

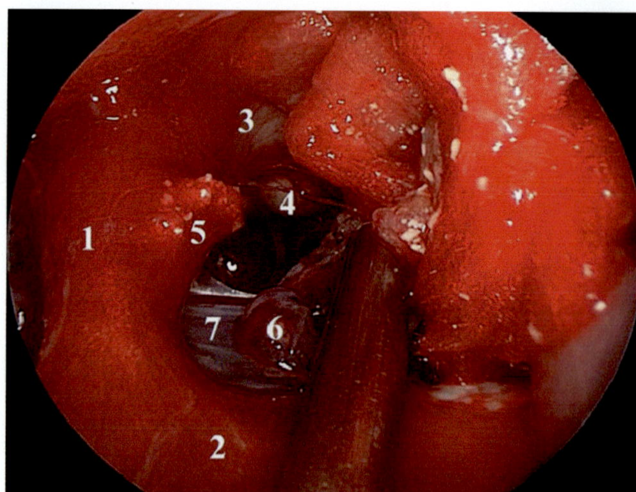

Fig. 5.38 The tumor was removed from the pituitary stalk. (1) Pituitary stalk, (2) pituitary gland, (3) third ventricle floor, (4) mammillary body, (5) origin point, (6) tumor, (7) Liliequist membrane

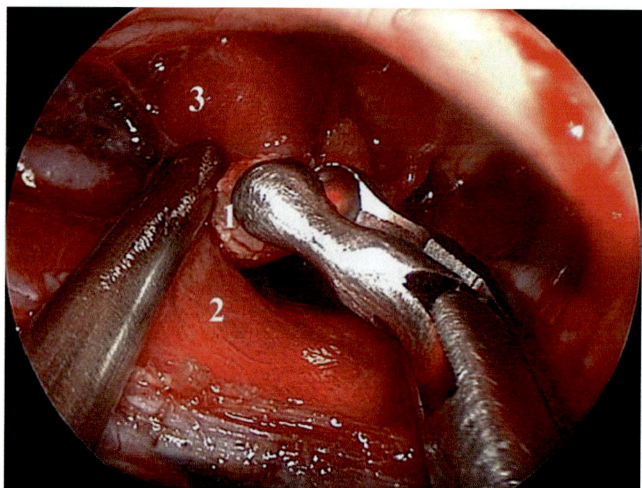

Fig. 5.39 The tumor at the point of origin was pulled out. (1) Tumor at the origin site, (2) pituitary gland, (3) pituitary stalk

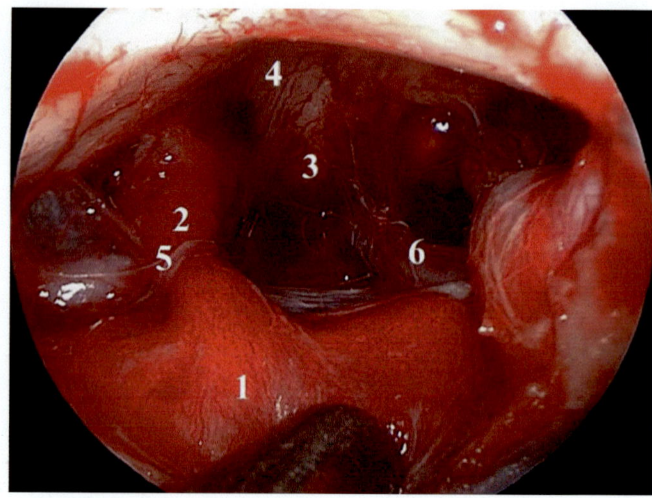

Fig. 5.40 The structures are well protected after the tumor is removed. (1) Pituitary gland, (2) pituitary stalk, (3) mammillary body, (4) third ventricle floor, (5) arachnoid sleeve of the pituitary stalk, (6) posterior communicating artery

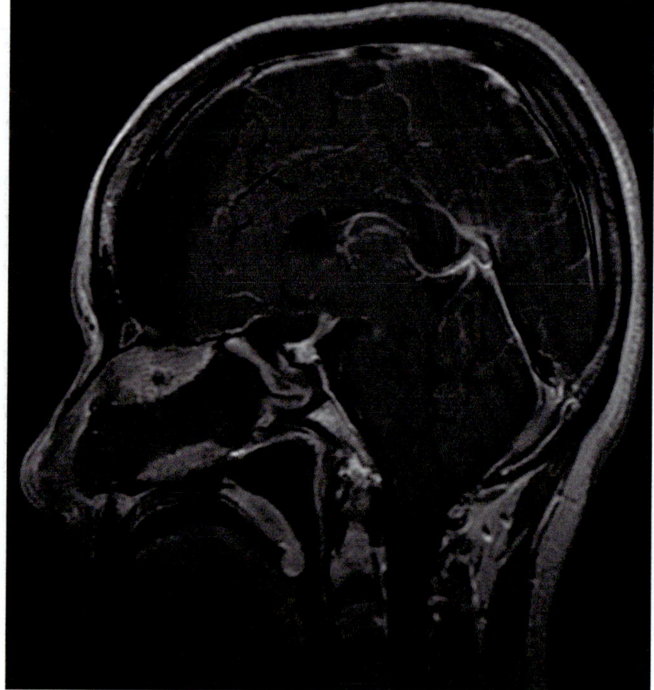

Fig. 5.41 Postoperative MRI showing that the pituitary stalk and pituitary gland were well protected and that the third ventricle floor remained intact

5.3.3 Case 2: A Case of T-Type Craniopharyngioma Occupying the Space of the Third Ventricle—Involving the Upper Part of the Pituitary Stalk (Figs. 5.42, 5.43, 5.44, 5.45, 5.46, 5.47, 5.48, 5.49, and 5.50)

5.3.4 Comment

This is a typical T-type craniopharyngioma case, mainly involving the hypothalamus and the upper part of the pituitary stalk. The tumor was located beneath the basal arachnoid membrane and outside the pia mater. Therefore, there was pia mater separation between the tumor and the third ventricle floor. As the tumor grows, the pia mater can be disrupted by the tumor, and finger-like invasions were found in the nervous layer of the third ventricle floor. However, the ependymal layer of the third ventricle floor was always intact. To wit, despite occupying the third ventricle space, the tumor remained located outside the third ventricle, so the term "third ventricle craniopharyngioma" or "intraventricular craniopharyngioma" requires further discussion.

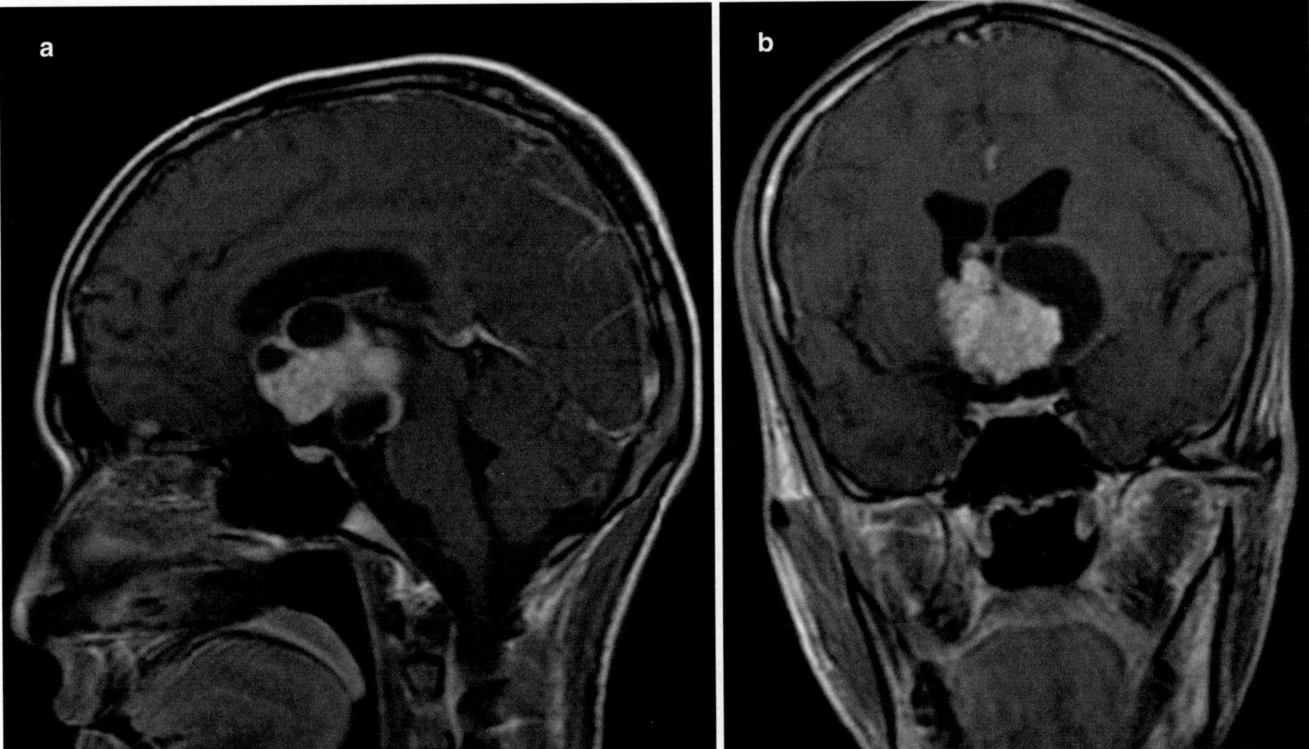

Fig. 5.42 A case of solid T-shaped craniopharyngioma (**a**, **b**). The tumor originates from residual Rathke's pouch precursor cells in the pars tuberalis adenohypophysis, occupying the space of the third ventricle. The lower part of the pituitary stalk and the pituitary gland are normal

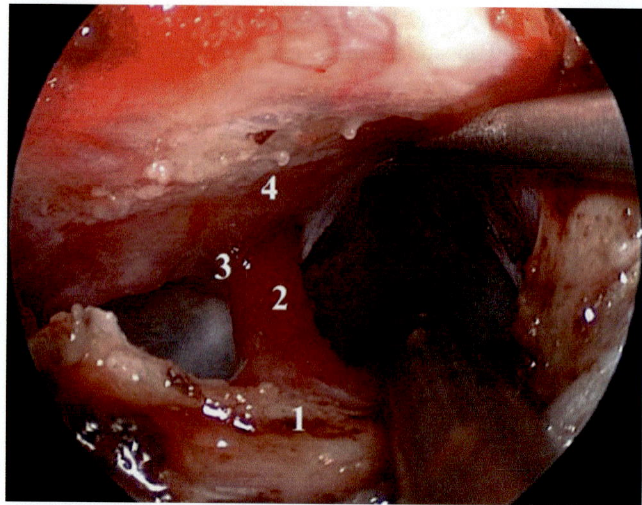

Fig. 5.43 The suprasellar arachnoid arising from the basement membrane of the arachnoid (BAM) envelops the pituitary stalk to form an arachnoidal sleeve (ASPS). The tumor is located in the arachnoid space; the lower part of the pituitary stalk and the pituitary gland are normal. (1) Pituitary, (2) pituitary stalk, (3) ASPS, (4) tumor

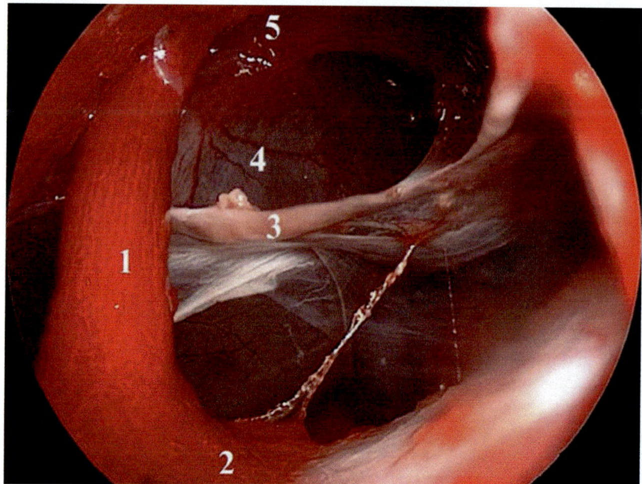

Fig. 5.44 Opening of the BAM and exposure of the tumor, showing that the tumor originated from the pars tuberalis adenohypophysis. (1) Pituitary stalk, (2) pituitary gland, (3) BAM, (4) tumor, (5) tumor origin

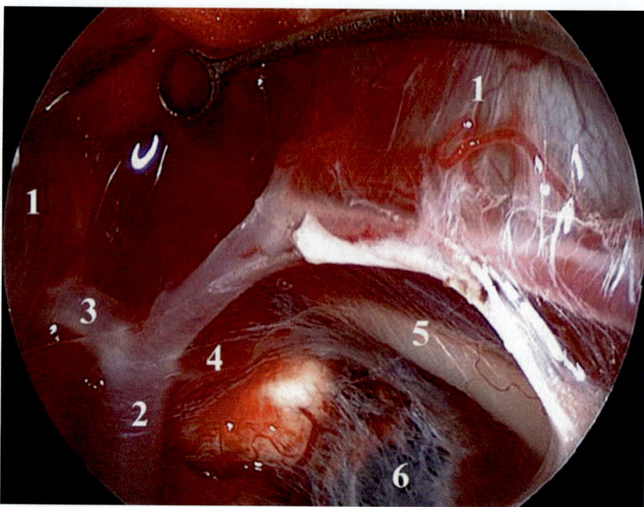

Fig. 5.45 The tumor involved the posterior cerebral artery and the interpeduncular cistern. (1) Tumor, (2) basilar artery, (3) right posterior cerebral artery, (4) left superior cerebellar artery, (5) ocular nerve, (6) Liliequist membrane

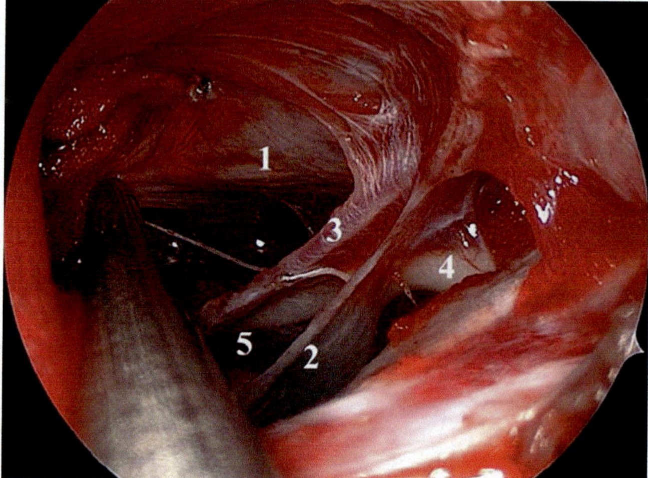

Fig. 5.46 Separation of the tumor from surrounding structures. (1) Tumor, (2) BAM, (3) left posterior cerebral artery, (4) ocular nerve, (5) Liliequist membrane

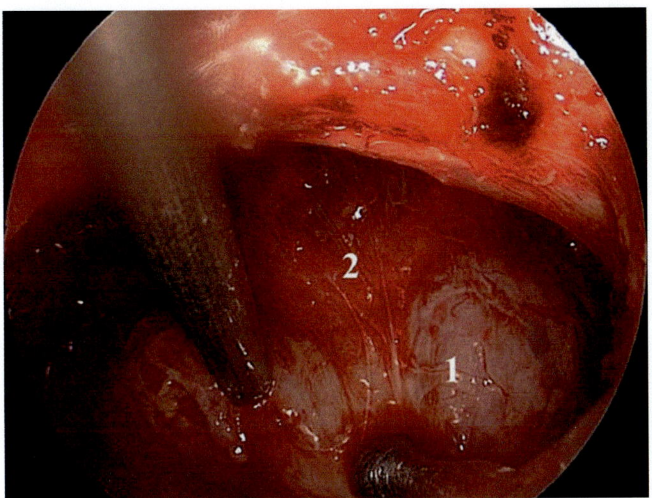

Fig. 5.47 Separation of the tumor from the third ventricle floor. The boundary between the tumor and the third ventricle floor is clear at the non-origin point. (1) Tumor, (2) third ventricle floor

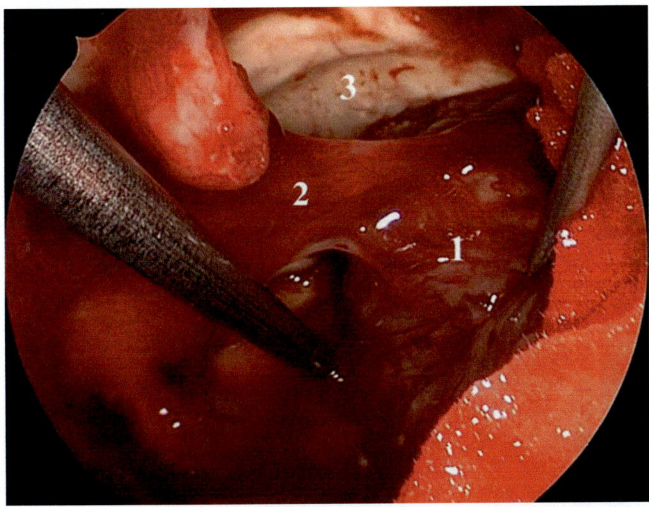

Fig. 5.48 At the point of origin, the boundary between the tumor and the third ventricle floor is unclear, requiring sharp separation. (1) Tumor, (2) origin point, (3) optic chiasm

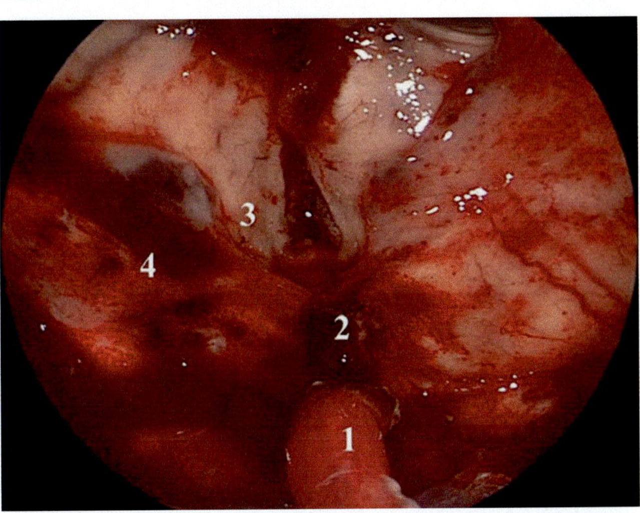

Fig. 5.49 Because the tumor involves the upper end of the pituitary stalk, the upper end of the pituitary stalk has been completely tumorized, and thus the continuity of the pituitary stalk cannot be preserved. (1) Normal lower pituitary stalk, (2) the junction between the pituitary stalk and third ventricle floor, (3) third ventricle, (4) tumor origin

5.3.5 Case 3: A Case of T-Type Craniopharyngioma Growing Through the Pituitary Stalk (Figs. 5.51, 5.52, 5.53, 5.54, 5.55, 5.56, 5.57, 5.58, 5.59, and 5.60)

5.3.6 Comment

This is a special case of T-type craniopharyngioma. The tumor originated from the pars tuberalis adenohypophysis and grew through the pituitary stalk. We hypothesized that the growth pattern of type T tumor is closely related to the thickness of the inner arachnoid layer near the pars tuberalis adenohypophysis and ASPS. When the inner arachnoid, pia mater, and ASPS are sufficiently dense to prevent tumor growth into the subarachnoid space and third ventricle, the tumor tends to grow through the pituitary stalk. The pituitary stalk tends to expand. Surgeons had to remove the pituitary stalk to ensure that the tumor was completely resected under

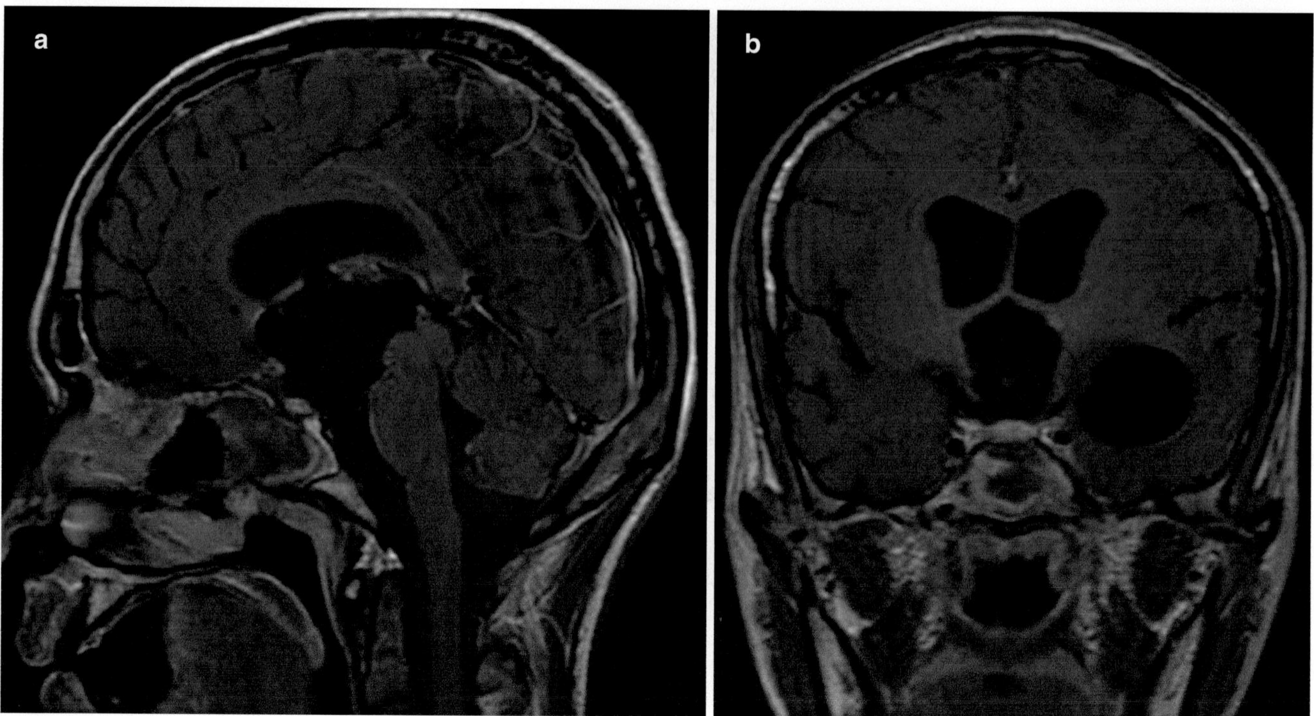

Fig. 5.50 Postoperative MRI (**a**, **b**) indicates that total tumor resection was achieved

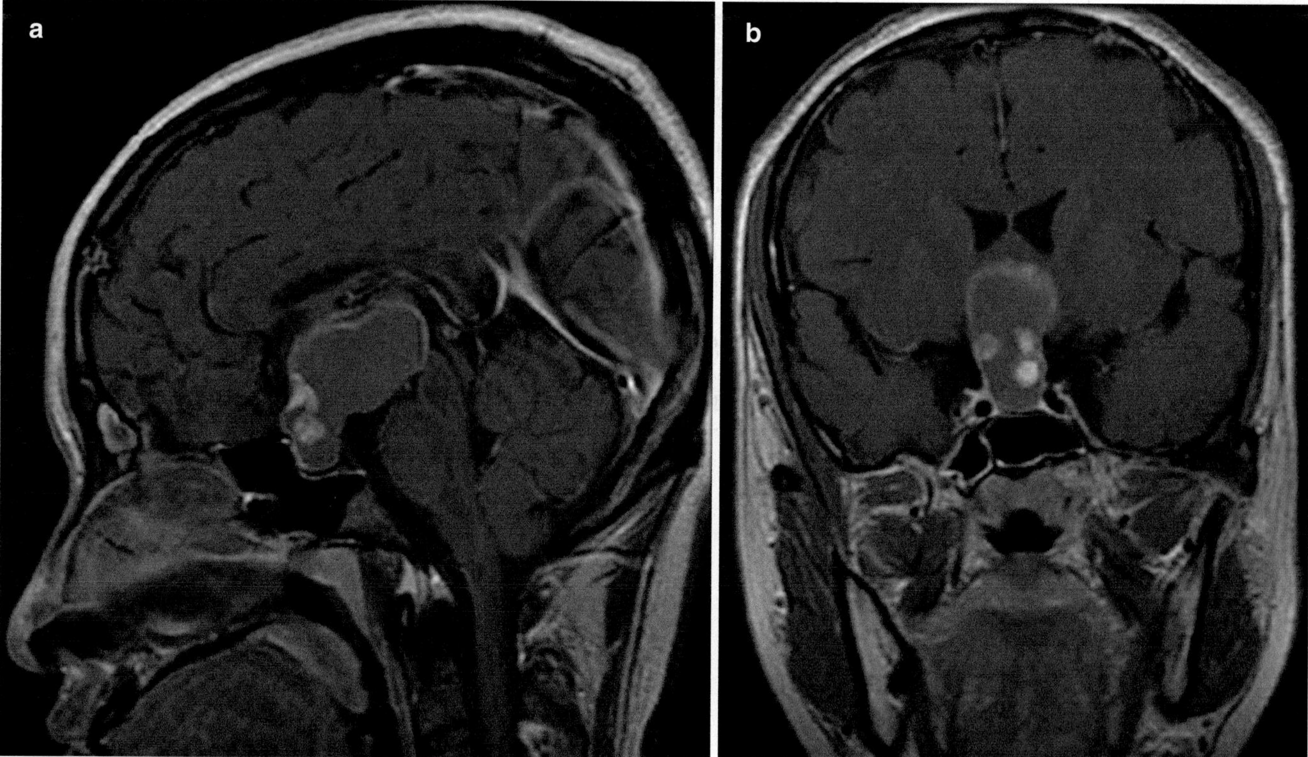

Fig. 5.51 A case of T-type craniopharyngioma. The tumor originates from the pars tuberalis adenohypophysis and grows through the pituitary stalk. The pituitary stalk cannot be seen on MRI

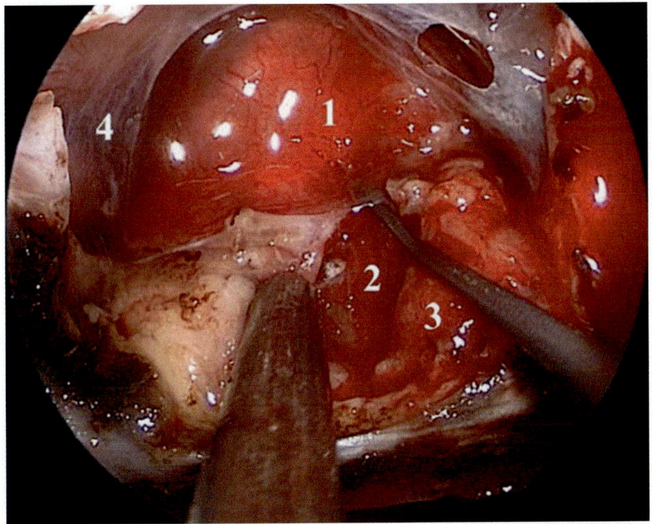

Fig. 5.52 The tumor is exposed after the dura is opened. The tumor originates from the pars tuberalis adenohypophysis and grows through the pituitary stalk, extending intra-sellarly. (1) Super-sellar tumor, (2) intra-sellar tumor, (3) pituitary gland, (4) arachnoid

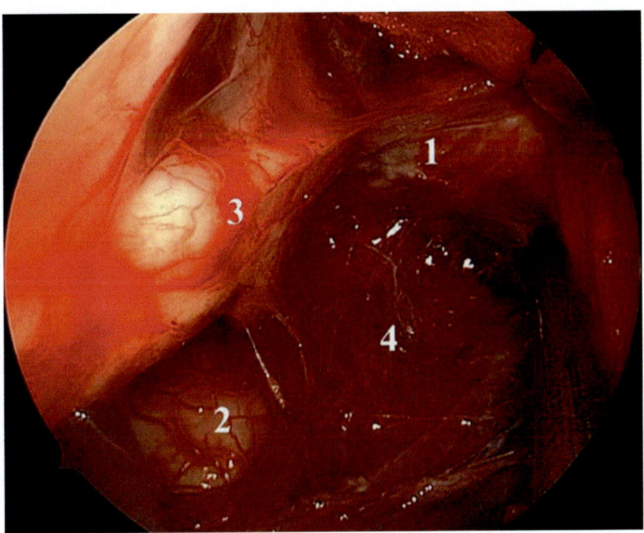

Fig. 5.54 Exploration of the upper border of the tumor. (1) Tumor, (2) brain stem, (3) optic chiasm, (4) interpeduncular cistern

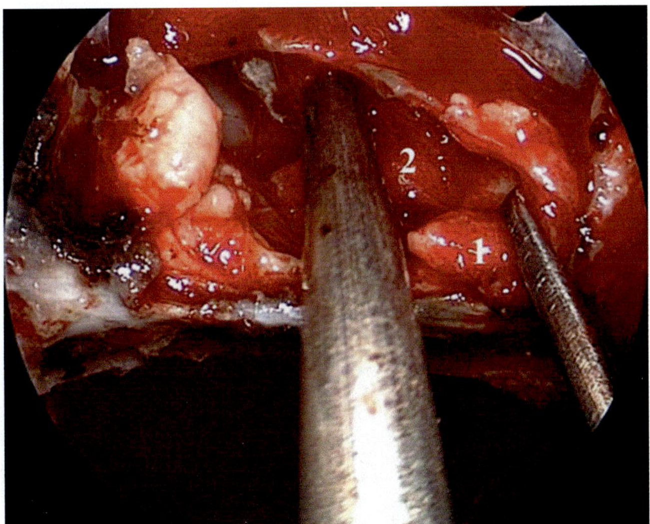

Fig. 5.53 Separation of the intra-sellar tumor and pituitary gland. The boundary between the tumor and pituitary gland is clear. (1) Pituitary gland, (2) tumor

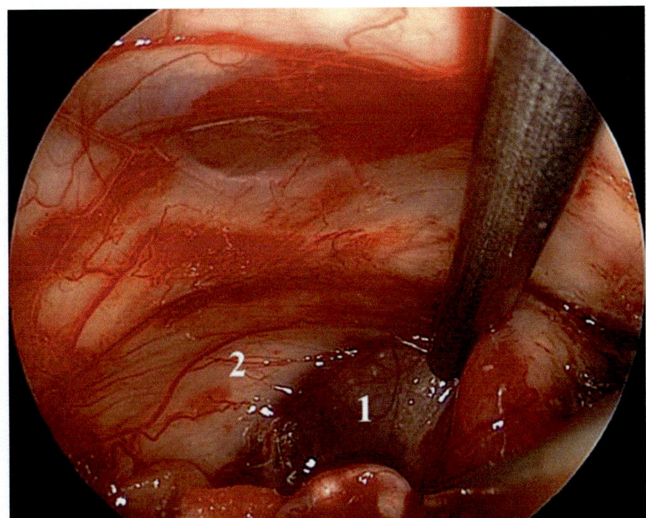

Fig. 5.55 Separation of the tumor from the third ventricle floor. At the non-origin point, the boundary is clear and easy to separate. (1) Tumor, (2) third ventricle floor

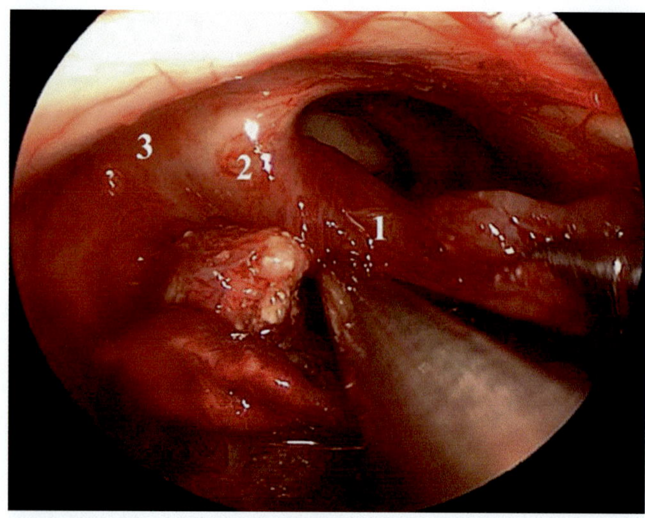

Fig. 5.56 Part of the tumor broke through the third ventricle floor, and there was no obvious boundary between the tumor and third ventricle floor. (1) Tumor, (2) boundary between the tumor and third ventricle floor, (3) third ventricle floor

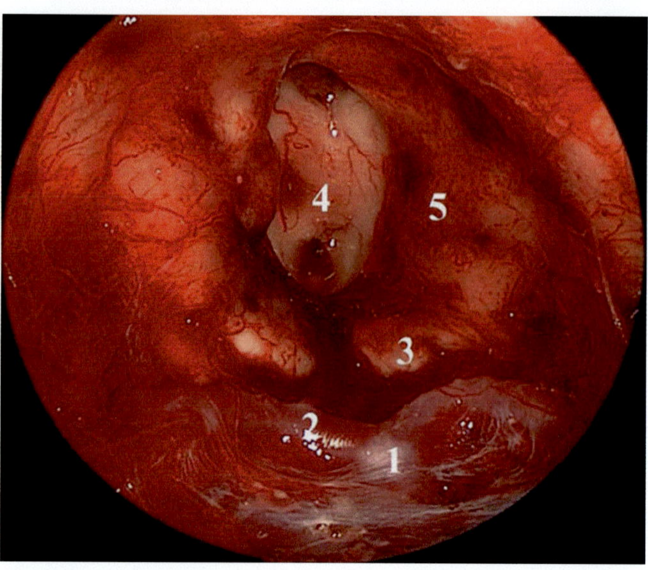

Fig. 5.58 After the tumor is totally removed, the structure is well protected. (1) Basilar artery, (2) right posterior cerebral artery, (3) mammillary body, (4) third ventricle, (5) tumor origin

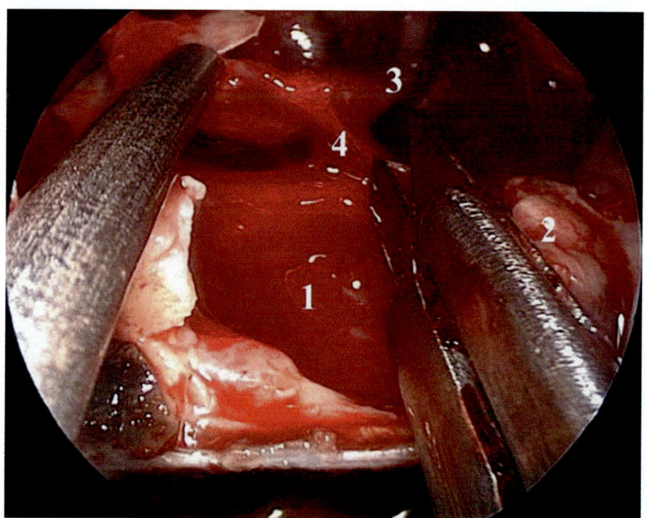

Fig. 5.57 The pituitary stalk is completely tumorized and cannot be retained, so the pituitary stalk is removed to ensure that the tumor is entirely removed. (1) Pituitary fossa, (2) Pituitary gland, (3) tumor, (4) tumorized pituitary stalk

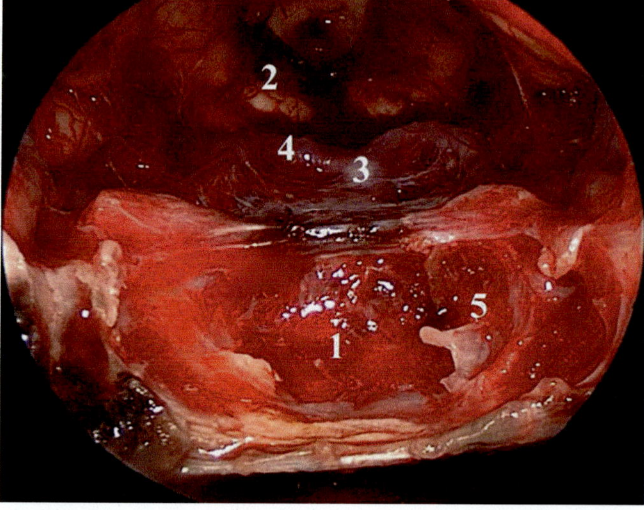

Fig. 5.59 The structure in the pituitary fossa is also well protected. (1) Pituitary fossa, (2) mammillary body, (3) basilar artery, (4) right posterior cerebral artery, (5) pituitary gland

endoscopy due to limited instruments. When performing surgery under a microscope, the pituitary stalk can sometimes be preserved after tumor resection.

5.3.7 Case 4: A Case of T-Type Papillary Craniopharyngioma Occupying the Space of the Third Ventricle (Figs. 5.61, 5.62, 5.63, 5.64, 5.65, 5.66, 5.67, 5.68, 5.69, 5.70, and 5.71)

5.3.8 Comment

This is a case of a T type of papillary craniopharyngioma. The origin is located in pars tuberalis adenohypophysis. Due to the expansion of the tumor, the pia mater between the tumor and the third ventricle floor may still disappear, and the tumor may involve the third ventricle floor, but does not break through the ependymal layer of the third ventricle. Type T tumor is the most complex and it is

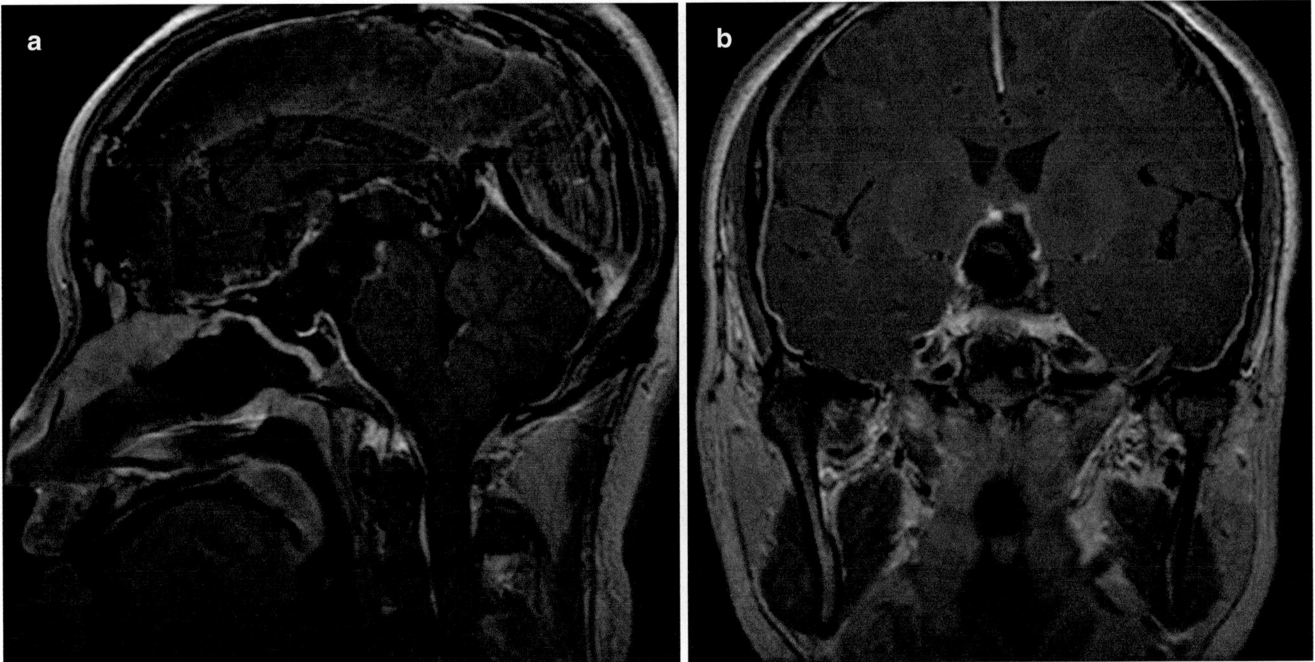

Fig. 5.60 Postoperative MRI (**a**, **b**) showing that total tumor resection was achieved

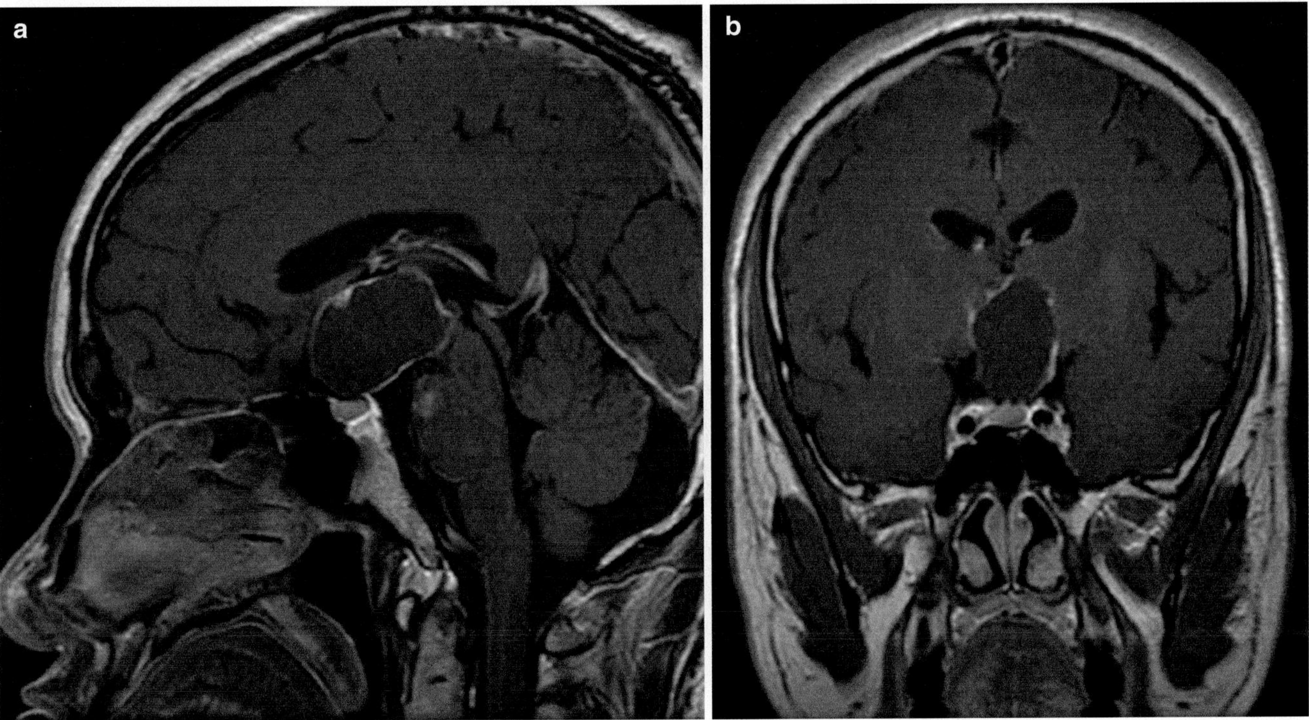

Fig. 5.61 MRI (**a**, **b**) showing that the small nodule is in the cystic wall, which is one of the typical imaging features of PCP. The pituitary stalk is invisible, while the pituitary gland is clearly visible. The tumor originates from the pars tuberalis adenohypophysis and grows downward

important to protect the third ventricle floor in this type during surgery. Both transcranial surgery and transsphenoidal surgery provide the oppotunity to protect the third ventricle floor, however, in our view, the outter layer of the third ventricle floor (facing the pia mater) is more likely protected in transcranial surgery, while the inner layer of the third ventricle floor (facing the ependyma) is more likely protected intranssphenoidal surgery. Whether this distinction would influence the long-term prognosis is not yet clear and requires further study.

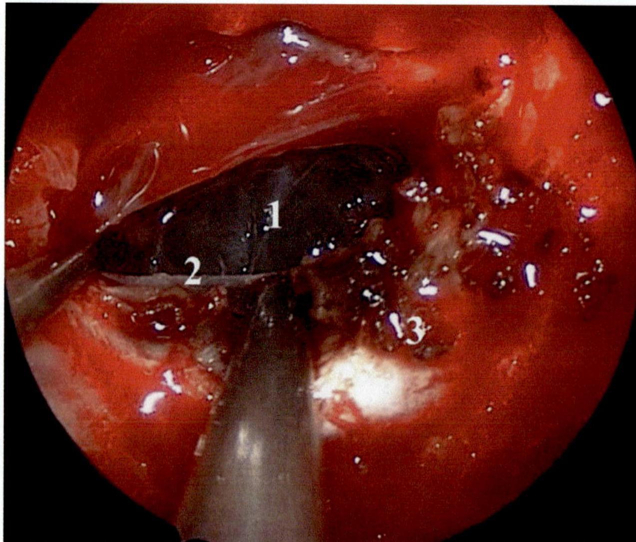

Fig. 5.62 The tumor is exposed after the arachnoid is opened. The tumor is located in the subarachnoid space. (1) Tumor, (2) arachnoid, (3) dura mater

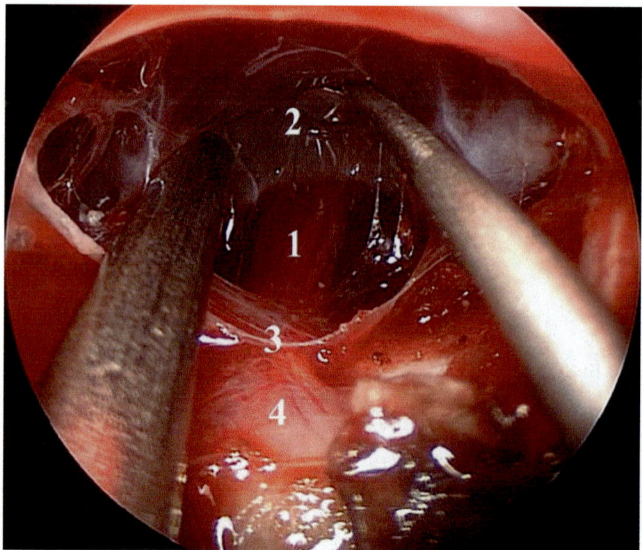

Fig. 5.63 The tumor originates from the pars tuberalis adenohypophysis. The lower part of the pituitary stalk and the pituitary gland are clearly visible. (1) Pituitary stalk, (2) tumor, (3) BAM, (4) pituitary gland

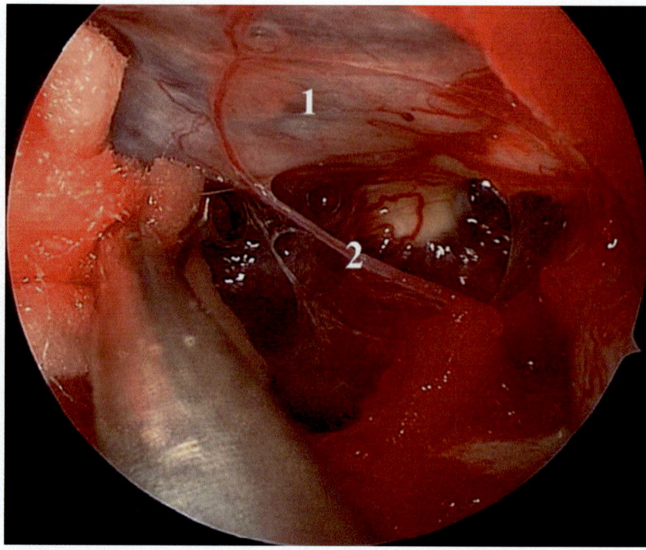

Fig. 5.64 The feeding vessel of the tumor is identified. (1) Tumor, (2) feeding vessel

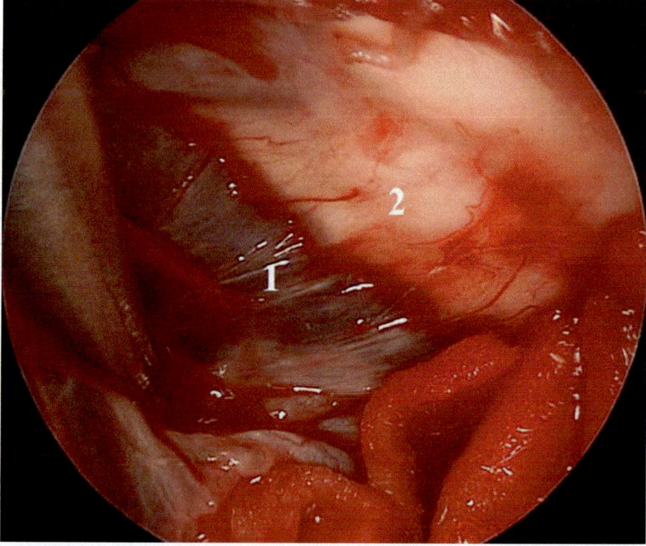

Fig. 5.65 In the non-origin part, the boundary between the tumor and third ventricle floor is clear. (1) Tumor, (2) third ventricle floor

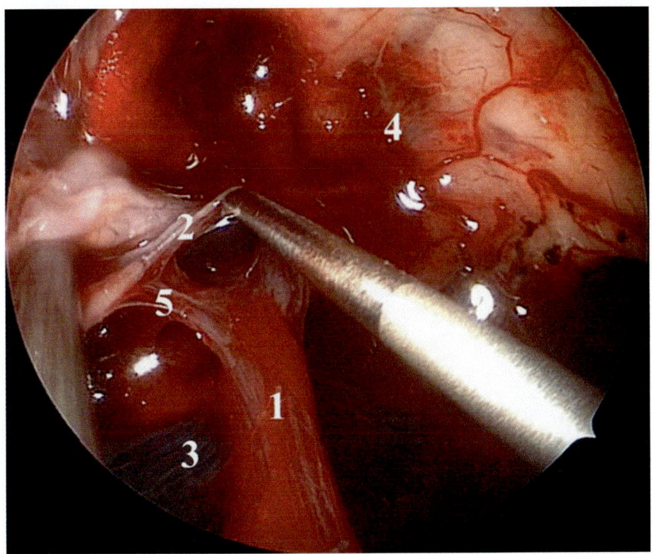

Fig. 5.66 Separation of the tumor from the pituitary stalk; inner arachnoid between the tumor and the pituitary stalk remains. (1) Pituitary stalk, (2) tumor, (3) Liliequist membrane, (4) third ventricle floor, (5) inner arachnoid

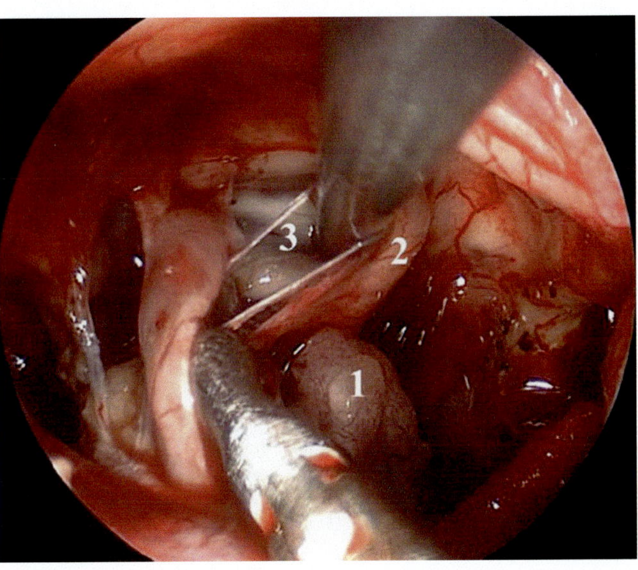

Fig. 5.68 The tumor at the origin part broke through the pia mater of the third ventricle floor, involving the third ventricle floor tissues, but did not break through the ependymal layer of the third ventricle. (1) Tumor, (2) third ventricle floor, (3) ependymal layer of the third ventricle

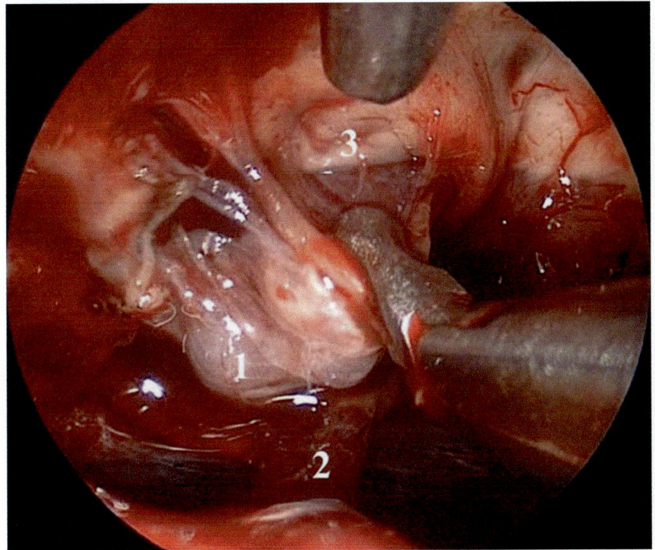

Fig. 5.67 Separation of the origin point of the tumor. (1) Tumor, (2) pituitary stalk, (3) third ventricle floor

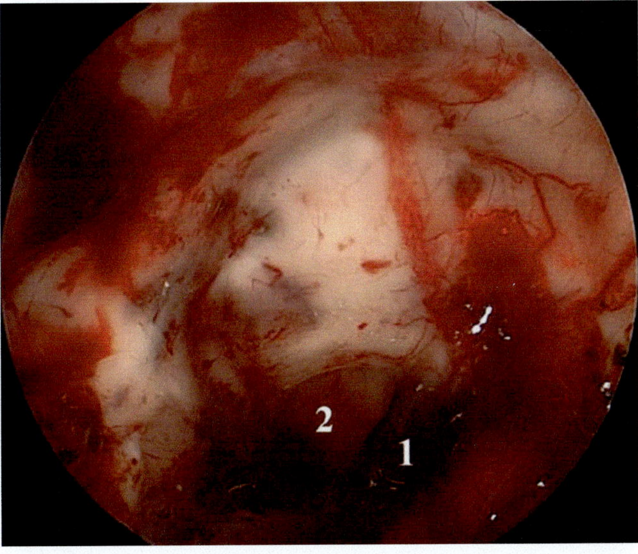

Fig. 5.69 After the tumor is completely resected, the third ventricle floor is partially opened. (1) Third ventricle floor, (2) third ventricle

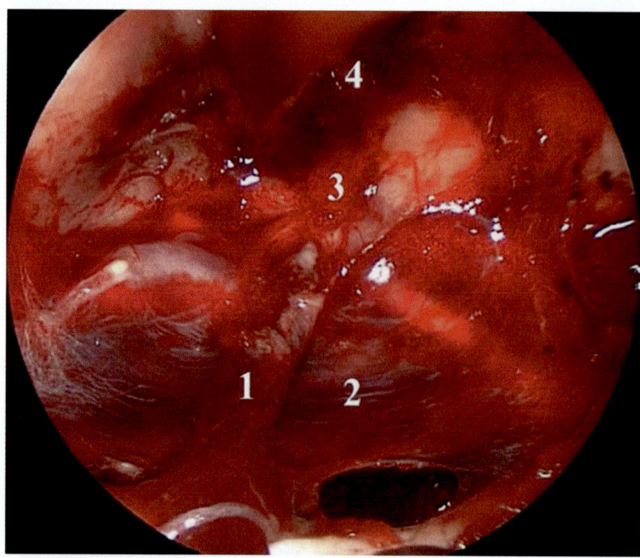

Fig. 5.70 After the tumor is removed, the structure is well protected. (1) Pituitary stalk, (2) Liliequist membrane, (3) mammillary bodies, (4) third ventricle floor

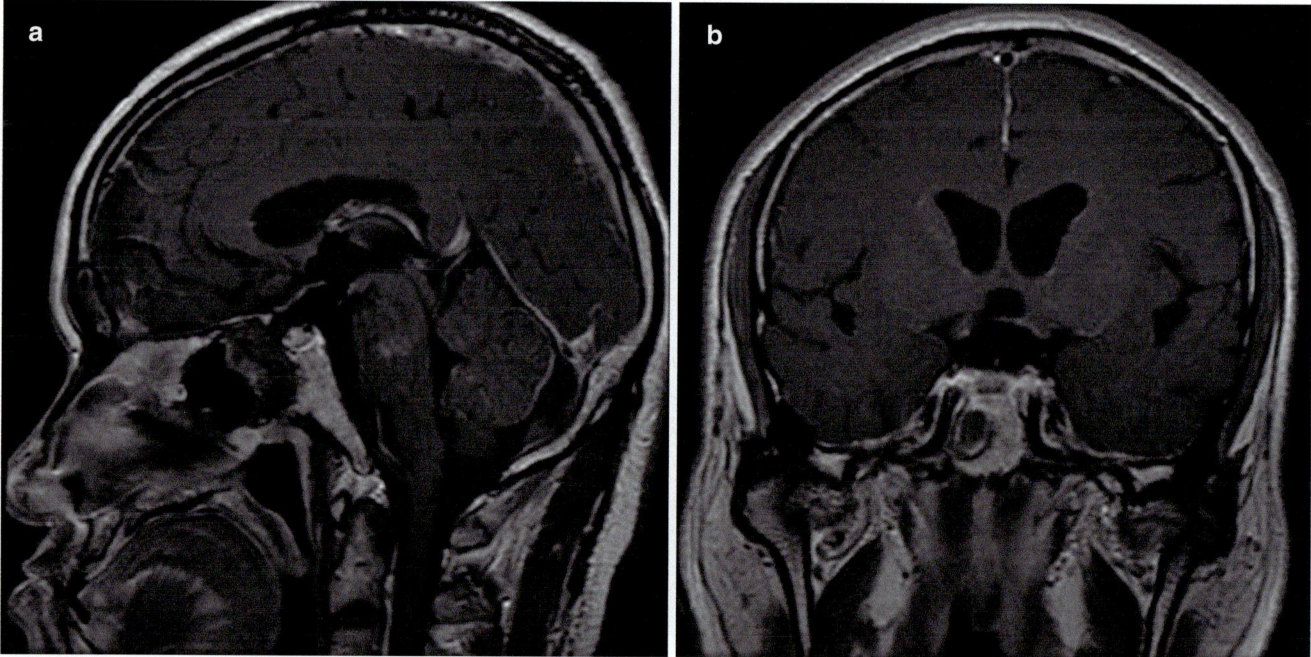

Fig. 5.71 Postoperative MRI (**a**, **b**) showing that the tumor is complete resected and the third ventricle floor and pituitary stalk are well protected

Surgical Treatment of Craniopharyngioma: Transcranial Approach

6

Jun Pan, Jun-xiang Peng, and Song-tao Qi

6.1 Introduction

6.1.1 Preface

Craniopharyngiomas may develop at any point along the pituitary–hypothalamus axis, from the sella turcica to the infundibularis partes of the third ventricle but they most commonly expand in the suprasellar cistern or within the third ventricle floor [1–3]. Tumors originate from along the path of embryonic development of Rathke's pouch out pia mater of the third ventricle. Tumors are usually classified according to the involving anatomical sites; however, large tumors may severely compress, distort, or involve neural tissue (third ventricular floor, pituitary stalk, and optic tract structures), making preoperative evaluation difficult even with excellent-quality neuroradiological studies [3–7]. In such a small area of the sellar region, therefore, accurate typing is sometimes difficult when the tumor is large. Here we propose a clinical classification system (QST classification system) based on both the tumor's original site and the relationship of the tumor to the suprasellar membranous structures (namely the diaphragma, the arachnoid membrane, and the pia mater) [1, 6–8].

The perfect use of this type requires a lot of clinical practice. The content of this chapter is to provide clinical cases with typical and complex growth patterns, so that readers can grasp the essence of the QST classification, thus improving the quality of surgery for craniopharyngioma.

The authors basic point of view is that because of the difficulty of reoperation, total resection is the primary goal in any case for surgical treatment of craniopharyngioma. Transcranial surgery still remains the essential treatment for craniopharyngiomas even though the extended endoscopic transnasal approaches (EEA) are increasingly used in the current state [5]. For a giant craniopharyngioma occupying multi-cistern spaces (very common in craniopharyngioma) and those with relapsed and refractory cases, transcranial surgery may become the last line of defense. Therefore, for craniopharyngioma, transcranial surgery has a wider range of indications, which should be regarded as the "mother technology" for surgical treatment of craniopharyngioma.

This chapter involves a lot of technical methods, the final surgical concept is: complete en bloc tumor resection technique, its significance is: to ensure a high total tumor resection rate, to maximize the identification and protection of the surrounding structure; useful to clarify the tumor and surrounding structures. Understanding the morphological relationship between tumor and the surrounding structures can also shorten the operation time of this complex tumor after proficiency.

6.2 Transcranial Surgical Treatment of Craniopharyngiomas

Surgical resection is the mainstay in craniopharyngioma management. Both extended endoscopic transnasal approaches (EEA) and transcranial approaches (TCA) were performed by neurosurgeons considered experts in the field in each approach. In the past decades, surgical approaches have improved dramatically. Firstly, the EEA has been increasingly used to manage craniopharyngiomas based on the improved view of the undersurface of the chiasm which is always being a blind spot during the transcranial approach. Secondly, in transcranial surgery, anterior interhemispheric midline approach has becoming the principal method in the management of craniopharyngioma (compared to Yasargil transsylvian approach) [3]. Even though, the selection criteria, the advantages and disadvantages of each approach still remain problematic.

In craniopharyngioma surgery, special attention must be paid in two facts:

1. There is indeed a considerable proportion of tumors that are completely unsuitable for transsphenoidal surgery. For example, tumors that have significant lateral extent

J. Pan (✉) · J.-x. Peng · S.-t. Qi
Department of Neurosurgery, Nanfang Hospital of Southern Medical University, Guangzhou, Guangdong, China

© Springer Nature Singapore Pte Ltd. 2020
S. Qi (ed.), *Atlas of Craniopharyngioma*, https://doi.org/10.1007/978-981-13-7322-0_6

into the middle or posterior fossa can't be well visualized by the endonasal approach.

2. For midline craniopharyngioma, viable neural tissue which contains hypothalamic nuclei may not be safely dissected through the transnasal approach if the tumors mainly occupy the third ventricle chamber (type T craniopharyngiomas).

In this chapter, the authors mainly discuss the operative nuances for removal of suprasellar craniopharyngioma via the transcranial approach. Every effort was made to maintain the intactness of normal nervous tissues, especially the infundibulum-pituitary stalk tract.

6.3 Surgical Technique for Transcranial Resection of Craniopharyngioma: Generalized Overview

As mentioned above, transcranial surgery is still dominant in the treatment of craniopharyngioma. The main reason is that craniopharyngiomas are naturally multi-cavity growth tumors, which block the full exposure of the tumor through the transsphenoidal approach. Another important reason is that craniopharyngioma is easy to relapse, and recurrent tumors often adhere to the vascular nerve structures, which may put the patient in a dangerous situation when choosing a transnasal route.

The transcranial approaches for craniopharyngioma surgery generally include two types: lateral approaches and midline approaches.

6.3.1 The Lateral Approaches

The lateral approach includes the classic frontotemporal approach (namely transsylvian approach), the sub-frontal approach, eyebrow keyhole approach, etc. It is worth emphasizing that the lateral fissure should be fully dissected during the abovementioned approaches. The bone window should be tailored according to the extent of the tumor involvement. For example, when the tumor significantly expanded into the posterior fossa, the bone window on the temporal side should be enlarged backwards and enable enough exposure of the posterior cranial fossa through the tentorial approach (Fig. 6.1).

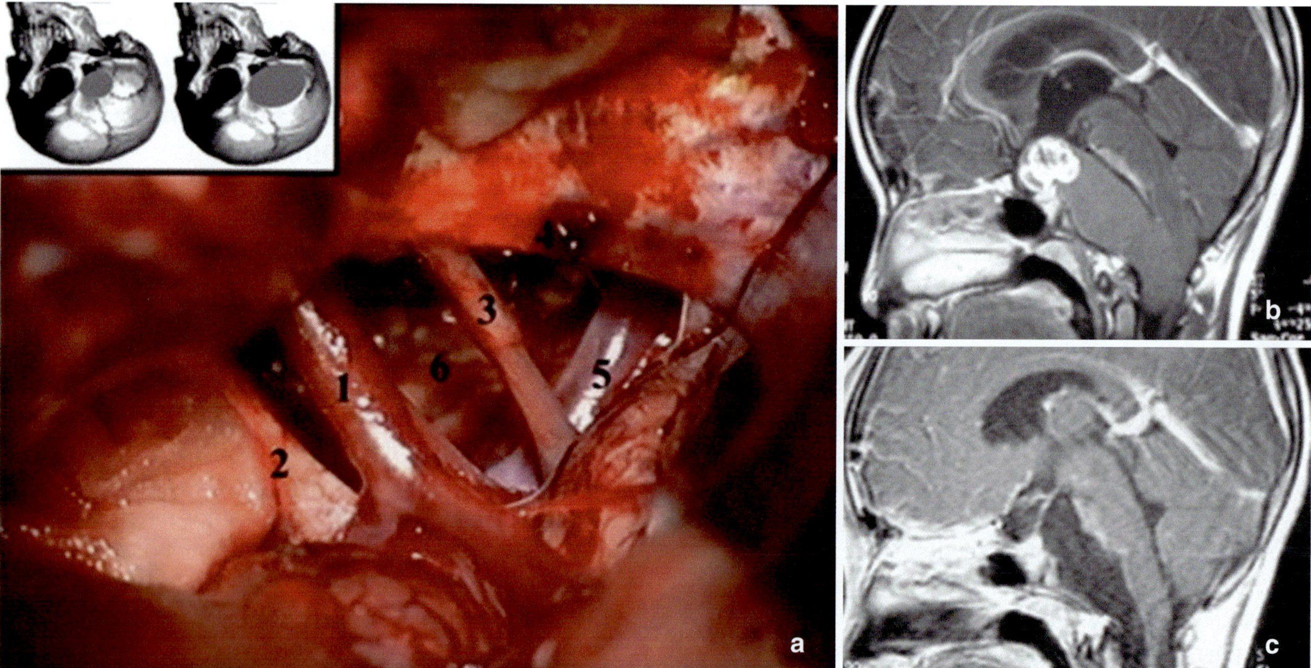

Fig. 6.1 This was a case of a 7-year-old boy. The tumor cyst expands to the mid-lower portion of the clivus. The operation uses a lateral fissure transtentorial approach. The posterior fossa tumor is fully exposed through the cerebellar hiatus. The schematic diagrams in the black box in the upper right corner show that the bone window is enlarged backwards to expose the posterior tumor part (gray shadow in the pictures). (**a**) Intraoperative picture showed the anatomy around right side of the cerebellar hiatus; (**b**, **c**) pre- and postoperative MR sagittal images. (1) Right-side ICA, (2) optic chiasm, (3) right-side oculomotor nerve, (4) tentorial margin, (5) basal artery, (6) tumor exposed through the cerebellar hiatus

6.3.2 The Midline Approaches

The midline approach mainly includes the frontobasal anterior interhemispheric approach and the interhemispheric transcallosal approach. Some scholars advocate the removal of the craniopharyngioma that invades the third ventricle through the transcallosal approach. However, the authors believe that this approach is difficult to dissect the tumor at the original site of infundibular tuberculum, so it is not described in this atlas.

The following focuses on the surgical techniques in the frontobasal anterior interhemispheric approach:

When the frontobasal anterior interhemispheric approach is used, the exposure of the tumor is mainly through two major surgical spaces: the prechiasmatic space and the lamina terminal space.

In this chapter, we mainly discuss two major surgical techniques in frontobasal anterior interhemispheric approach: (1) drilling of tuberculum bone to increase prechiasmatic space and intrasellar tumor exposure; (2) detachment of anterior communicating artery to increase space at the lamina terminal.

6.3.3 Increase Intrasellar Tumor Exposure by Drilling Bone at the Tuberculum Sellae

The prechiasmatic space is sometimes narrow in craniopharyngioma. Some patients belong to prefixed optic chiasm (the short optic nerve, anatomical variation), and more patients are due to the retrochiasmatic tumor (type T tumors). Drilling the bones of the tuberculum sellae and the sphenoidal platform can increase the space for surgical manipulation and reduce the traction on the optic chiasm. More importantly, through bone removal, the intrasellar tumor can be exposed under direct vision. It is particularly meaningful for the removal of type Q tumor (subdiaphragmatic CP), which can improve the total resection rate and of the possibility of pituitary stalk preservation (Fig. 6.2).

6.3.4 Division of the Anterior Communicating Artery to Exposure of Cistern at the Lamina Terminal

Lamina terminal space is the main corridor for T-type craniopharyngioma through the anterior interhemispheric approach. The lamina terminal is often crowded by the blood vessels of the anterior communicating artery complex. Therefore, dividing of AcoA becomes the choice. Dividing of the artery will provide adequate exposure of the lamina terminal space, making the surgical manipulation more convenient and safer (Fig. 6.3).

Because of the difference in anatomical development, the vascular architecture of the anterior communicating artery complex is diverse (Fig. 6.4). Therefore, it is important to evaluate the vascular structure of the anterior communicating artery before and during the operation for the division of the artery.

The evaluation methods mainly include: (1) preoperative angiography to understand the development of bilateral A1 and A2 segments and the morphology of the anterior communicating artery; (2) intraoperative microscopic exploration of the development of bilateral anterior cerebral arteries; (3) intraoperative experimental blockade using temporary aneurysm clip, and the blood supply of bilateral A2 segments and the perforating vessels were observed. If necessary, intraoperative phthalocyanine green angiography is a useful method (Figs. 6.5 and 6.6). It is worth emphasizing that dividing of anterior communicating artery is not a necessary step in the treatment of T-type craniopharyngioma through the trans-laminal terminal approach. In addition to assessing its feasibility, the growth characteristics of the tumor itself are more important factor. In the authors experience, only those cases where the tumor is located in a high position in the direction of the third ventricle (for example, 2/3 of the tumor exceeds the anterior communicating artery complex, the tumor significantly exceeds the anterior commissure, etc.) are the potential indication of the artery division.

6.4 Illustrate Cases

Here, we will discuss three types of tumors (type QST), which were removed using transcranial approaches; the surgical procedures and techniques for each type of tumor will be described and illustrated.

6.4.1 Type Q

6.4.1.1 Case 1

Medical History This was the case of a 9-year-old girl with a 12-month history of headache and decreased vision for 1 month. Her height was 115 cm, which is lower than average for her age and sex by 2 SD, and she was under the third percentile of average height for Chinese girls. Endocrinological examination revealed hypo-thyroxine and growth hormone axis and increased levels of prolactin (31 ng/μL).

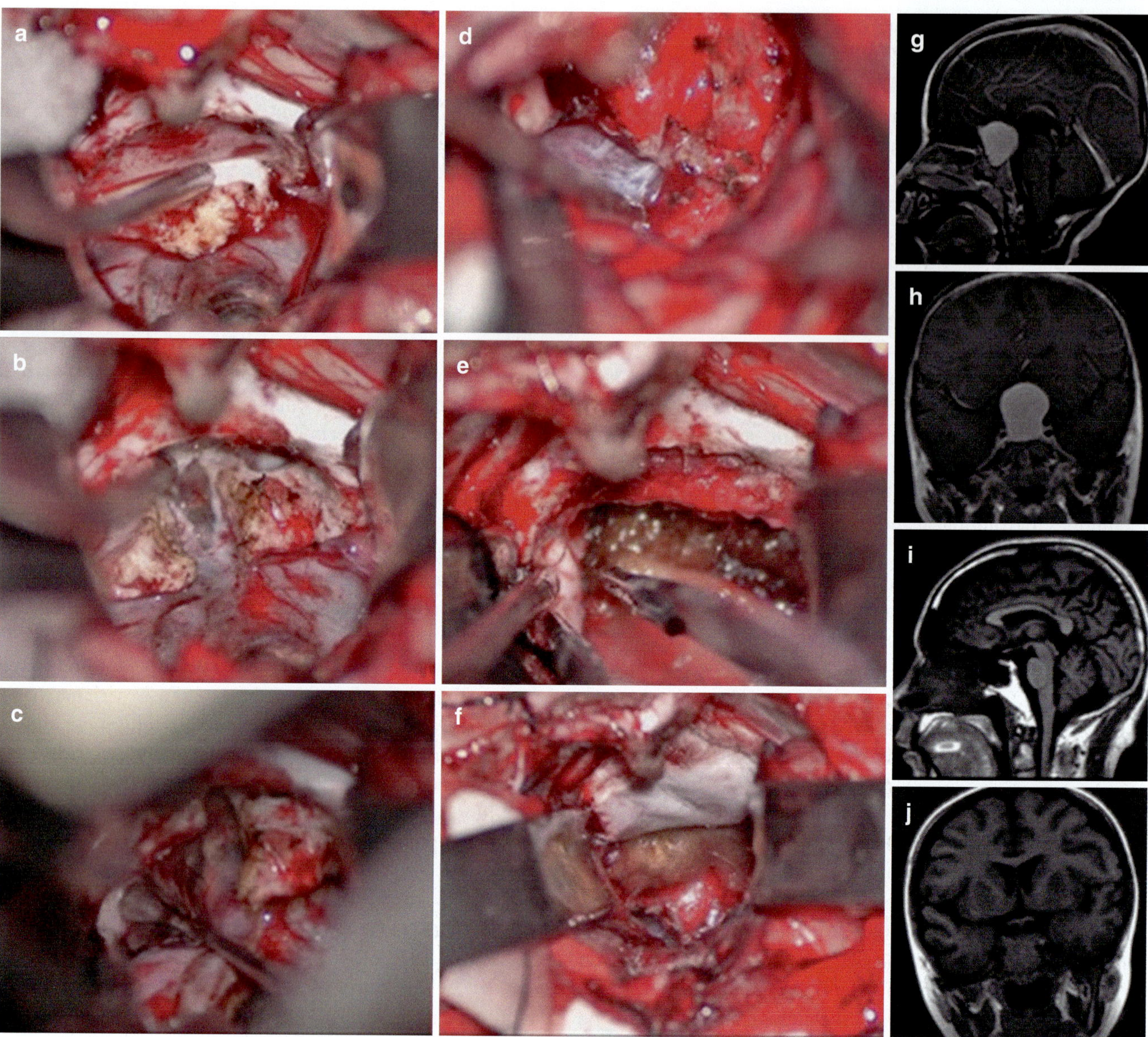

Fig. 6.2 The picture shows the surgical procedure for tuberculum sellae removal to increase exposure of the intrasellar tumor. This technique was used in a patient with a 3-year-old boy who harboring a type Q craniopharyngioma. Although this type of tumor is suitable for endoscopic transsphenoidal transtuberculum approach, we used a transcranial anterior interhemispheric approach. By removing bone at the tuberculum sellae, the tumor was totally removed while retaining the continuity of the pituitary stalk and neurohypophysis. The left two columns showed the bone removal and the procedure to dissect tumor along the tumor boundary, as well as the procedure repairing the sellae bone defection. Right column is the MR scan of the child before and after surgery. As to show the reservation of the pituitary stalk, we specially selected the sagittal sequence which clearly shows the structure of the pituitary stalk (white arrow on the figure **i**). (**a**) After tumor exposure through anterior interhemispheric fissure, a curved incision was made on the dual covering tuberculum sellae, (**b**) after drilling of the bone of tuberculum sellae, an incision was made longitudinally at the dural fold to expose the tumor boundary underneath diaphragm. (**c**) The tumor was separated along the interface between the tumor wall and the dura mater (dilated diaphragm), which ensures complete resection of the tumor and preservation of the pituitary stalk fibers that fuse with the dilated diaphragm, (**d**) the picture showed the thinned and dilated pituitary stalk, diaphragm, and intrasellar pituitary gland and neurohypophysis after tumor resection. (**e**) Bone defect at the sella was repaired by using a small piece of autologous muscle, (**f**) dura defect of the diaphragm was covered with artificial dura to prevent possible recurrence of the tumor from expanding intracranially. (**g–j**) Pre- and postoperative MR images showed total tumor removal and the preservation of the pituitary stalk

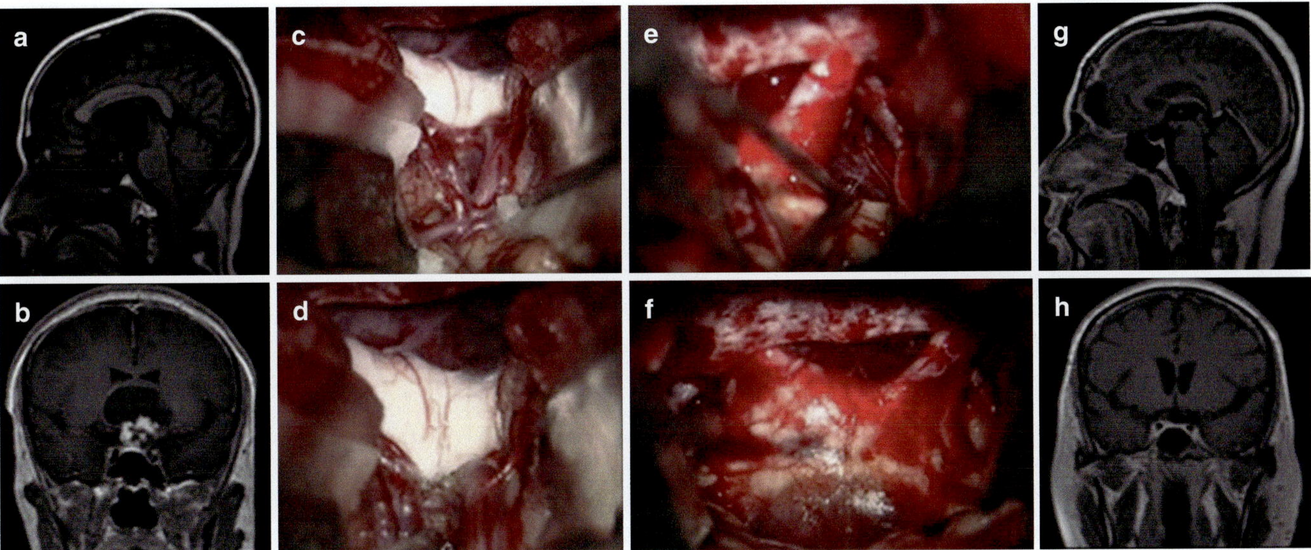

Fig. 6.3 This was a case of a 27-year-old male patient with craniopharyngioma. The left pictures were the preoperative sagittal and coronal MR scan (**a**, **b**). The intraoperative pictures showed the structure of the lamina terminal cistern after the longitudinal fissure is opened. Division of the anterior communicating artery provided a sufficient surgical space (**c**–**f**). The right pictures showed the postoperative sagittal and coronal MR scans suggesting total tumor resection, and the lateral wall of the third ventricle was preserved (**g**, **h**)

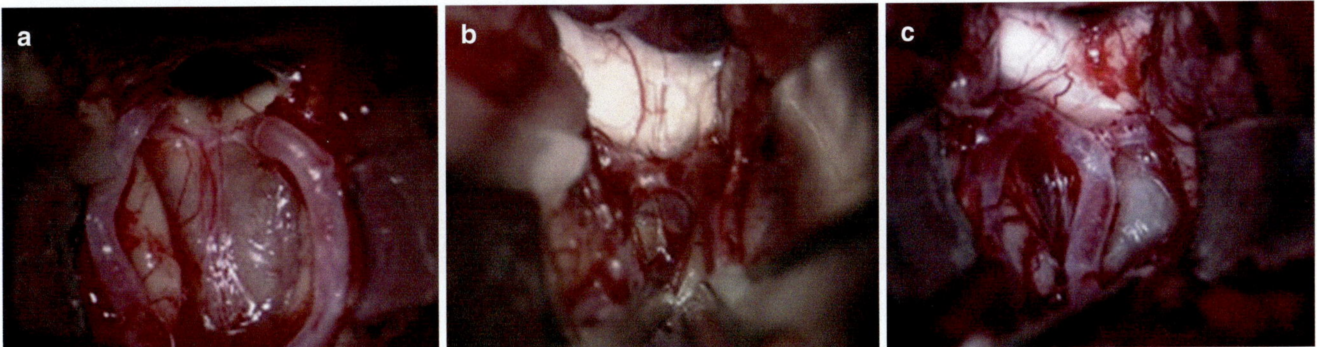

Fig. 6.4 The differences in anatomical development of the anterior communicating artery complex in patients with craniopharyngioma

Analysis Before Surgery The tumor was a typical type Q tumor, and the patient's primary complaint was vision disturbance, and she presented with growth retardation.

Neuroimaging Surgical consideration: Type Q tumor growth began below the diaphragm and arachnoid. The suprasellar part was covered by the diaphragma sellae (DS) and arachnoid above the DS, and therefore this kind of tumor is considered the optimal tumor type for the transsphenoidal approach. However, there are several difficulties associated with selection of the transsphenoidal approach for the management of this type Q tumor (Fig. 6.7).

1. The suprasellar part of the tumor breaks through the diaphragma sellae into the anterior cranial fossa, which might present a significant challenge to GTR.
2. The PS always inflates and fuses with the tumoral cystic walls. The absence or interruption of the PS is very often associated with posterior pituitary gland anomalies and hormonal dysfunction. As a result, these tumors are difficult to treat surgically with the transsphenoidal approach with preservation of the PS and pituitary function.

The midline interhemispheric approach was selected for gross total or maximum possible safe resection and to main-

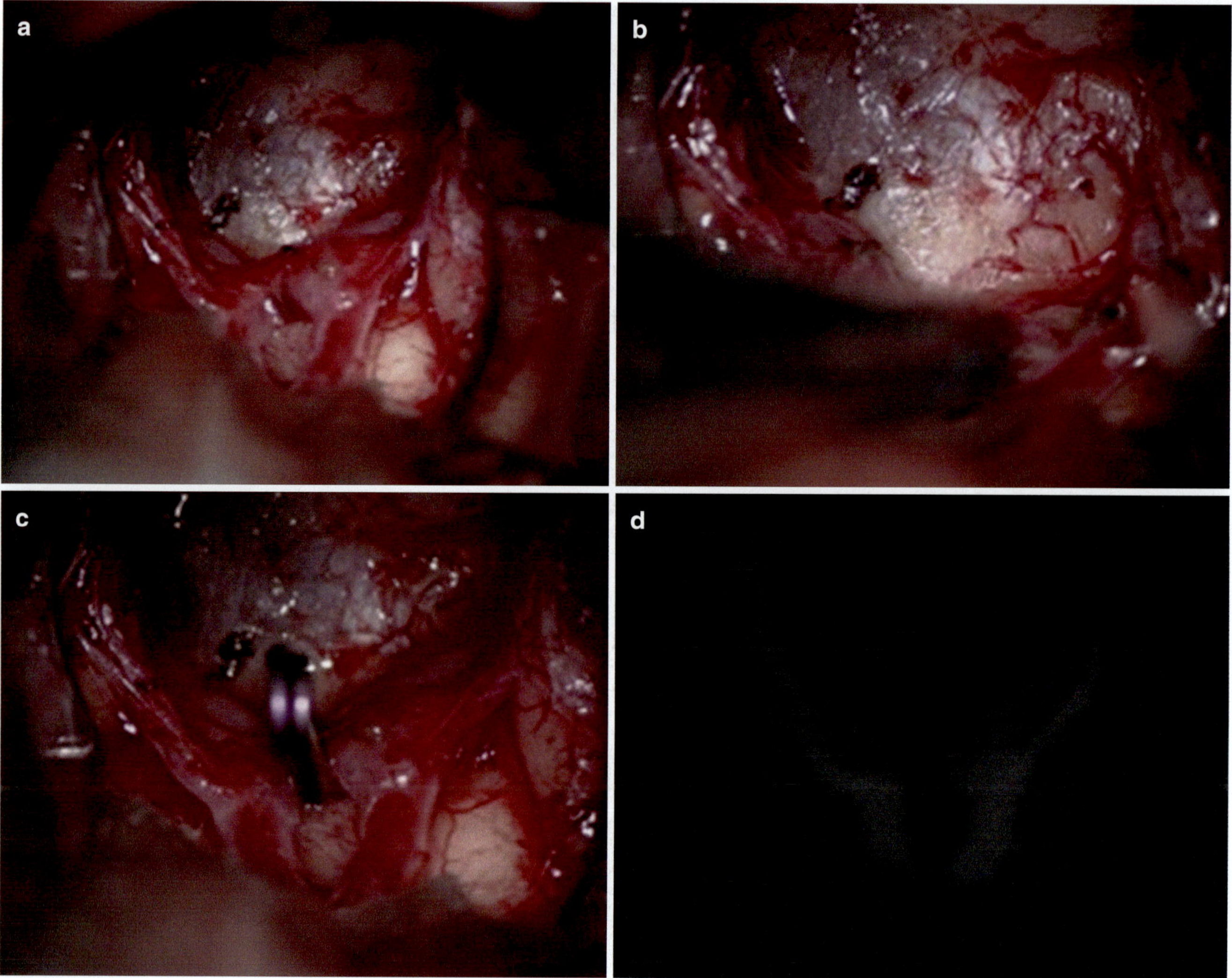

Fig. 6.5 This was a case of a 34-year-old man with recurrent craniopharyngioma. After temporary blockage of the anterior communicating artery (**c**), the indocyanine green angiography showed that bilateral A1 and A2 were well filled (**d**). The ascending pictures showed the extent of the laminal terminal cistern before and after the division of the anterior communicating artery (**a**, **b**). Division of the vessel provides adequate exposure of the lamina terminal cistern

tain the intactness of normal nervous tissues, especially the infundibulum-pituitary stalk tract. The ultimate goal of surgery is to pursue a certain quality of life while removing the tumor, specifically the endocrine function dominated by the hypothalamic-hypophyseal axis.

The operative steps involving craniotomy utilized for the removal of type Q craniopharyngiomas can be summarized as follows: (1) standardized skull base craniotomy (frontobasal interhemispheric craniotomy), (2) separation of the tumor from suprasellar structures and the stretched, attenuating DS, (3) resection of the bone at the tuberculum sellae to provide direct vision on the intrasellar tumor portion, (4) T-shaped incision of the elevated DS, and (5) tumor dissection along the true capsule while attempting to preserve the neurohypophysis and continuity of the PS.

Intraoperative Findings Figures 6.8, 6.9, 6.10, 6.11, 6.12, 6.13, 6.14, and 6.15.

Perioperative Treatment Postoperative MRI (10a–c) obtained after 24 months revealed total tumor removal with preservation of the pituitary stalk (Fig. 6.16). Endocrinological detection performed 6 months after surgery indicated no new hormone deficiencies. The PRL level was normal, although the levels of several sexual hormones remained low.

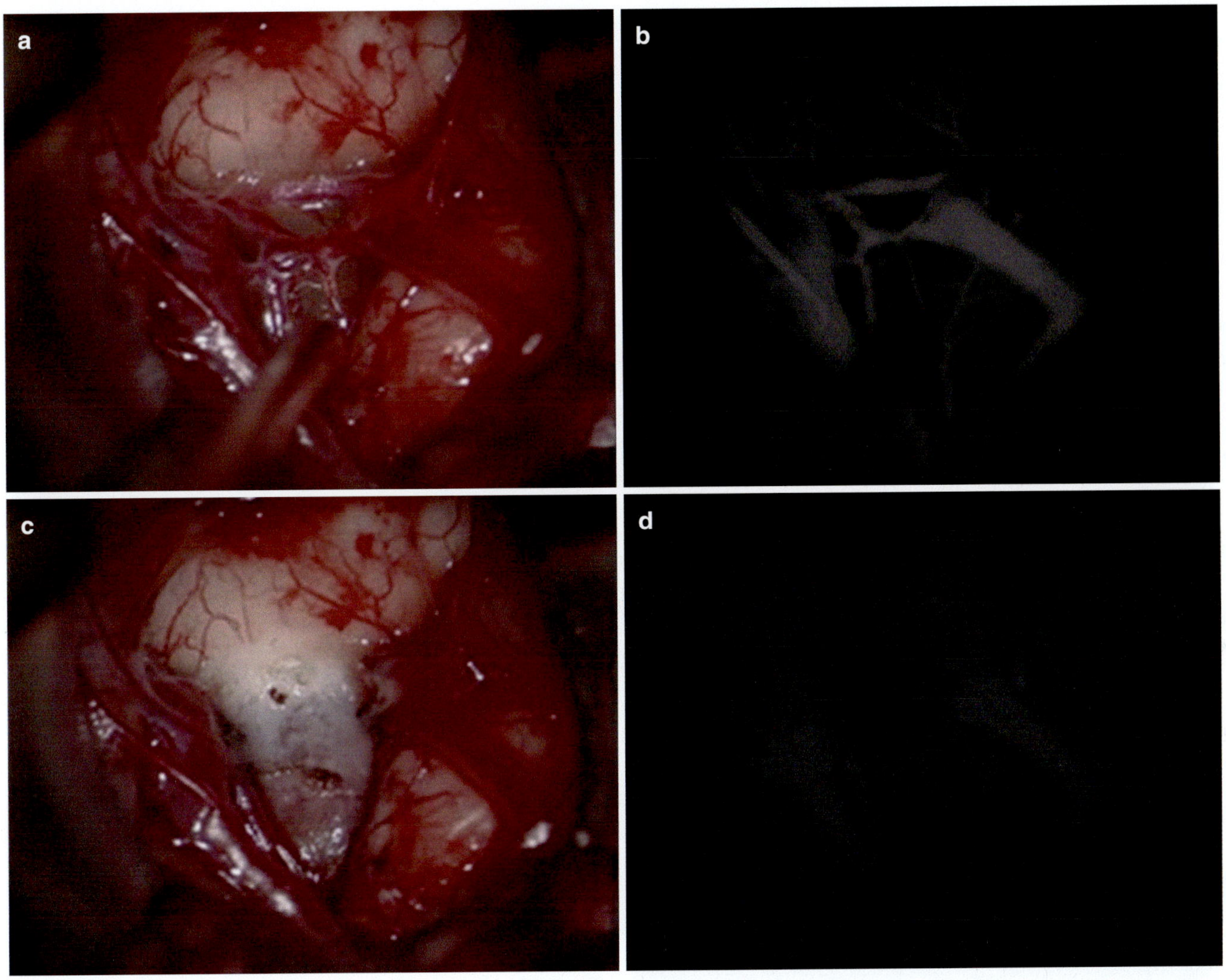

Fig. 6.6 This was a case of a 5-year-old girl with craniopharyngioma. Intraoperative findings showed the dual trunk anterior communicating artery. The right pictures showed the filling of the indocyanine green angiography before and after division of the anterior communicating artery

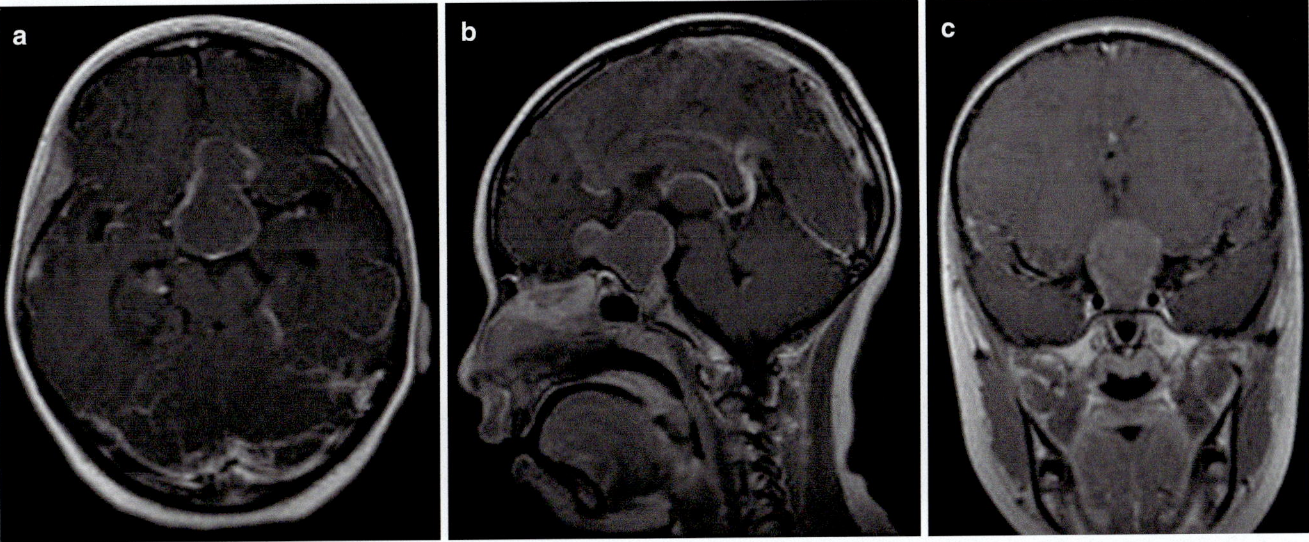

Fig. 6.7 Presurgical axial (**a**), sagittal (**b**), and coronal (**c**) studies revealed a large intra- and suprasellar, predominantly cystic mass with enlargement of the pituitary fossa and a rounded, symmetrical cystic suprasellar extension; on the sagittal and axial views, the suprasellar tumor cyst had expanded anteriorly to the anterior cranial fossa. No obstructive hydrocephalus was observed on presurgical radiological images

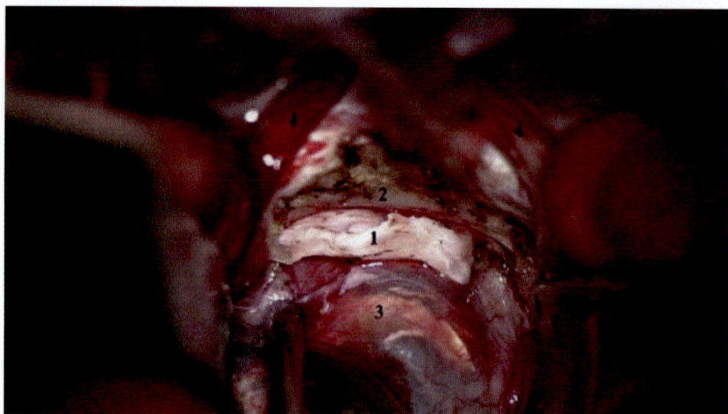

Fig. 6.8 After careful dissection of the anterior interhemispheric cistern, the planum sphenoidale, bilateral optic nerves, and prechiasmatic cistern were exposed. The tumor was dissected mainly through the prechiasmatic space. Dura mater was arc-shapely incised to remove the bone at the planum sphenoidale and tuberculum sellae and expose the intrasellar space. (1) Dual flap of the planum sphenoidale, (2) bone of the planum sphenoidale, (3) tumor, (4) bilateral olfactory nerves

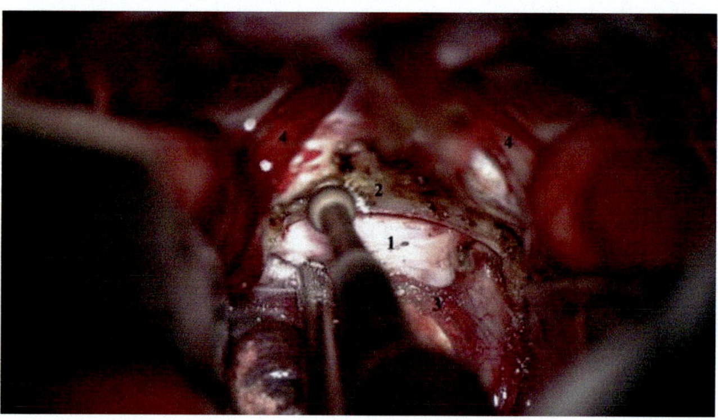

Fig. 6.9 A high speed drill was used to remove the bone at the planum sphenoidale in order to expose the intrasellar tumor portion. (1) Dual flap of the planum sphenoidale, (2) bone of the planum sphenoidale, (3) tumor, (4) bilateral olfactory nerves

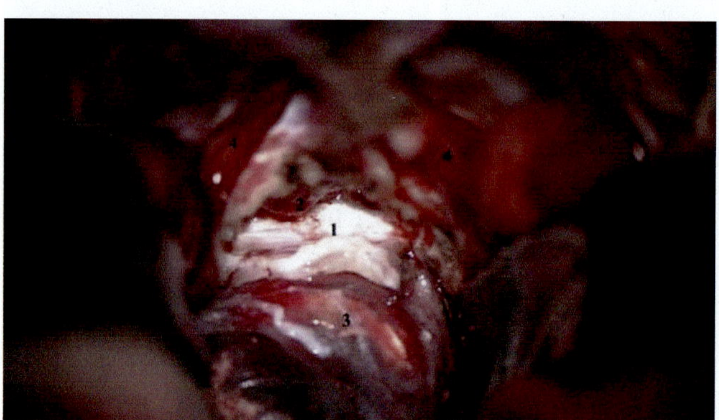

Fig. 6.10 After bone removal, the dural fold anterior to the pituitary fossa was exposed. (1) Dual fold of the planum sphenoidale, (2) sphenoid sinus mucosa, (3) tumor, (4) bilateral olfactory nerves

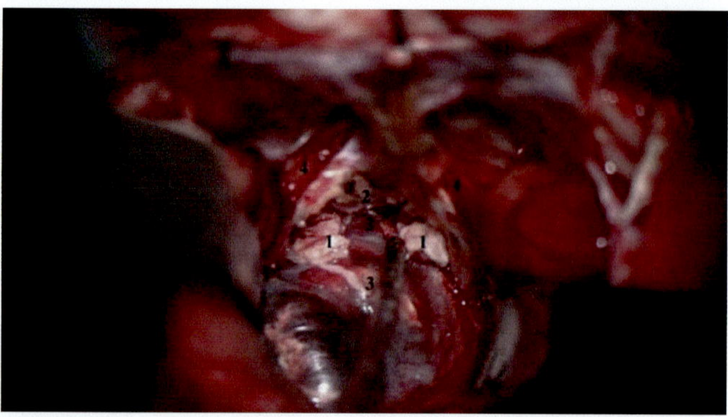

Fig. 6.11 A "T-shaped" incision was made on the diaphragm to expose the tumor wall underlining the diaphragmatic cover. (1) Dual fold of the planum sphenoidale, (2) sphenoid sinus mucosa, (3) tumor wall, (4) bilateral olfactory nerves

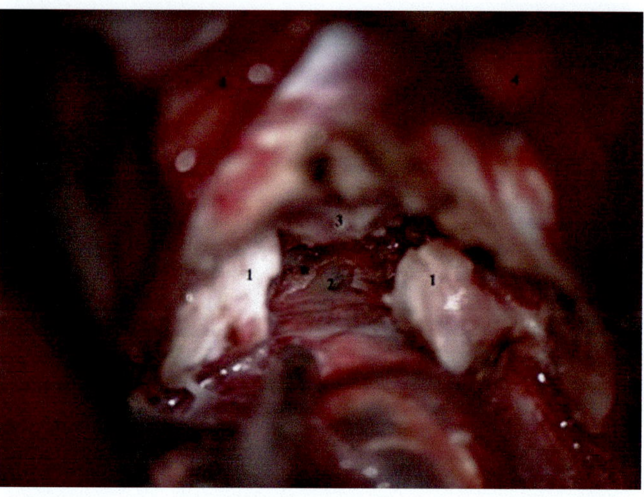

Fig. 6.12 After careful dissection, the boundary of the intrasellar tumor was identified; there was thinning membranous separation (black asterisk) between the stretched diaphragm and tumor wall, considered to be the remnant of the pituitary gland. (1) Dual fold of the planum sphenoidale, (2) tumor, (3) sphenoid sinus mucosa, (4) bilateral olfactory nerves

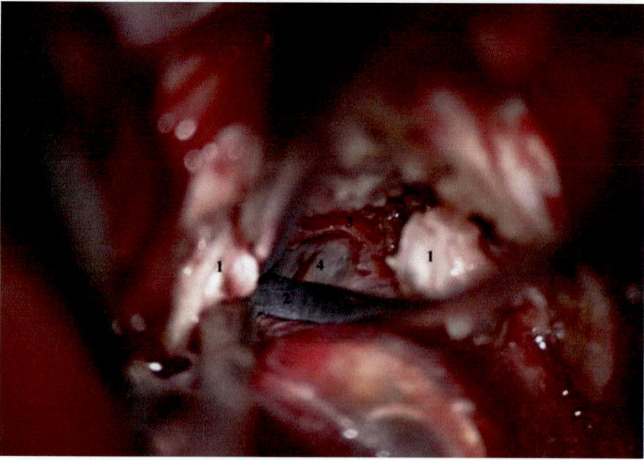

Fig. 6.13 The intrasellar tumor portion was dissected along the real tumor cystic wall to facilitate GTR and to preserve the pituitary stalk. (1) Dual fold of the planum sphenoidale, (2) tip of the stripper, (3) sphenoid sinus mucosa, (4) intrasellar tumor wall

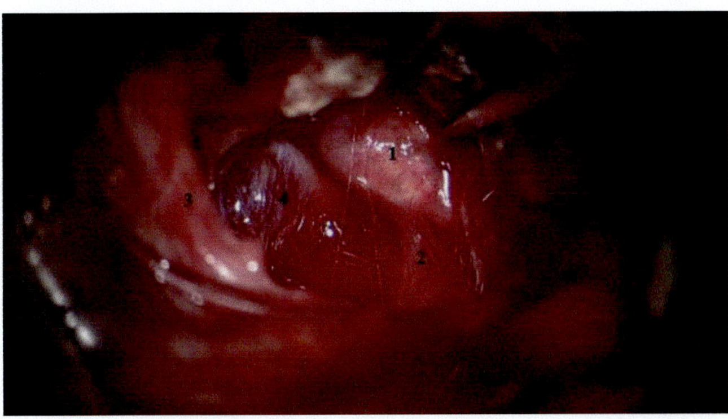

Fig. 6.14 The distal portion of the PS diverged and fused with the upper posterior part of the tumor capsule and elevated diaphragma sellae (DS). (1) Diaphragma sellae, (2) proximal part of the PS, (3) left optic nerve, (4) Liliequist membrane

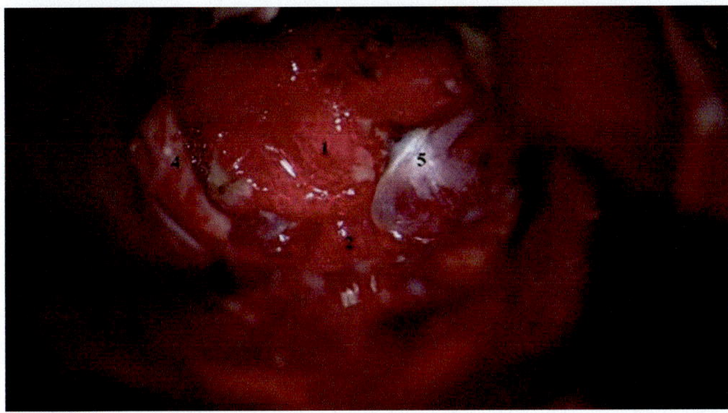

Fig. 6.15 After total tumor removal, continuity of the hypothalamus–pituitary stalk axis was preserved. The intact proximal segment of the pituitary stalk was identified. Note that the pituitary stalk and part of the diaphragm were preserved. (1) Diaphragma sellae, (2) proximal part of the PS, (3) remaining neurohypophysis, (4) left optic nerve, (5) Liliequist membrane

Long-Term Follow-Up The patient's visual symptoms had recovered by the time of the last official follow-up, which was conducted at 24 months postoperatively. Her diabetes insipidus (DI) recovered gradually. She was able to attend school and did not require hormone replacement therapy at the time of the last follow-up study.

6.4.1.2 Case 2

Medical History This was the case of a 6-year-old male patient with a 12-month history of intermittent headache and vomiting. He also exhibited growth failure, emaciation, and partial hypopituitarism. He presented with visual deterioration (right eye: 0.4, left eye: 0.08) and bitemporal hemianopia.

Physical and Experimental Examination The patient's routine blood and urine analysis results were normal; however, he had low levels of plasma thyroxine and free thyroxine (fT4). An insulin stimulation test for cortisol and growth hormone (GH) revealed subnormal responses.

Radiological Images Before Surgery A predominantly cystic intra- and suprasellar mass was identified both on CT and MRI (Fig. 6.17). The anterior communicating (AcoA) and anterior carotid arteries (ACA) formed a snowman shape at the top of the cystic tumor. On enhanced MRI, the cystic tumor wall was significantly enhanced roundly. On a coronal scan, a solid tumor was observed on the right side of the pituitary fossa near the medial wall of the CS. No obstructive hydrocephalus consequent to the tumor growth pattern and expansion was observed.

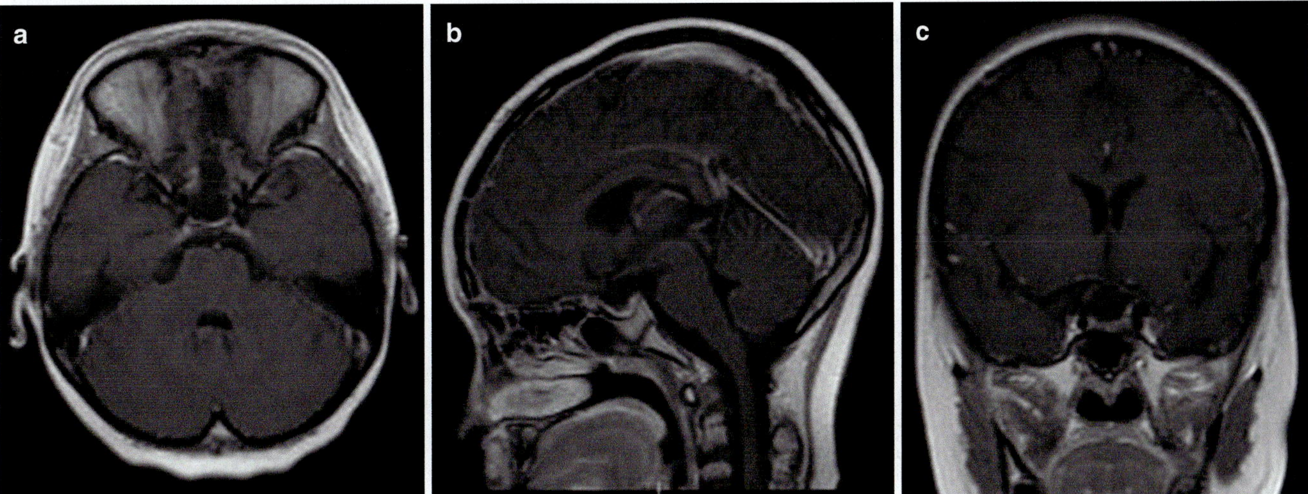

Fig. 6.16 A postoperative MRI study after 2 years confirmed total tumor removal and maintenance of an intact third ventricle floor and preserved pituitary stalk

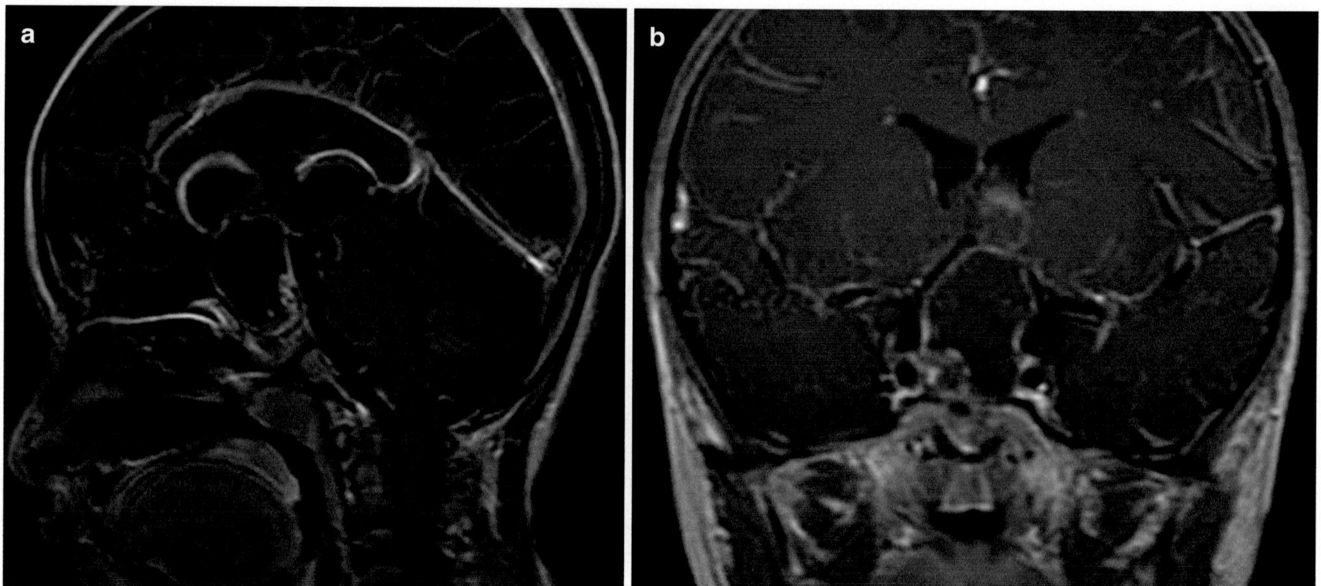

Fig. 6.17 Presurgical magnetic resonance images indicating a predominantly cystic tumor in the suprasellar region with upward expansion of a daughter cyst behind the anterior communicating artery. The cystic wall and solid part of the tumor were enhanced significantly (reproduced with permission from Qi (Ed.), *Craniopharyngioma*, People's Medical Publishing House, ISBN 978-7-117-26463-1, 2018)

Analysis Before Surgery

1. Surgical and topographic tumor classification: Type Q tumor (intra- and suprasellar Id-CP).
2. Relationship with the AcoA: The AcoA complex was displaced upwards.
3. Tumor growth began below the diaphragm and arachnoid. The suprasellar part was covered by the diaphragma sellae and arachnoid above the DS.
4. Surgical excision should be the first-line therapy. A frontobasal interhemispheric approach was ultimately selected to reach the lesion.

Intraoperative Findings After general anesthesia induction, the patient was placed in the supine position with the head fixed in a Mayfield three-pin head-holder. The head was extended slightly downward (approximately 15°), allowing the frontal lobe to spontaneously fall downward because of gravity during surgery. A standard frontobasal interhemispheric craniotomy (FIH) was performed (Fig. 6.18). A square of forehead periosteum was maintained for further frontal sinus repair. The bone flap extended beyond the median line, with the lowest margin as near as possible to the nasion. The mucosa inside the frontal sinus was removed carefully after opening the bone window. The bone of the posterior sinus wall was removed and drilled to increase exposure. Next, bone wax with antibiotic powder was used to fill the sinus cavity completely and reduce the risk of intracranial infection. A curved incision was made to open the bilateral dura mater beside the superior sagittal sinus; this incision was made close to the skull base. Subsequently, the anterior part of the superior sagittal sinus was ligated, followed by removal of the cerebral falx. The dural flap was turned rearward.

Dissection of the Interhemispheric Fissure A self-retaining retractor was used to retract the bilateral frontal lobe. The bilateral frontal lobes were separated along the interhemispheric corridor and the cerebrospinal fluid (CSF) was drained to the extent possible. Occasionally, dissection of the frontal interhemispheric fissure is much more complex than that used in a lateral transsylvian approach, especially in patients with increased intracranial pressure (ICP). Continuous lumbar CSF drainage during dissection is a valid method of ICP release. The planum sphenoidale, optic chiasm, and cisterna lamina terminalis were exposed in a stepwise fashion after allowing the frontal lobe to fall.

Tumor Removal The enlarged prechiasmatic space was the major corridor for surgical manipulation. Because of diaphragmatic septation, the suprasellar cystic tumor could be separated via slight pulling from the circle of Willis vascular ring. In this case, the suprasellar cystic tumor protruded in front of the AcoA complex to form a snowman sign (Fig. 6.17). However, this type of snowman sign can be separated easily via intracystic decompression while following the cystic wall interface. At the posterosuperior part of the tumor, the proximal PS could be exposed. The distal PS fused with the tumor capsule at the border of the diaphragmatic foramen. Here, the pituitary appeared to be inflated as an umbrella rather than displaced by compression, and thus

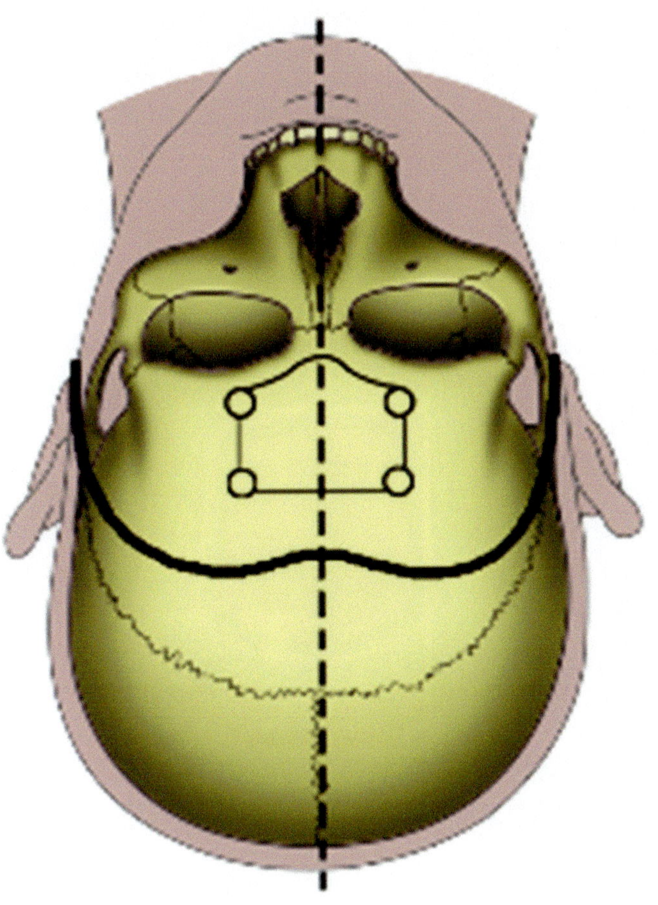

Fig. 6.18 Illustrations of the operating position and incision via a frontobasal interhemispheric approach (reproduced with permission from Qi (Ed.), *Craniopharyngioma*, People's Medical Publishing House, ISBN 978-7-117-26463-1, 2018)

it was difficult to preserve PS continuity. As a result, the distal segment of the PS was seceded where the stalk and tumor capsule had fused. Upon total separation of the suprasellar tumor cyst, a circular incision was made in the diaphragm at the bony opening of the pituitary fossa to locate the true subdiaphragmatic tumor capsule. Following this interface, the intrasellar part of the tumor was removed in a stepwise manner. When separating bilateral tumor walls, brisk venous bleeding is often encountered from the bilateral CS. This can be readily controlled via gentle packing with a small piece of Gelfoam (Fig. 6.19).

Pathology Study A typical adamantinomatous CP was identified on the pathological slides.

Postoperative course: The third VF remained intact (Fig. 6.20). Postoperatively, the patient developed mild transient DI. Hyponatremia was the major manifestation of electrolyte disturbance. The symptoms were relieved with fluid and electrolyte replacement. Endocrinological detection revealed evidence of panhypopituitarism. The patient's visual function recovered significantly.

6.4.1.3 Case 3

Medical History This was the case of an 8-year-old female patient. She had undergone a prior craniotomy via a right pterional approach to address a significant reduction in visual acuity at a local hospital in December 2011. However, a follow-up series of MRIs indicated tumor recurrence. The patient subsequently had intermittent vomiting and constant headache.

Physical and Experimental Examination No significant positive symptoms were observed except right eye blindness.

Radiological Images Before Surgery The MRI scan conducted in December 2011 indicated a typical Id-CP in the intra- and suprasellar regions. This lesion was mixed cystic-solid, and the optic chiasm was displaced upward. Postsurgical MRI indicated subtotal tumor removal with residual intrasellar tumor. Follow-up MRI in April 2012 indicated intrasellar tumor recurrence. In September 2012, MRI indicated that this significant recurrent tumor remained an Id-CP with upward displacement of the optic chiasm. However, the tumor was not treated until the patient presented in our department in March 2013. CT indicated an extensive and expanding tumor in the sellar region, anterior basement of the cranial fossa, and upper clivus that also occupied the third ventricular cavity. Broad punctate calcification was observed. MRI revealed a huge mixed cystic-solid tumor in the intra- and suprasellar regions with extensive extension and external growth. The solid part of the tumor was significantly enhanced on T1-weighted enhanced MRI. The ACA and AcoA were entrapped by the cystic tumor. As a result, the tumor exhibited a lobular tumor shape (Fig. 6.21).

Analysis Before Surgery This was a case of recurrent CP, and the notable morphological features should be emphasized. Before the primary surgery, the tumor was a typical case of Id-CP. However, the natural "protective membranous structures" such as the diaphragm and suprasellar arachnoid were destroyed by surgery so that no such interface obstructed the invagination of the recurrent tumor into the nervous tissue layer. MRI performed before the secondary surgery indicated tumor penetration through the PS and growth toward the nervous tissue layer of the infundibulum and third VF, leading to severe hypothalamic involvement.

Intraoperative Findings Although the primary surgery destroyed the normal membranous structures that covered the tumor surface, the inner arachnoid layer continued to separate the tumor from the surrounding neurovascular structures. During surgery, this interface was followed to avoid injury. The most important locations were the site of origin and PS. Intrasellar recurrence is the most frequent issue, and therefore identification of the pituitary capsule was necessary to ensure total intrasellar tumor removal. After total tumor removal, the floor of the pituitary fossa

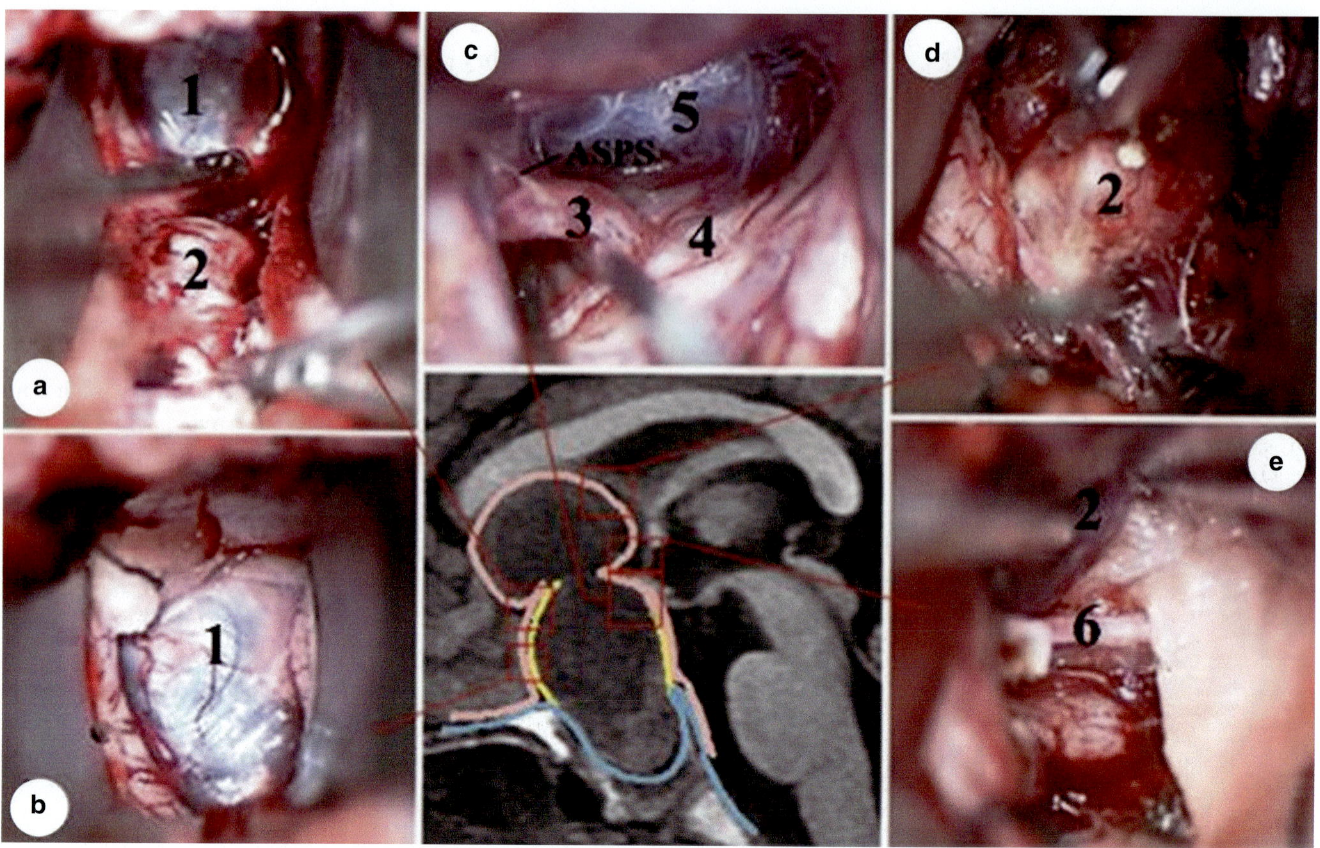

Fig. 6.19 Tumor exposure via the frontobasal interhemispheric approach. (**a**) The bilateral frontal lobes and hemispheric fissure were visible after completing the craniotomy. (**b**) The suprasellar tumor capsule along with the evaluated DS was identified through the prechiasmatic space. (**c**) Intraoperative photographs showing the tumor–stalk relationship; the lower part of the stalk had fused with the superoposterior part of the tumor capsule. The third ventricle floor (third VF) remained intact. (**d**, **e**) The protruding suprasellar tumor encased the anterior communicating artery (AcoA) complex, necessitating sharp dissection to release. (1) Infradiaphragmatic tumor portion, (2) dome of the tumor protruding from the diaphragma sellae, (3) pituitary stalk, (4) third ventricular floor, (5) Liliequist membrane, (6) anterior communication artery. Abbreviations: *ASPS* arachnoid sleeve of pituitary stalk (reproduced with permission from Qi (Ed.), *Craniopharyngioma*, People's Medical Publishing House, ISBN 978-7-117-26463-1, 2018)

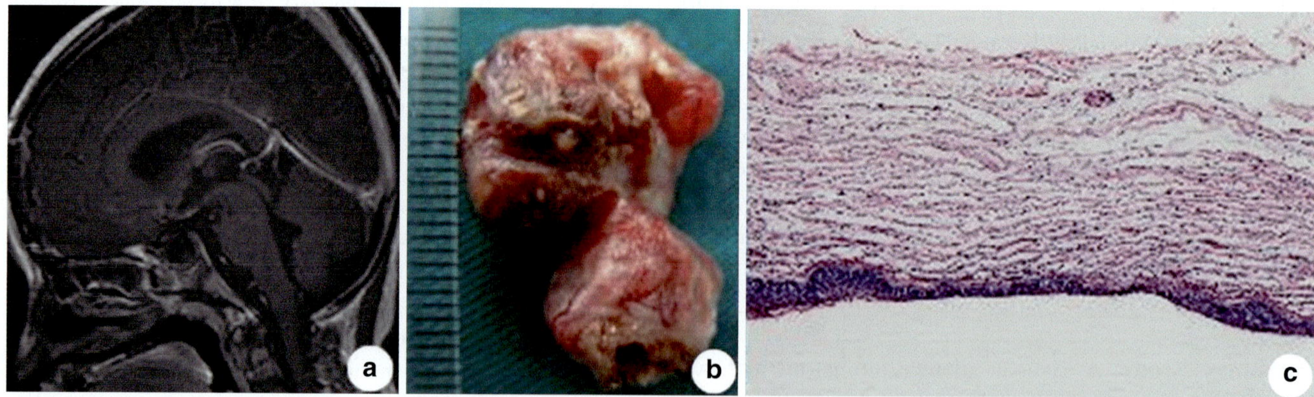

Fig. 6.20 Postoperative sagittal T1-weighted magnetic resonance image confirming total tumor removal (**a**). The tumor was removed completely en bloc (**b**). Pathological examination (**c**) revealed that the tumor was covered by a layer of fiber tissue, resembling the structure of the diaphragma sellae (reproduced with permission from Qi (Ed.), *Craniopharyngioma*, People's Medical Publishing House, ISBN 978-7-117-26463-1, 2018)

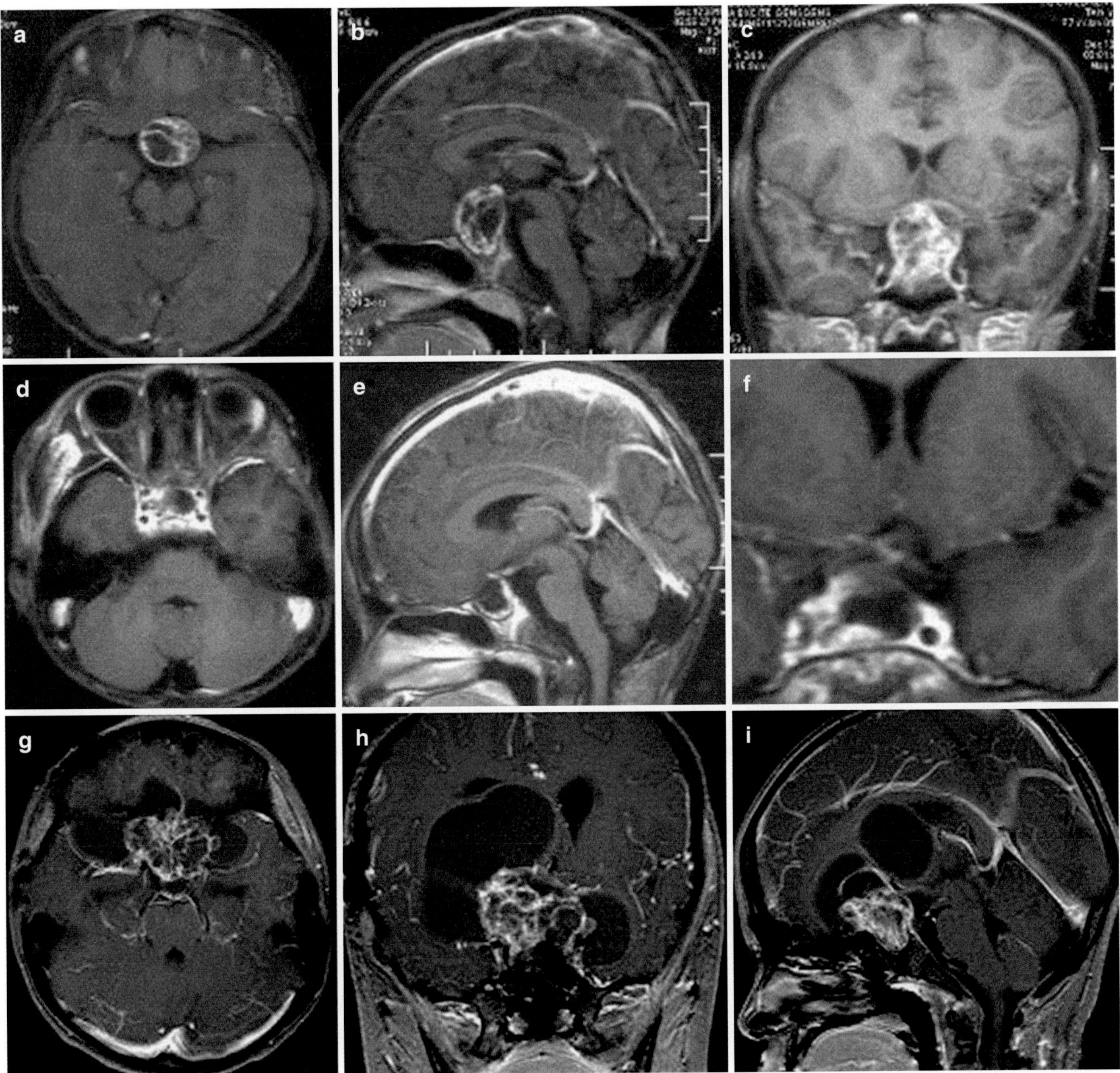

Fig. 6.21 Radiological images of this patient. (**a–c**) Magnetic resonance imaging (MRI) before the first craniotomy surgery. (**d–f**) MRI after the first surgery. (**g–i**) MRI before the second surgery (reproduced with permission from Qi (Ed.), *Craniopharyngioma*, People's Medical Publishing House, ISBN 978-7-117-26463-1, 2018)

was smooth and contained the neurohypophysis. The involved PS was ruptured to avoid additional recurrences (Figs. 6.22 and 6.23).

Perioperative Treatment The patient developed severe water and electrolyte imbalance disorder and required fluid and sodium substitution and adjustment. Postsurgical endocrinological detection indicated panhypopituitarism. The patient's right eye was completely blinded.

Long-Term Follow-Up After a 1.5-year follow-up, the patient's right eye remained blind. However, vision in the patient's left eye was restored. She continued receiving oral prednisone, thyroxin, and desmopressin to treat panhypopituitarism and permanent DI. Her BMI increased from a presurgical value of 15.7–20.

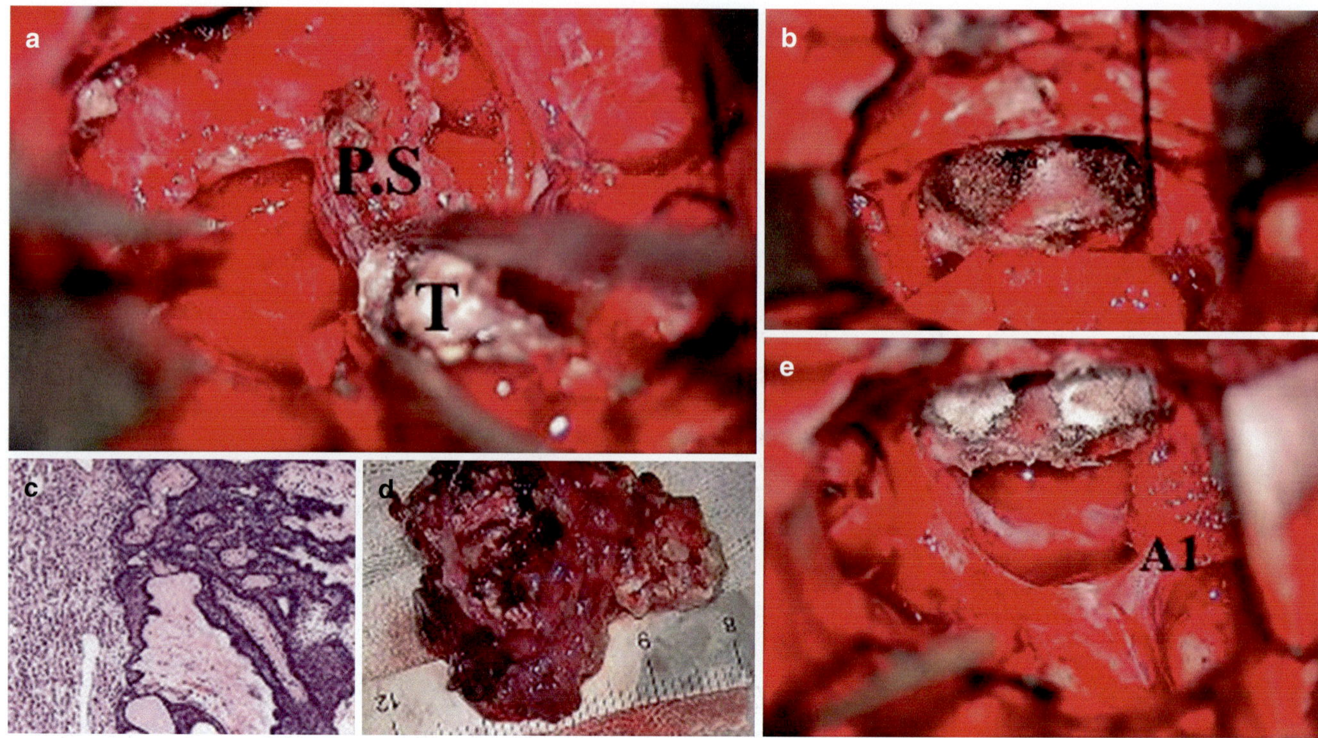

Fig. 6.22 Intraoperative findings. (**a**) The posteriorly located pituitary stalk, which exhibited severe tumor involvement, was identified after dissecting the suprasellar and intrasellar tumor. (**b**) After total tumor removal, the smooth pituitary fossa floor was visible. (**c**) Pathological examination (**c**) of the intrasellar tumor part showed the tightly adhered interface between the tumor and adenohypophysis, which was believed to be the cause of hypopituitarism of this tumor type. (**d**) Through an opening in the cystic wall, punctate calcification could be observed on the wall of the removed tumor. (**e**) After tumor removal, the sellar neurovascular structures were exposed (reproduced with permission from Qi (Ed.), *Craniopharyngioma*, People's Medical Publishing House, ISBN 978-7-117-26463-1, 2018)

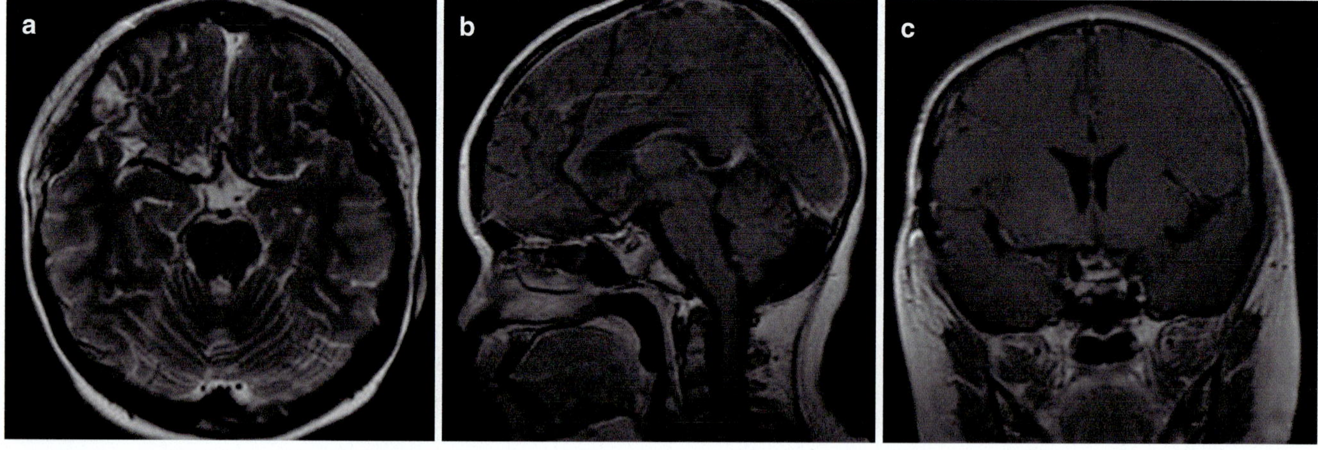

Fig. 6.23 Postoperative magnetic resonance image confirmed total tumor removal (reproduced with permission from Qi (Ed.), *Craniopharyngioma*, People's Medical Publishing House, ISBN 978-7-117-26463-1, 2018)

6.4.1.4 Case 4

Medical History This was the case of a 5-year-old male patient with a 1-year history of intermittent headaches that had progressively worsened during the last 2 weeks.

Physical and Experimental Examination The patient exhibited growth retardation and bitemporal hemianopia but no other positive physical signs. Endocrinological detection indicated hypopituitarism. Deficiencies in fT4, T3, sexual hormones, and GH were present. The PRL level was slightly increased.

Radiological Images Before Surgery CT indicated a suprasellar round, cystic tumor with egg-shell calcification that had caused obstructive hydrocephalus. MRI revealed a predominantly cystic lobulated tumor in the intra- and suprasellar regions. Part of the cystic tumor had protruded through the enlarged first space. The optic chiasm was displaced upward, and the tumor had entrapped the AcoA (Fig. 6.24).

Analysis Before Surgery A frontobasal interhemispheric approach was selected to remove the tumor. Although the tumor had protruded through the diaphragm to the suprasellar ventricular region, it remained covered by the arachnoid. Therefore, the tumor could be removed via an extra-axial route.

Membranous Structures and Hierarchical Layers See the schematic Fig. 6.25.

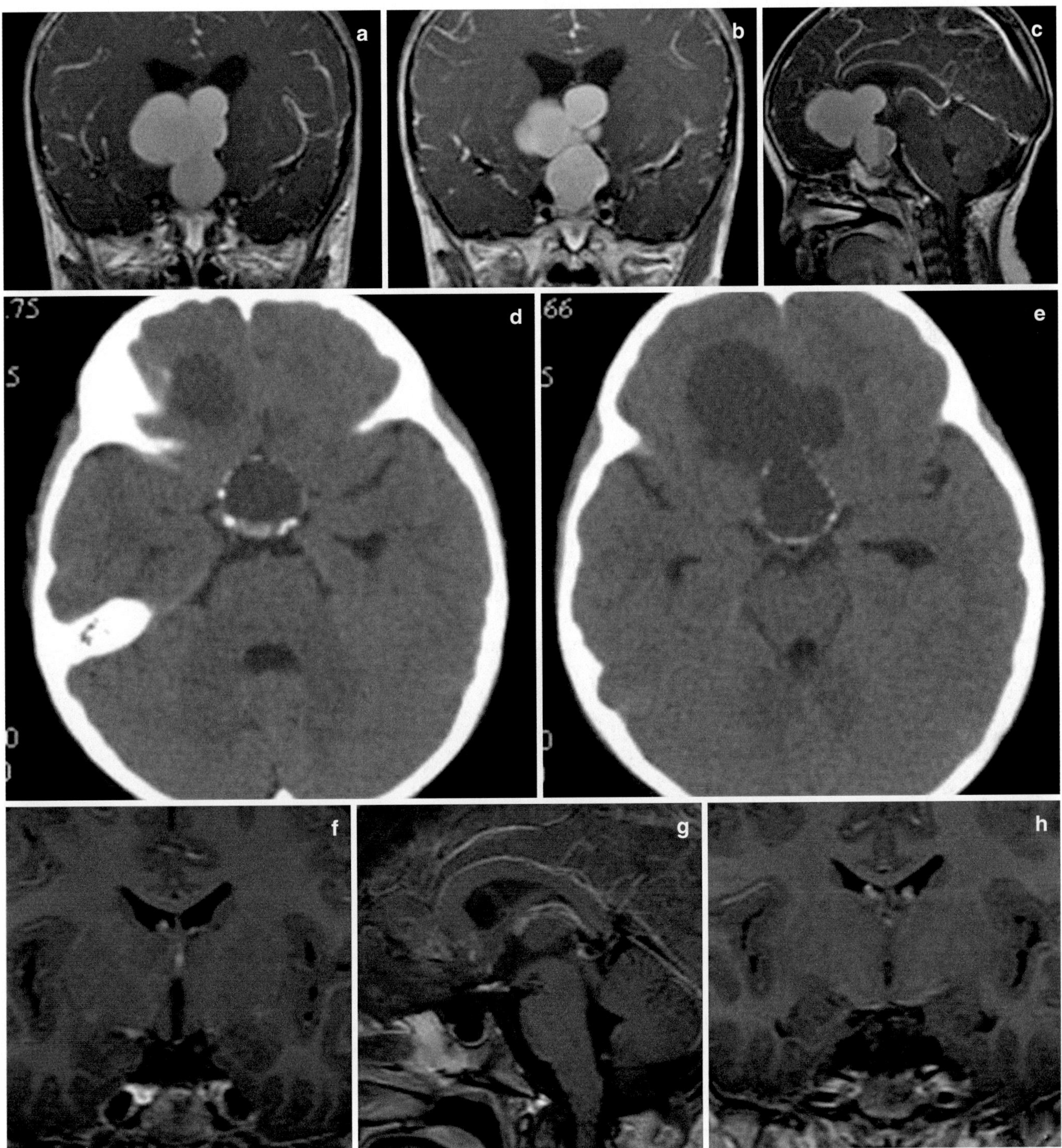

Fig. 6.24 Presurgical and postsurgical radiological images. (**a**–**e**) Presurgical computed tomography and magnetic resonance imaging (MRI) data. (**f**–**h**) Postsurgical MRI data (reproduced with permission from Qi (Ed.), *Craniopharyngioma*, People's Medical Publishing House, ISBN 978-7-117-26463-1, 2018)

Intraoperative Findings The tumor dome was covered by the arachnoid and attenuated diaphragm, allowing easy separation from the surrounding suprasellar neurovascular structures. The main three steps are illustrated in the following intraoperative pictures during tumor removal: (1) exposure and dissection of the tumor boundary in the suprasellar optic-chiasm cistern (Fig. 6.26), (2) dissection and removal of the cystic tumor part that protruded from the diaphragm and involved the anterior communicating artery complex and the third ventricle (Fig. 6.27), (3) removal of the intrasellar tumor portion and reconstruction of the diaphragma sellae (Fig. 6.28).

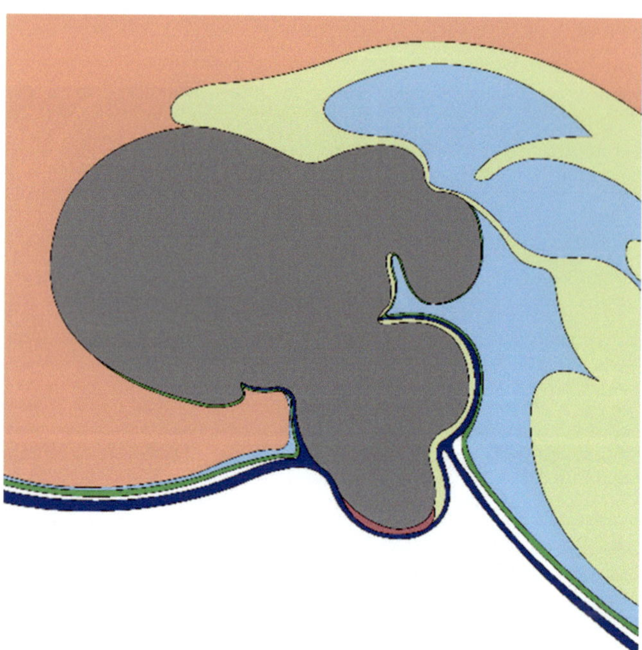

Fig. 6.25 Schematic figure showing the tumor morphology and relationships with the surrounding structures. Blue line: dura mater (diaphragm and sellar floor dura); green line: arachnoid mater (reproduced with permission from Qi (Ed.), *Craniopharyngioma*, People's Medical Publishing House, ISBN 978-7-117-26463-1, 2018)

Perioperative Treatment Pathological analysis proved the diagnosis of adamantinomatous CP. Postsurgical endocrinological detection indicated panhypopituitarism.

Long-Term Follow-Up No tumor recurrence was detected after a 6-year follow-up period. At the last follow-up study, the patient had a body mass index (BMI) of 19.33, compared with the presurgical BMI of 14.2, indicating significant weight gain. However, no other hypothalamic dysfunction such as cognitive deficits or memory impairment was evident.

6.4.2 Type S

6.4.2.1 Case 1

Medical History This was the case of a 31-year-old female patient with headache and decreased visual accuracy in both eyes for 6 months. She had irregular menstruation and amenorrhea for 2 years.

Physical and Experimental Examination Physical examination revealed no significant positive results except for temporal hemianopia of the right eye and decreased vision in both eyes. Moreover, endocrinological testing before surgery indicated increased PRL level (45 ng/μL) and normal

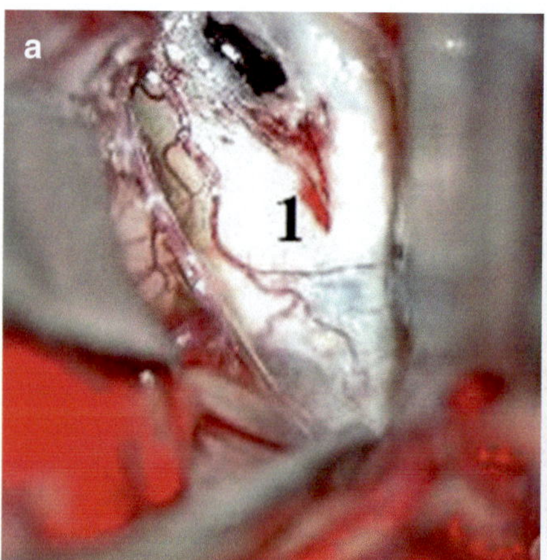

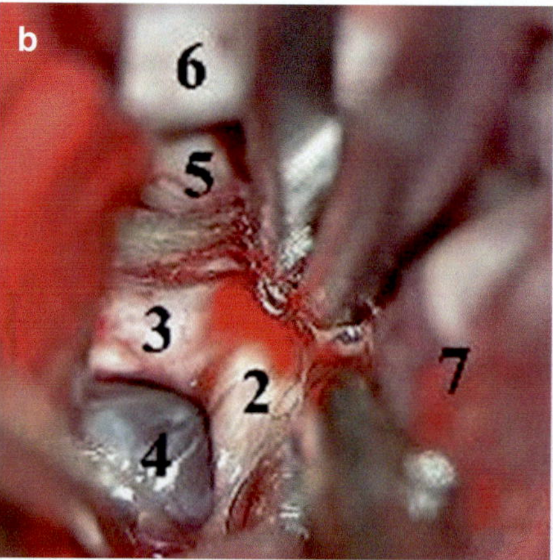

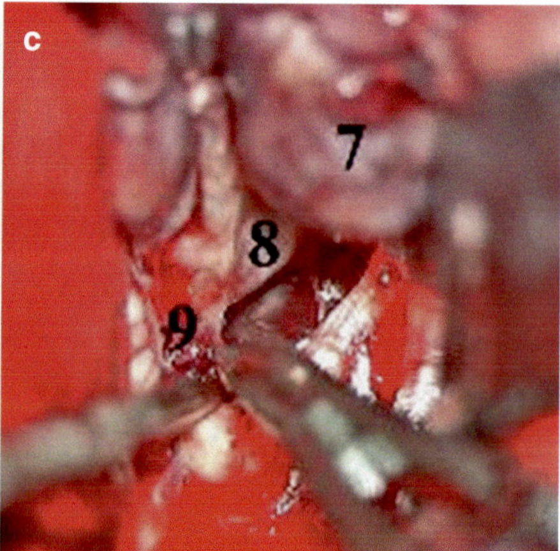

Fig. 6.26 Intraoperative findings. (**a**) The diaphragm-covered tumor was exposed by interhemispheric fissure dissection. After reducing the cystic fluid, the suprasellar arachnoid was used as a surgical interface to separate the tumor and surrounding neurovascular structures. (**b**) The left-side tumor boundary at the dorsum sellae was exposed, and the contralateral side was dissected in the same manner. The posterior end of the Liliequist membrane was found to be intact and separated the tumor from the posterior circulation. (**c**) At the posterosuperior part of the tumor, the remaining proximity pituitary stalk was exposed. (1) Tumor capsule exposed from the anterior chiasma space, (2) left-side tumor boundary at the dorsum sellae, (3) dorsum sellae covered by the dura mater, (4) Liliequist membrane, (5) intrasellar tumor, (6) planum sphenoidale, (7) upper part of the tumor capsule, (8) right side of the tumor boundary, (9) proximal pituitary stalk (reproduced with permission from Qi (Ed.), *Craniopharyngioma*, People's Medical Publishing House, ISBN 978-7-117-26463-1, 2018)

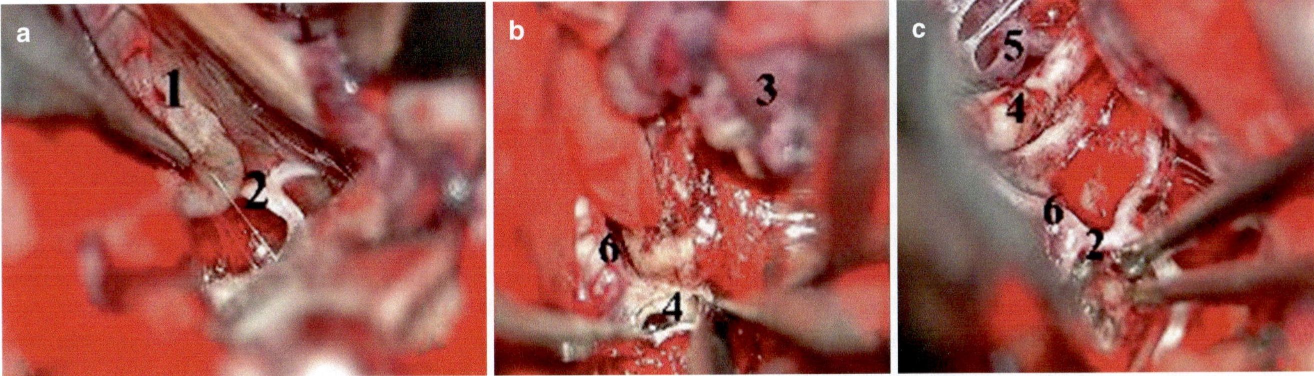

Fig. 6.27 Removal of the suprasellar tumor capsule. (**a**) The ipsilateral anterior carotid artery was exposed and protected. (**b**) Part of the tumor had protruded beyond the lamina terminalis; opening the terminalis permitted entry into the third ventricular cavity. (**c**) The anterior communicating artery complex and optic chiasm were exposed and protected. (1) Tumor capsule beyond the lamina terminalis, (2) anterior communicating artery complex exposed from the anterior chiasma space, (3) upper part of the tumor capsule, (4) opening of the lamina terminalis, (5) apex of the basilar artery, (6) left side of the anterior carotid artery (reproduced with permission from Qi (Ed.), *Craniopharyngioma*, People's Medical Publishing House, ISBN 978-7-117-26463-1, 2018)

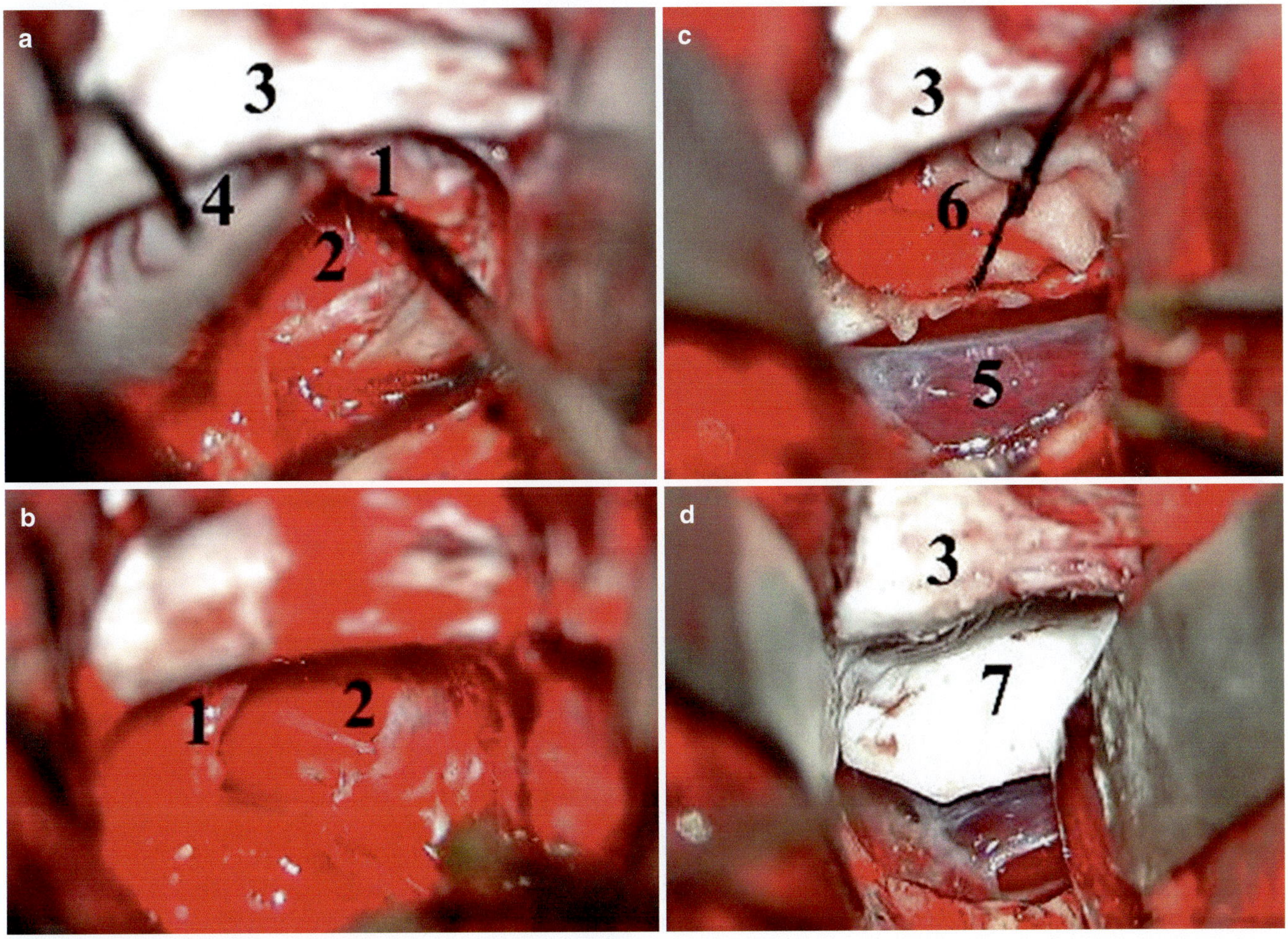

Fig. 6.28 Removal of the intrasellar tumor part. (**a**) The intrasellar tumor was dissected along the interface between the tumor and compressed neurohypophysis. (**b**) After removal of intrasellar tumor, a thin layer of tissue became visible, considered to be the remaining neurohypophysis. (**c**) A gelatin sponge was used to control bleeding from the bilateral cavernous sinuses. The entire pituitary stalk except for the tuberoinfundibular part of the hypothalamus was inflated by the tumor, and the involving pituitary stalk was resected along with the tumor capsule. (**d**) Artificial dura mater was used to repair diaphragmatic defects after tumor removal. Ensure that possible recurrent tumor is blocked under the diaphragma sellae and can be removed through the transsphenoidal route. (1) Intrasellar tumor part, (2) remaining neurohypophysis, (3) planum sphenoidale, (4) suction head displacing tumor capsule, (5) Liliequist membrane, (6) cotton sheet to compress the gelatin sponge, (7) artificial dura mater to cover the diaphragmatic defect (reproduced with permission from Qi (Ed.), *Craniopharyngioma*, People's Medical Publishing House, ISBN 978-7-117-26463-1, 2018)

hormone levels on the remaining hypothalamic–pituitary axis (Fig. 6.29).

Surgical Consideration The site of tumor origin was considered to be located in the upper segment of the pituitary stalk. The normal pituitary stalk was displaced caudally to the left side of the tumor. The main tumor body was located exclusively in the suprasellar subarachnoid cisternal spaces around the pituitary stalk (PS). The cystic tumor involved several subarachnoid cisterns, including the chiasmatic cistern, exterior and interior carotid artery cisterns (right side), and interpeduncular cistern. The right-side internal carotid artery (ICA) and its branches as well as cranial nerve III were surrounded by the tumor, which required sharp surgical dissection. Thus, a right-side frontolateral approach was applied to tumor removal.

Intraoperative Findings Figures 6.30, 6.31, 6.32, 6.33, 6.34, 6.35, and 6.36.

Perioperative Treatment Endocrinological detection indicated significant decreases in the free T4 and thyroid-stimulating hormone (TSH) levels. Disordered water and electrolyte balances were detected and treated as usual; however, this patient experienced these symptoms over the long term because of the longer time required to separate the pituitary stalk from the tumor calcification.

Long-Term Follow-Up Total tumor removal was proven during a 2-year follow-up period (Fig. 6.37). After surgery, the patient developed transient oculomotor nerve palsy, which recovered during the follow-up period. However, regarding the endocrinological evaluation, the menstrual dis-

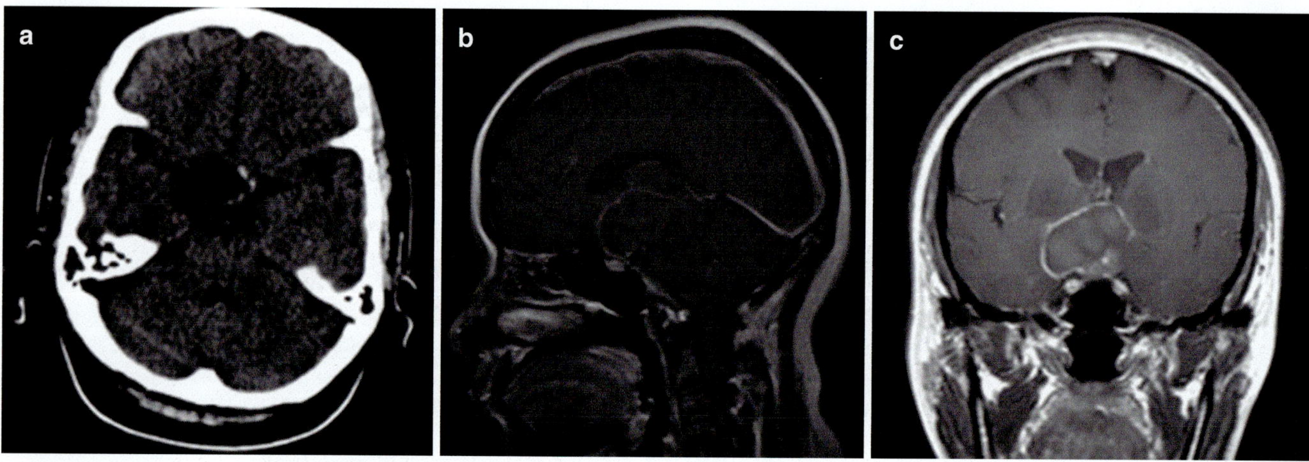

Fig. 6.29 Presurgical radiological images of the present case. (**a**) CT scan before surgery indicated a suprasellar lesion with slight calcification along the tumor wall. (**b**, **c**) Sagittal and coronal MR images showing that the tumor mainly occupied the subarachnoid chiasma cistern and expanded backward to the prepontine cistern

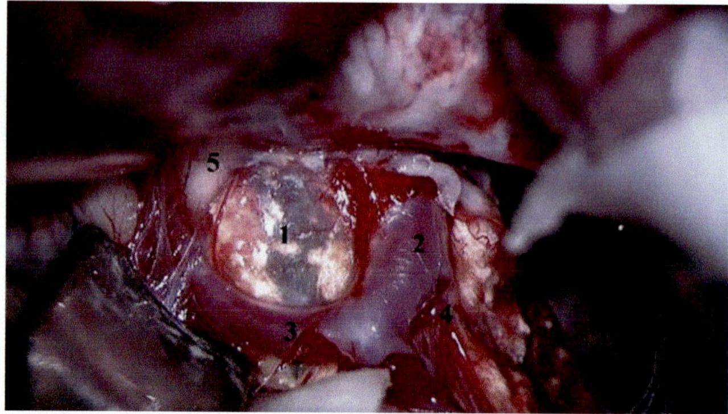

Fig. 6.30 A right-side frontolateral approach was selected. After dissecting the lateral fissure, the suprasellar tumor was exposed. The calcified tumor had adhered tightly to the right side of the internal carotid artery (ICA) and its branches, thus presenting significant challenges to surgical removal. (1) Tumor exposed from the optic-carotid space, (2) right-side ICA, (3) ACA, (4) right-side PCA and anterior choroidal artery, (5) optic nerve

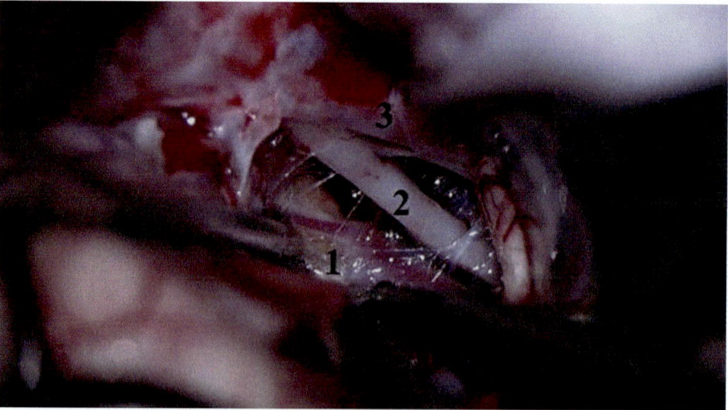

Fig. 6.31 Intraoperative photograph showing that through the lateral space of the ICA (ICA-oculomotor nerve space), the lateral boundary of the tumor was exposed. Note the perforator vessel from the PCA adhering to the tumor wall. (1) Tumor, (2) oculomotor verve (right side), (3) tentorial margin

order and low thyroxine level persisted. Prednisone and levothyroxine tablets were administered as substitutive treatment. Her weight increased slightly without other hypothalamic dysfunctions such as obesity.

6.4.2.2 Case 2

Medical History This was the case of a 27-year-old female patient who presented with decreased visual accuracy in the right eye for 3 months. She did not experience headache, nausea and vomiting, polyuria, or polydipsia.

Physical and Experimental Examination Physical examination revealed no significant positive symptoms except for temporal hemianopia and decreased vision in the right eye.

Radiological Images Before Surgery Computed tomography (CT) indicated a suprasellar lesion with round enhancement but without significant calcification. Magnetic resonance imaging (MRI) revealed a suprasellar cystic tumor (2.5 × 2.0 cm) located beneath the optic chiasm. The prechiasmatic space was enlarged. A normal pituitary stalk was identified behind the tumor (Fig. 6.38).

Analysis Before Surgery

- *Patient's general condition*: Only minor and partial hypopituitarism was observed during endocrinological detection, and no hypothalamic dysfunction was found. The visual defect was limited and reversible.

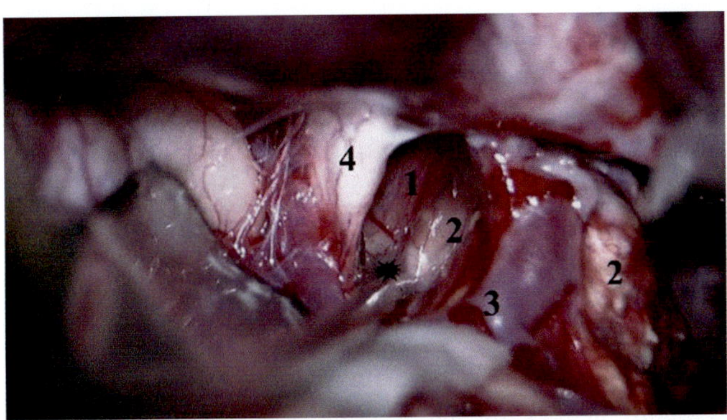

Fig. 6.32 Through the second surgical space (ICA-optic space), the observed tumor was entirely located outside the ventricular cavity. At the ventral optic chiasm, the tumor adhered tightly to the tuberoinfundibular part of the pituitary stalk, which was considered to be the site of origin (black asterisk). (1) Pituitary stalk, (2) tumor exposed from the inside (the optic-carotid space) and outside (lateral space) of the ICA spaces, (3) right side of the ICA, (4) right side of the optic chiasm

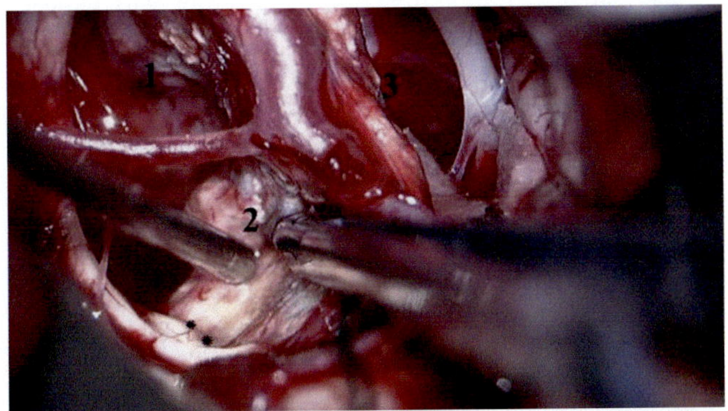

Fig. 6.34 The main corridors used for manipulation are the space between the carotid artery and chiasm, bifurcation of the ICA, and space at the lateral to the internal carotid artery. The calcified tumor had adhered tightly to the floor of the third ventricle (black asterisks), thus presenting significant challenges to surgical removal. (1) Space between the optic chiasm and internal carotid artery, (2) space at the bifurcation of the internal carotid artery, (3) space between the ICA and oculomotor nerve (third nerve)

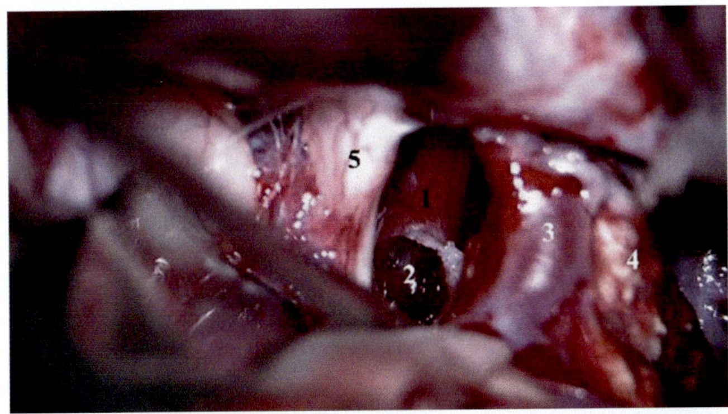

Fig. 6.33 Through the ICA-optic space, the pituitary stalk is observed. There was no arachnoidal interface at the infundibular site of tumor origin, necessitating sharp dissection. Anatomical preservation of the pituitary stalk was pursued. (1) The distal portion of the pituitary stalk, (2) defect on the pituitary stalk at the tumor origin, (3) ICA, (4) tumor boundary at the right side, (5) right optic nerve

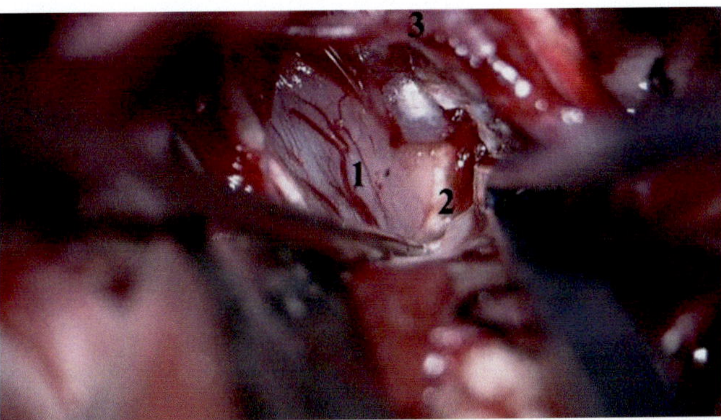

Fig. 6.35 Intraoperative picture showing the intactness of the third ventricle floor after tumor dissection. (1) Intact third ventricle floor after tumor dissection, (2) the tumor adhered to the third ventricle floor, (3) bifurcation of the internal carotid artery

- *Surgical aims*: (1) Total tumor removal, (2) attempted preservation of hypothalamus–infundibulum-pituitary axis continuity to the extent possible.
- *Surgical techniques*: This was a typical case of type S tumor that originated from the subarachnoid segment of the pituitary stalk. The lesion predominantly occupied the chiasmatic arachnoidal cistern with external growth from the third ventricle floor (third VF). Most of the pituitary stalk was intact except for the site of tumor origin. The basilar membranous arachnoid covered the tumor surface and provided an interface between the tumor and adjacent neurovascular structures. Given the tumor's cisternal occupation, an extra-axial route was selected. Although a transnasal endoscopic would be a suitable route for this tumor, a transsylvian approach using a keyhole technique also satisfied tumor resection. The tumor was exposed using a right-side transsylvian approach with a relatively small bone window. For membranous structures and hierarchical layers, see the schematic figure (Fig. 6.39).

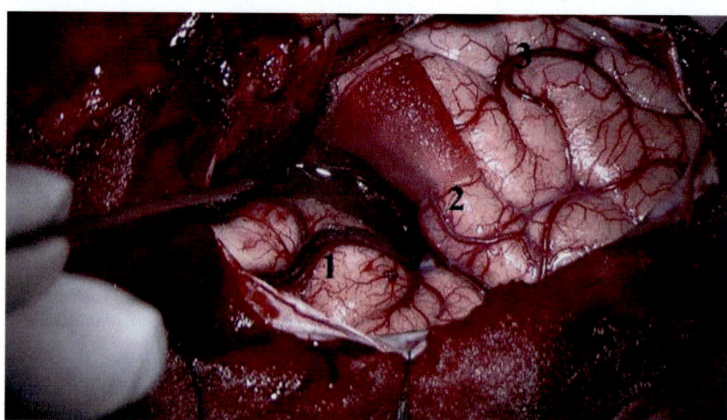

Fig. 6.36 Dural window after tumor removal: the bone window had expanded posteriorly to the temporal lobe, facilitating exposure of the lateral boundary of the tumor. (1) Frontal lobe exposed after craniotomy, (2) temporal lobe, (3) bone expansion to the temporal lobe

Intraoperative Findings A right transsylvian approach was selected because of the decreased vision in the right eye. After dissecting the lateral fissure, the suprasellar tumor was exposed. Significant arachnoidal septation existed between the tumor and optic nerves. The site of tumor origin was located at the lower arachnoid sleeve segment of the pituitary stalk (Fig. 6.40).

Perioperative Treatment For this patient, perioperative treatment included close monitoring of intake and output volumes as well as electrolyte levels. Intramuscular or oral antidiuretic hormone (ADH; desmopressin) was used in accordance with the urine volume and blood sodium level to help the patient transition through the period of profuse urination.

Long-Term Follow-Up MRI was used intermittently to evaluate the extent of tumor removal and indicate tumor recurrence. This patient was proven to remain free of tumor recurrence during the 6-year follow-up period. Her decreased vision and visual field defects were completely reversed. She experienced no other symptoms except for a menstrual disorder, suggesting a clinical cure.

6.4.2.3 Case 3

Medical History This was the case of a 4-year-old girl with 6-month history of intermittent headache and dizziness, 3-month history of polyuria and polydipsia, and 1-month history of double vision and muscle weakness.

Physical and Experimental Examination The abductive function of the left eyeball was abnormal. The left limb muscle force was weakened and the patient had an unsteady gait. No significant positive results were detected in the physical examination. Presurgical endocrinological detection indicated hypopituitarism. Plasmid hormone detection indicated

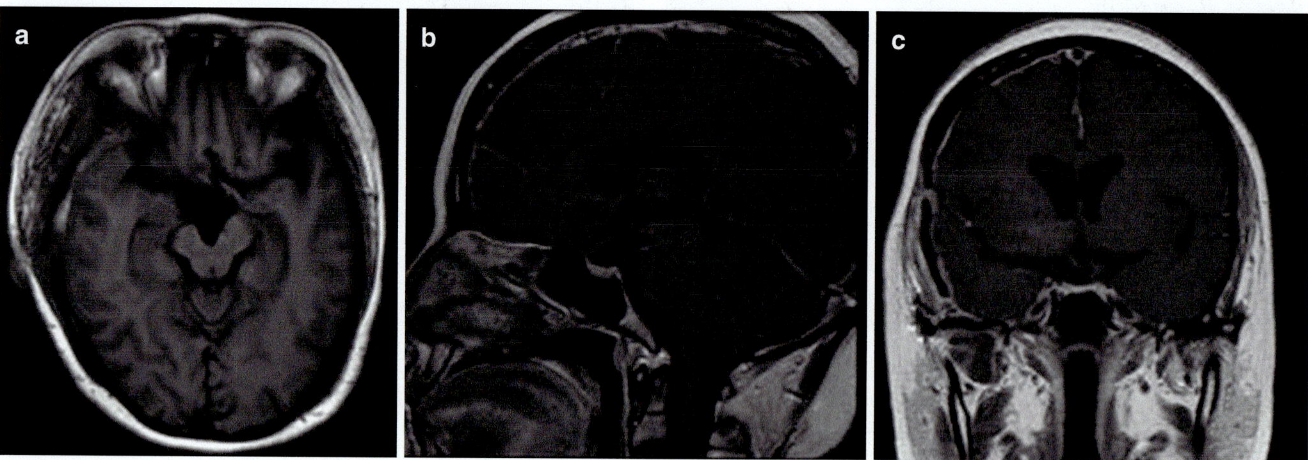

Fig. 6.37 The tumor was completely removed, and the pituitary stalk was anatomically preserved

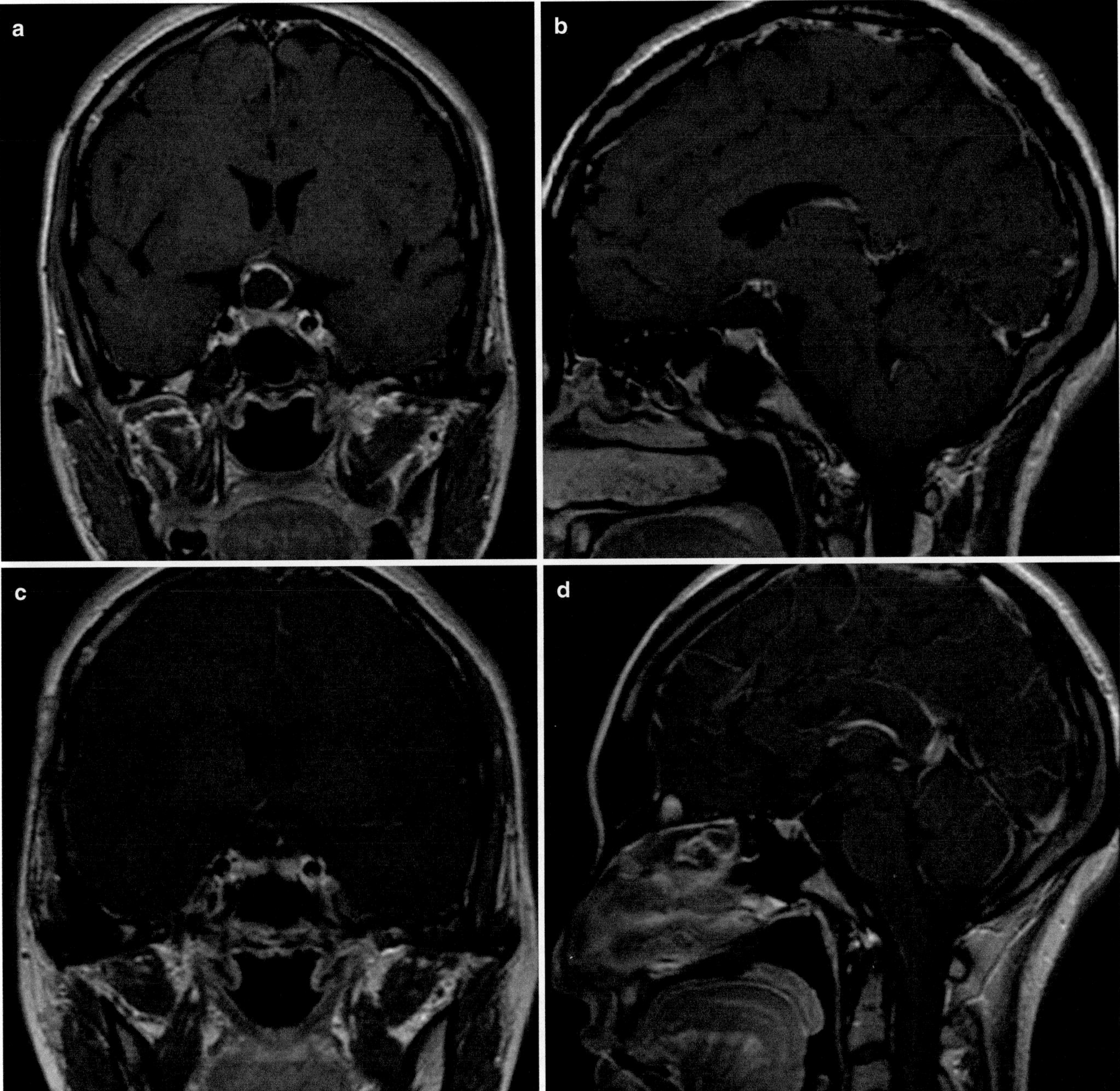

Fig. 6.38 Presurgical and postsurgical magnetic resonance imaging (MRI) of the present case. (**a**, **b**) Sagittal and coronal MR images indicating that the tumor mainly occupied the prechiasmatic subarachnoid cistern space. The site of tumor origin was located in the middle segment of the pituitary stalk. (**c**, **d**) Postsurgical MRI revealed total tumor removal with good pituitary stalk preservation

a near-normal level of thyroxine and below-normal levels of GH/adrenocorticotropic hormone (ACTH) axis hormones. Endocrinological detection indicated significant decreases in the levels of multiple sexual hormones.

Preoperative Radiological Images (Fig. 6.41) Presurgical MRI indicated a predominantly cystic tumor that possibly had originated from the posterior pituitary stalk with backward extension. The tumor occupied the suprasellar cistern, prepontine cistern, interpeduncular cistern, and the right side of the ambient cistern. Posteriorly, it even reached the superior side of the cerebellum. The brain stem was displaced rightward. Laterally, the tumor expanded leftward and reached the sylvian fissure cistern (Fig. 6.42).

Analysis Before Surgery

- *Patient's general condition*: A young child with extensive tumor expansion. In addition to hypopituitarism, the patient had significant cranial nerve palsy. The tumor had also expanded toward the interpeduncular space with

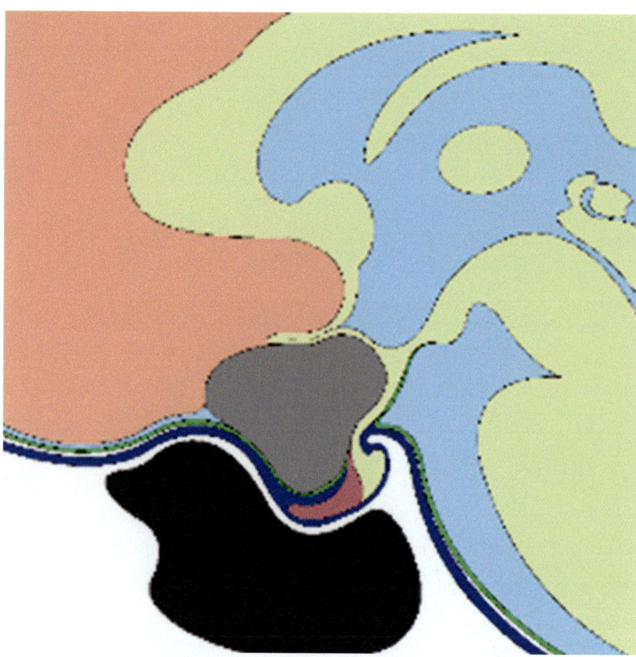

Fig. 6.39 Schematic figure revealing the tumor morphology and its relationship with the surrounding structures. Blue line: dura mater (diaphragm and sellar floor dura); green line: arachnoid mater

obvious third VF displacement, indicating a close relationship between the site of tumor origin and the infundibulum and third VF.

- *Surgical aim*: Despite the huge tumor size and extensive involvement, the surgical aim remained total tumor removal. The tumor had adhered to and surrounded the neurovascular structures, necessitating treatment according to the intraoperative conditions. Preservation of anatomical continuity of the third VF-infundibulum-PS was attempted.
- *Surgical difficulty*: (1) The huge tumor had adhered to and surrounded vital neurovascular structures. Therefore, the entire tumor could not be exposed via a single incision, leading to the possibility of blind spots during surgical manipulation. (2) The third VF was lifted significantly in the interpeduncular cistern, indicating close association of the tumor with the infundibulum and third VF. Moreover, a general skull base approach could not provide good exposure of this location, especially for the tumor side contralateral to the approach. (3) The patient was young with a poor tolerance for surgery. Before surgery, extensive communication was needed between clinicians and the patient's parents.

Membranous Structures and Hierarchical Layers After originating from the pars distal infundibular part of the PS, the tumor expanded extensively to the interpeduncular space, retroclivus, prepontine cistern, and cerebellopontine angle (CPA) region. Meanwhile, the cystic tumor extended along the left-side ambient cistern with tentorial margin involvement and reached the pineal region. Despite extensive involvement, the tumor remained inside the subarachnoid cistern. Theoretically, an arachnoidal interface between the tumor and neurovascular structures could be used to safely dissect the tumor cystic wall (Fig. 6.43).

Intraoperative Findings A left-side frontotemporal approach combining the supra- and infratentorial approaches was selected. The bone flap was modified and enlarged to expose the temporal lobe skull base (see Fig. 6.41).

Perioperative Treatment After surgery, endocrinological detection indicated no new hormone deficiencies except for a slight decrease in TSH. The transient abducens nerve palsy, left-side hemiparesis, diabetes insipidus, and electrolyte imbalance were relieved after treatment. The huge tumor caused a subdural hygroma that decreased after conservative treatment.

Long-Term Follow-Up No tumor recurrence occurred during a 2-year follow-up period. The patient gradually recovered central nervous system function. His diabetes insipidus was significantly relieved. The patient continued to use prednisone and Euthyrox tablets as a substitutive therapy for hormone deficiency.

6.4.2.4 Case 4

Medical History This was the case of a 10-year-old girl with decreased vision and double vision for more than 2 weeks.

Physical Examination and Laboratory Examination The patient's consciousness was normal, physical examination showed no visual acuity in the right eye, the visual acuity of the left eye was significantly decreased, and there was no other obvious positive sign.

Endocrine examination showed a slight increase in PRL levels and a decrease in GH levels (1.96 ng/L).

Preoperative Imaging Preoperative MRI showed solid lesions at the suprasellar region. The pituitary stalk was obviously displaced to the posterior aspect of the tumor. The tumor extended from the upper chiasma cistern to the adjacent cerebral cisterns. The left side entered the internal carotid artery cistern, the oculomotor cistern, and even the lateral fissure. The front extended to the under surface of the frontal lobe through the anterior optic space. The rear extended through the dorsum sellae to the interpeduncular prepontine cisterns. Enhanced MRI showed substantial enhancement of the solid tumor part. The main body of the tumor expanded in front of the optic chiasm. Coronal MRI showed cystic lesions that expanded bilaterally and protruded into the left lateral fissure (Fig. 6.44).

Preoperative Analysis

- *General condition of the patient*: The patient had severe visual impairment, but the complaints were mild, and the

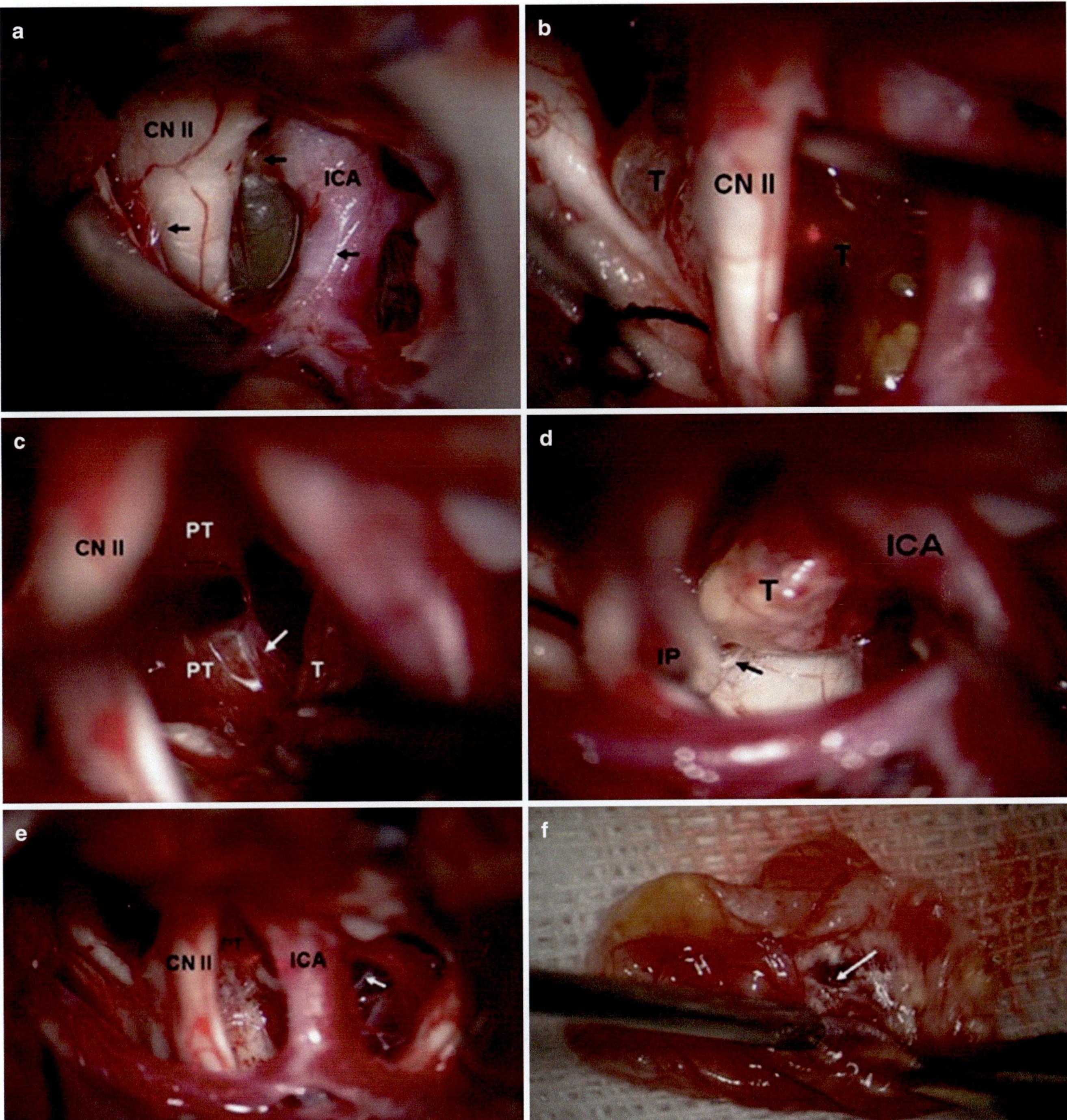

Fig. 6.40 Intraoperative findings. (**a–e**) A significant arachnoidal interface existed between the tumor, internal carotid artery, and bilateral optic nerves. The tumor was safely separated along this interface. (**f**) The tumor was removed completely en bloc. The white arrow indicates the arachnoid membrane around the tumor

parents reported that the symptoms were present for only 2 weeks. It reflects the visual impairment, which is easily aggravated and neglected in children, and it is noticed when the visual acuity is seriously damaged. The physical examination showed no other positive signs except for decreased visual acuity in both eyes and diplopia. Regarding the endocrine examination, GH levels were decreased, and GH levels <5 ng/L in children are generally considered to be insufficient for growth hormone, but the gold standard for objective evaluation is the insulin hypoglycemia stimulate test.

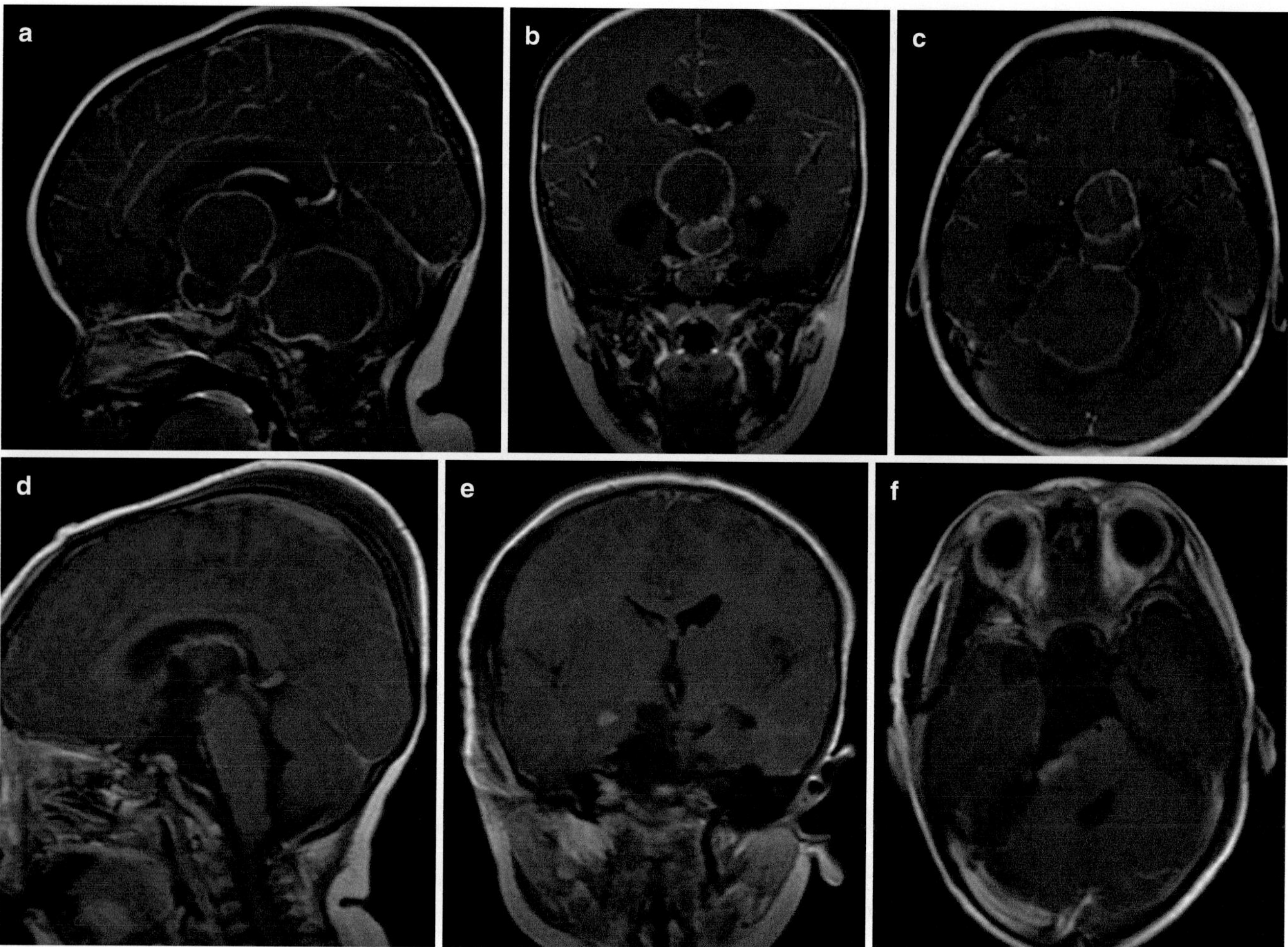

Fig. 6.41 Presurgical MRI (**a**–**c**) revealed a huge subarachnoid cisternal craniopharyngioma with expansion mainly to the retroclivus and posterior cranial fossa. From the site of origin at the chiasmatic cistern and around the pituitary stalk, the tumor capsule compressed the third ventricle floor significantly by extending into the adjacent basal cistern, ultimately involving multiple cisterns. Postsurgical MRI (**d**–**f**) revealed total tumor removal

- *Difficulties in operation*: The tumor was huge and expanded from the optic-chiasm cistern to the olfactory cistern and the frontal surface of the frontal anterior space through the optic chiasm, which surrounds the optic chiasm and the anterior communicating artery complex. Furthermore, this was a predominantly solid tumor. Lateral internal carotid artery cistern expansion may form adhesion to local perforating vessels and the oculomotor nerves and develop backward through the dorsum sellae to the interpeduncular space. The left internal carotid artery and its branches, as well as the oculomotor nerves, were surrounded by the tumor, so it was necessary to sharply dissect the tumor. The tumor calcification adhered tightly to the pituitary stalk and may also adhere to the left carotid artery.
- *Surgical purpose:* Total removal of the tumor and preservation of the integrity of the hypothalamus–infundibulum-pituitary axis.
- *Surgical plan*: This was a typical type S case growing mainly in extraventricular subarachnoid cerebral cistern. Although the tumor was extremely large, its surface was still covered with a layer of arachnoid membrane and pia structures, which separated the tumor from the surrounding nerve vessels and other structures. Lateral expansion of the tumor may have resulted in insufficient exposure of the extended transsphenoidal approach. Therefore, a frontal basal interhemispheric approach was selected to remove the tumor through the extra-axial route.

Intraoperative Findings After dissecting the anterior interhemispheric fissure, the tumor involving the anterior cranial fossa and lamina terminalis cistern was exposed. The lateral border of the tumor was separated along the arachnoid interface through the enlarged prechiasmatic space (Fig. 6.45).

Postoperative Neuroimaging (Fig. 6.46)

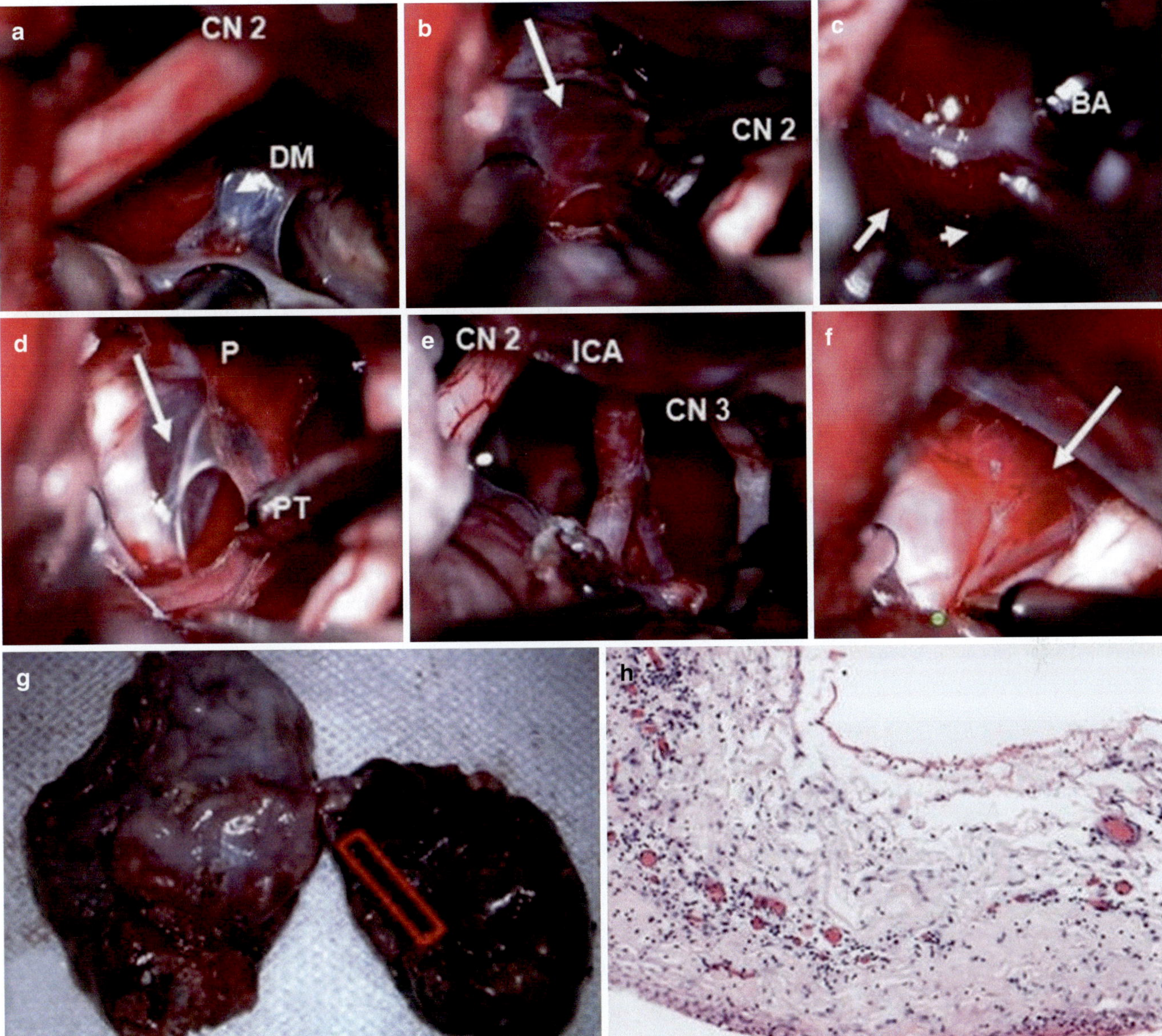

Fig. 6.42 The tumor was removed via a right-side frontotemporal combined supra- and infratentorial approach. Intraoperative images show the various aspects of the tumor; the tumor adhered tightly to, but did not infiltrate, the third ventricle floor (**a**–**f**). The white arrow indicates the arachnoid membrane around the tumor. Pathological examination of different materials derives different results; at the tumor's originating site, the tumor tissue is tightly bound to peripheral glia (**g**). However, the distant tumor wall within the cisterns appears as a single layer of tumor cells and loose connective tissue fibers (**h**)

Perioperative Treatment Endocrine examination showed that the growth hormone and corticosteroid axis were low. There was water–electrolyte balance disorder, which improved after treatment.

Long-Term Follow-Up The patient had transient oculomotor palsy symptoms but recovered gradually during the follow-up period. Hormone replacement was discontinued during the follow-up period.

A 2.5-year follow-up MRI (Fig. 6.46) confirmed complete tumor resection. The patient's weight was slightly elevated, and there were no symptoms of other hypothalamic dysfunctions such as obesity. After 3 years, the patient's hormone test results were basically normal, and the endocrine function recovered well.

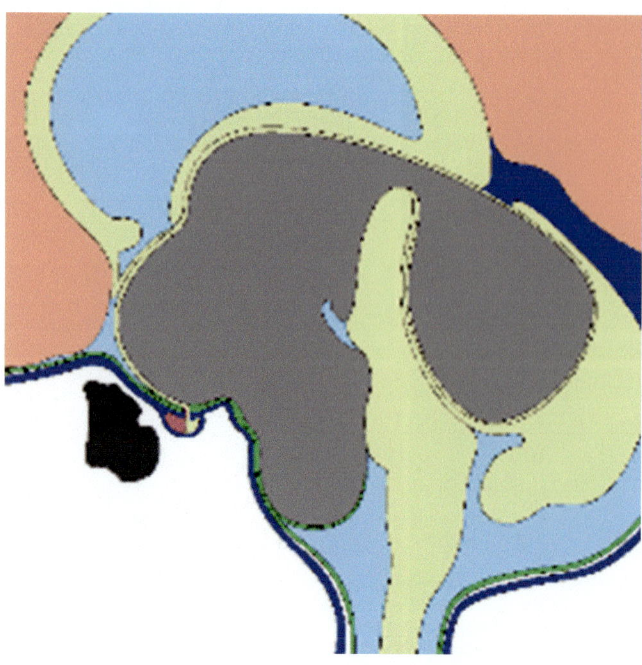

Fig. 6.43 Schematic figure showing the tumor morphology and relationships with the surrounding structures. Blue line: dura mater (diaphragm and sellar floor dura); green line: arachnoid mater

6.4.3 Type T

6.4.3.1 Case 1

Medical History This was the case of a 5-year-old girl. She presented with increased appetite for 1 month and hyperpyrexia for 1 week.

Physical examination showed decreased visual accuracy in both eyes. Endocrinological detection indicated a slight increase in PRL (28.7 ng/mL) and decreased GH (0.644 ng/mL) and IGF-1 (85.59 ng/mL) level; she did not undergo stimulate test due to her young age and critical preoperative condition. The other hormone levels were normal. Preoperative weight and height were 27 kg and 130 cm, respectively (Figs. 6.47 and 6.48).

Surgical Consideration In contrast to subdiaphragmatic (type Q) tumors and some suprasellar extraventricular (type S) tumors with upward involvement into the third ventricle chamber and a so-called pseudo-intraventricular location (tumors with an apparent third ventricle location that in fact originate from a suprasellar extra-axial position), in most

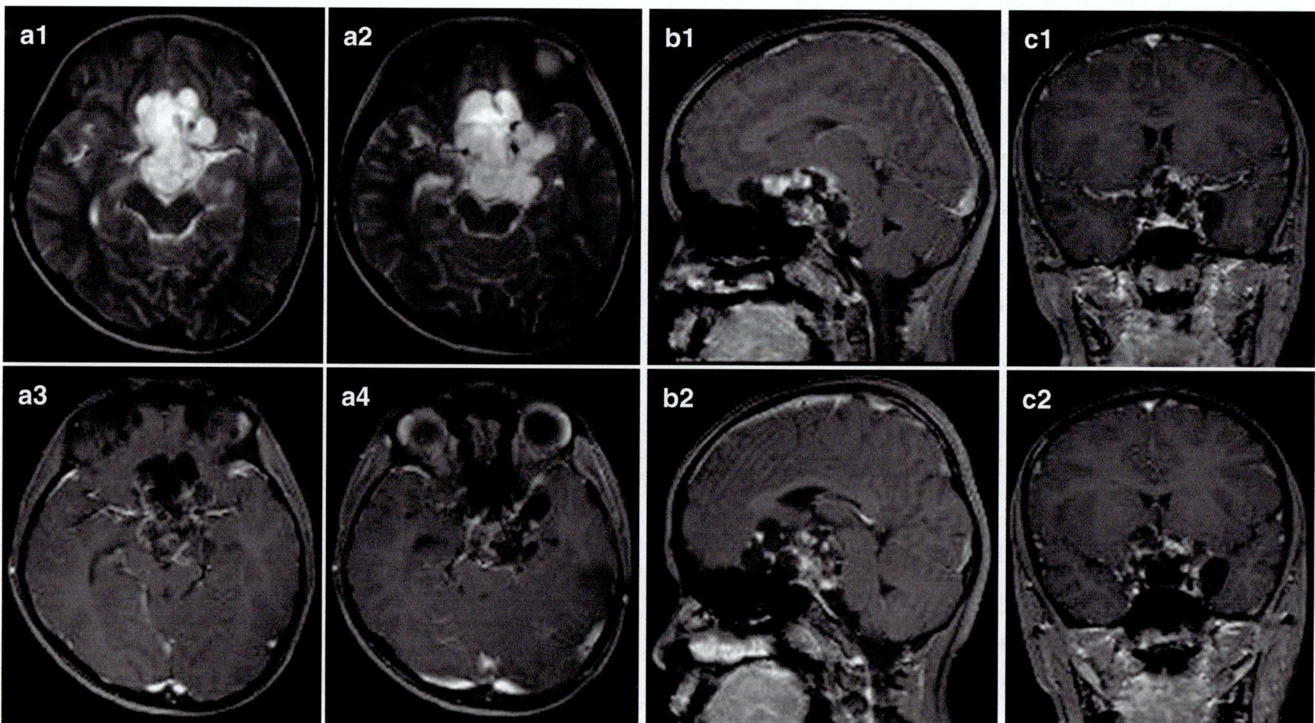

Fig. 6.44 Preoperative MRI. (**a**1–4) Preoperative axial T1 and T2 weighted images showing the extent of tumor involvement. (**b**1–2) Sagittal scan showing that the tumor occupied the interpeduncular fossa and expanded to the upper clivus, adjacent to the posterior circulation vessel in prepontine cistern through the Liliequist membrane. (**c**1–2) Coronal scan showing that the tumor surrounded the left internal carotid artery and the anterior communicating artery complex, extending into the left lateral fissure (reproduced with permission from Qi (Ed.), *Craniopharyngioma*, People's Medical Publishing House, ISBN 978-7-117-26463-1, 2018)

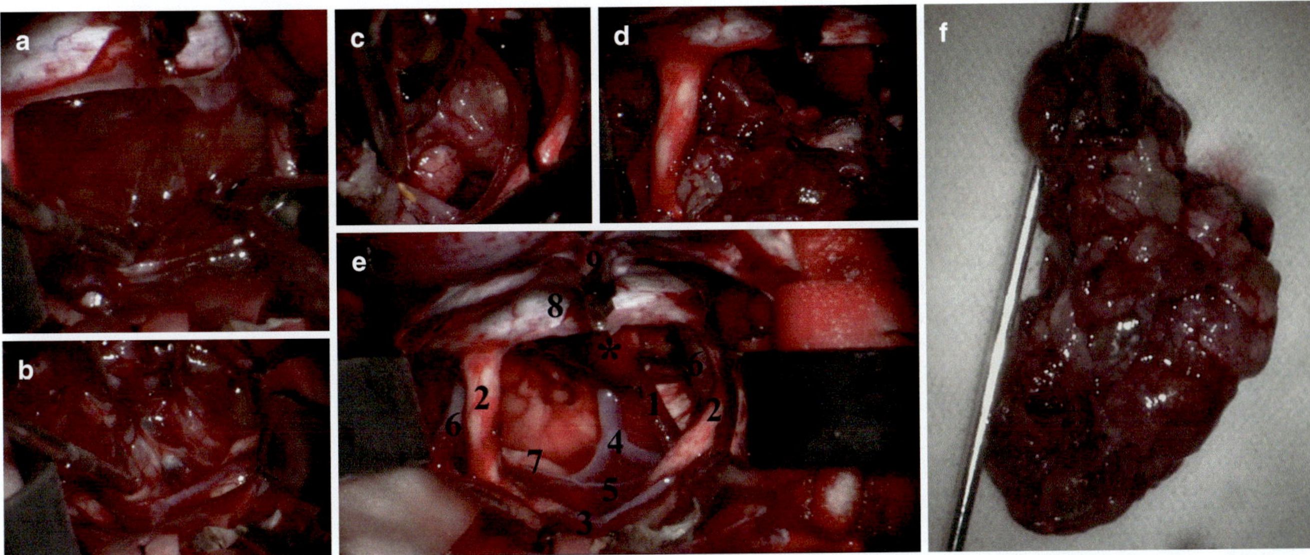

Fig. 6.45 Interoperative findings (via the frontobasal anterior interhemispheric approach). (**a**) The anterior interhemispheric fissure is dissected to expose the enlarged prechiasmatic space and tumor. (**b**) The tumor surrounding the optic chiasm and the anterior communicating artery was dissected along the basal arachnoid membrane. (**c**) The arachnoid boundary between the tumor and the distal part of the pituitary stalk is clear. (**d**) The distal segment of the pituitary stalk within the cistern and the normal pituitary gland (the black asterisk in the figure) are exposed. (**e**) After total tumor resection, the structures of the optic nerve, pituitary gland, and Willis ring were well protected. (**f**) The tumor was dissected in en bloc manner. (1) Pituitary stalk, (2) optic nerve, (3) anterior communicating artery, (4) apex of the basilar artery, (5) Liliequist membrane, (6) internal carotid artery, (7) oculomotor nerve (left side), (8) planum sphenoidale, (9) crista galli (reproduced with permission from Qi (Ed.), *Craniopharyngioma*, People's Medical Publishing House, ISBN 978-7-117-26463-1, 2018)

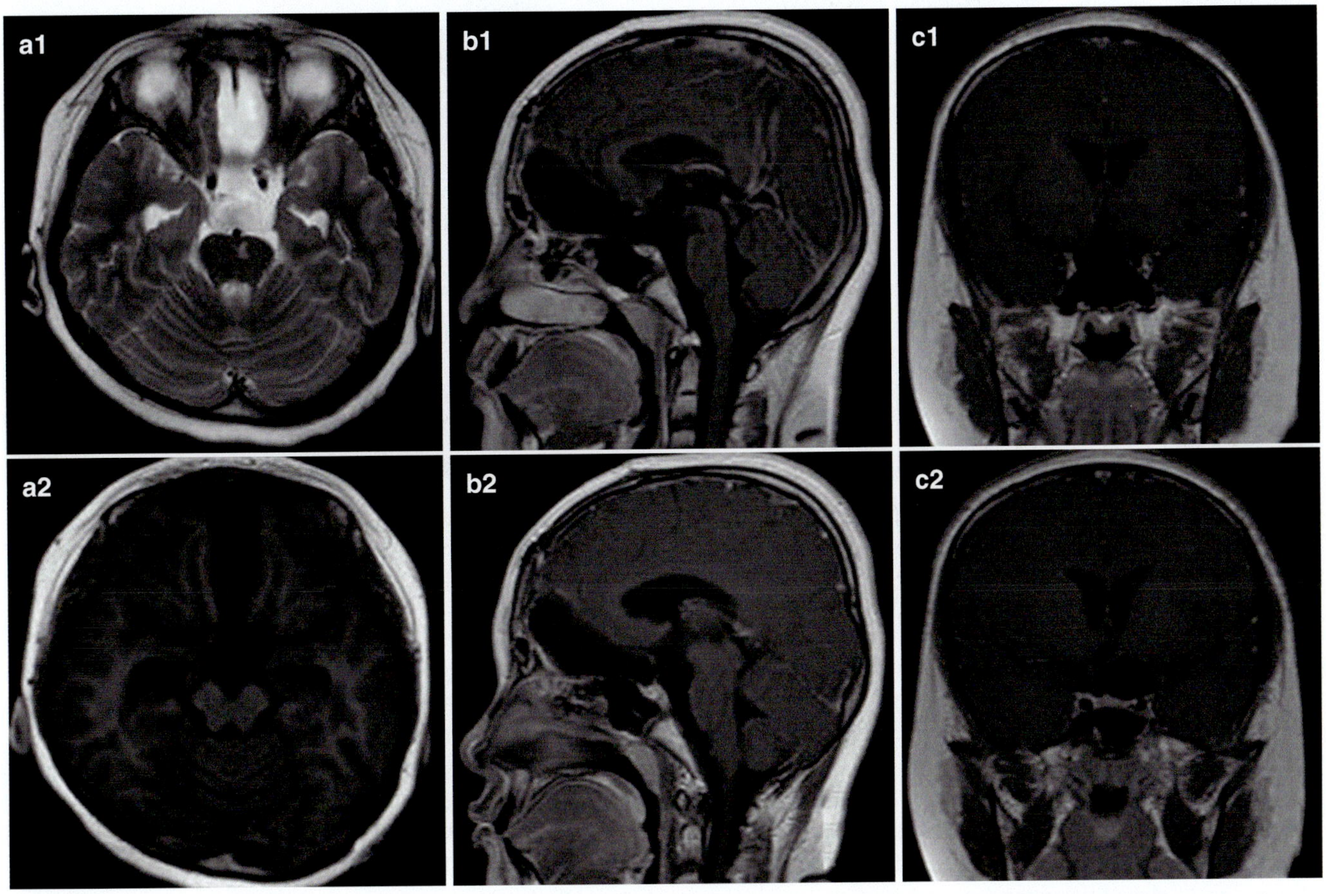

Fig. 6.46 Follow-up MR study revealed total tumor resection; the shape of the suprasellar cistern was roughly restored (**a**1–2), sagittal (**b**1–2) and coronal images showed the retained displaced pituitary stalk and normal pituitary gland (reproduced with permission from Qi (Ed.), *Craniopharyngioma*, People's Medical Publishing House, ISBN 978-7-117-26463-1, 2018)

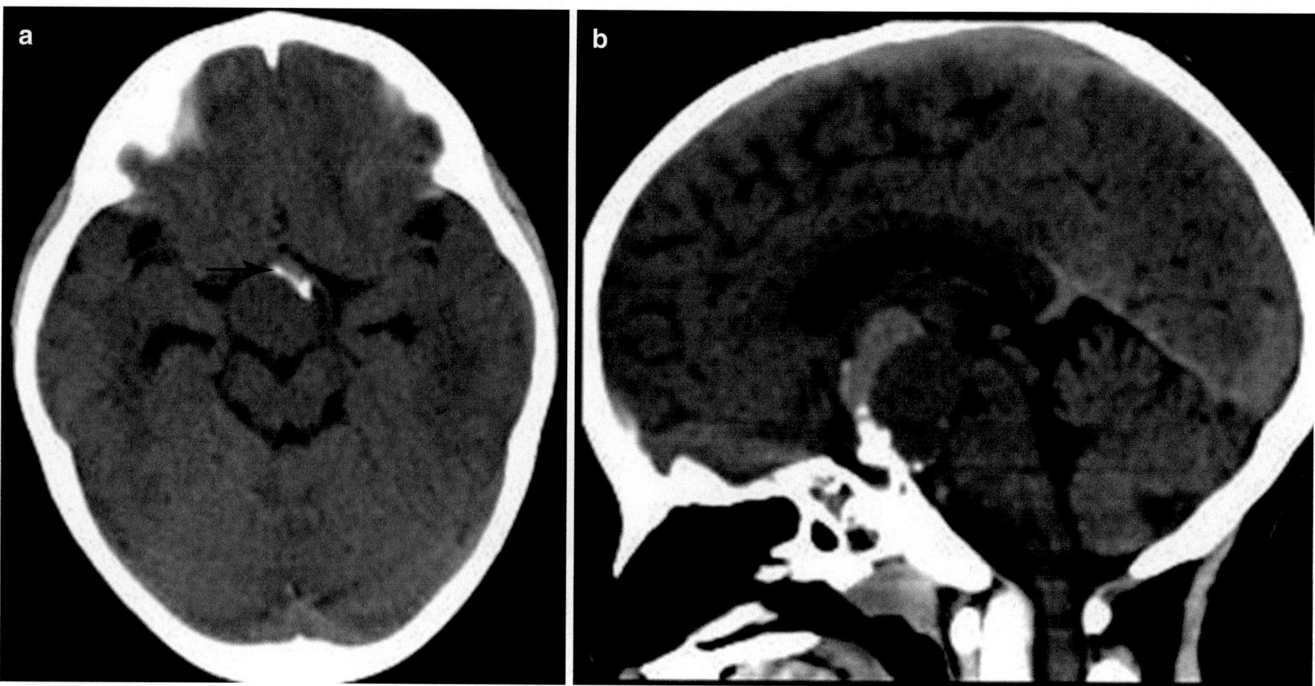

Fig. 6.47 Axial and sagittal computed tomography (CT) scan indicated a mixed cystic-solid lesion occupying the suprasellar region along with an egg-shell calcification on the cystic wall (black arrow on **a**)

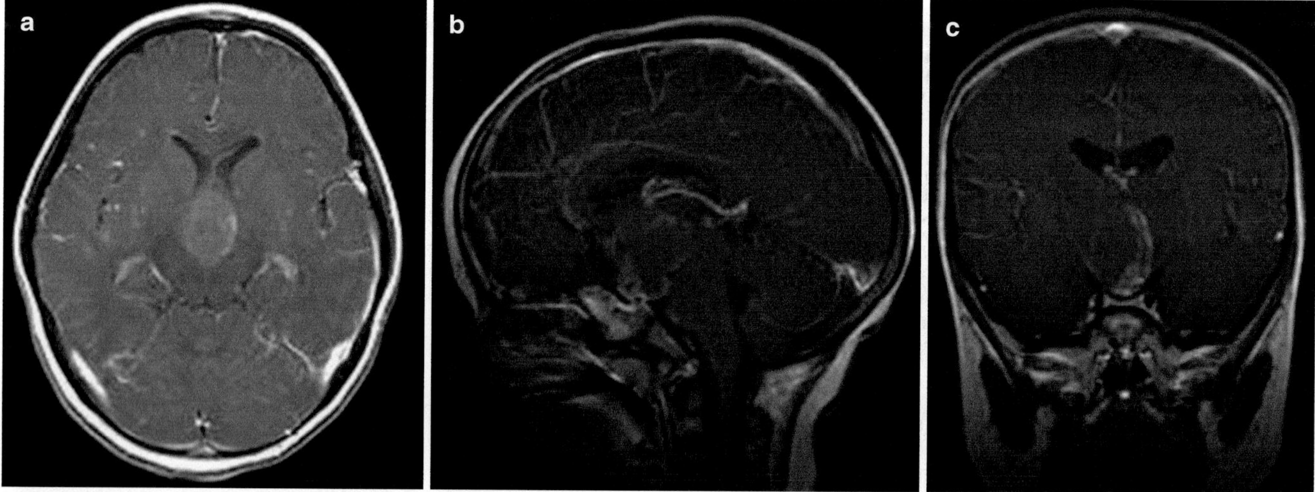

Fig. 6.48 Axial (**a**), sagittal (**b**), and coronal (**c**) views in preoperative MRI indicating a predominantly cystic tumor in the suprasellar region with invagination into the third ventricular floor and occupation of the third ventricle cavity. The distal segment of the pituitary stalk could be clearly identified both on sagittal and coronal views on MR images. It was a typical type T tumor, the original site of tumor is pars distal part of pituitary stalk near tuberoinfundibular region

cases of type T tumor, the normal nerve tissues of the third ventricle walls (containing viable hypothalamic tissue) remain in a lower position and attached to the basal tumor pole.

Approach Selection Surgical resection of type T tumor presents specific problems due to deep localization and risk of damage to the optic pathways and hypothalamic structures. The trans-lamina terminalis (LT) route is commonly used in resection of type T tumors. It offers more direct access to the anterior part of the third ventricle where the tumor lies adherent in the region of the tuber cinereum. The lamina terminalis is accessible either along the medial part of a frontotemporal approach or via an anterior interhemispheric approach. When a lateral approach is used to access the lamina terminalis, the oblique angle at which the lamina terminalis is viewed renders it difficult to see the posterior part of the third ventricle and hence, contributes to difficulty in opening the entire lamina terminalis. Tumors with wide and tight adherence to the third ventricle wall and/or floor such as that in the present case cannot be safely dissected through the lateral approach, as there is lack of direct vision of the posterior part of the third ventricle. In contrast, the anterior interhemispheric approach provides a good view of the entire lamina terminalis. Tumors can be removed either through the space anterior to the AcoA or, more often, through the bilateral A2 space, in cases where the AcoA is located close to the optic chiasm. The AcoA can be safely divided in some cases when it limits operative exposure. In this type T case, we selected the anterior interhemispheric approach to remove the tumor.

Intraoperative Findings Figures 6.49, 6.50, 6.51, 6.52, 6.53, and 6.54.

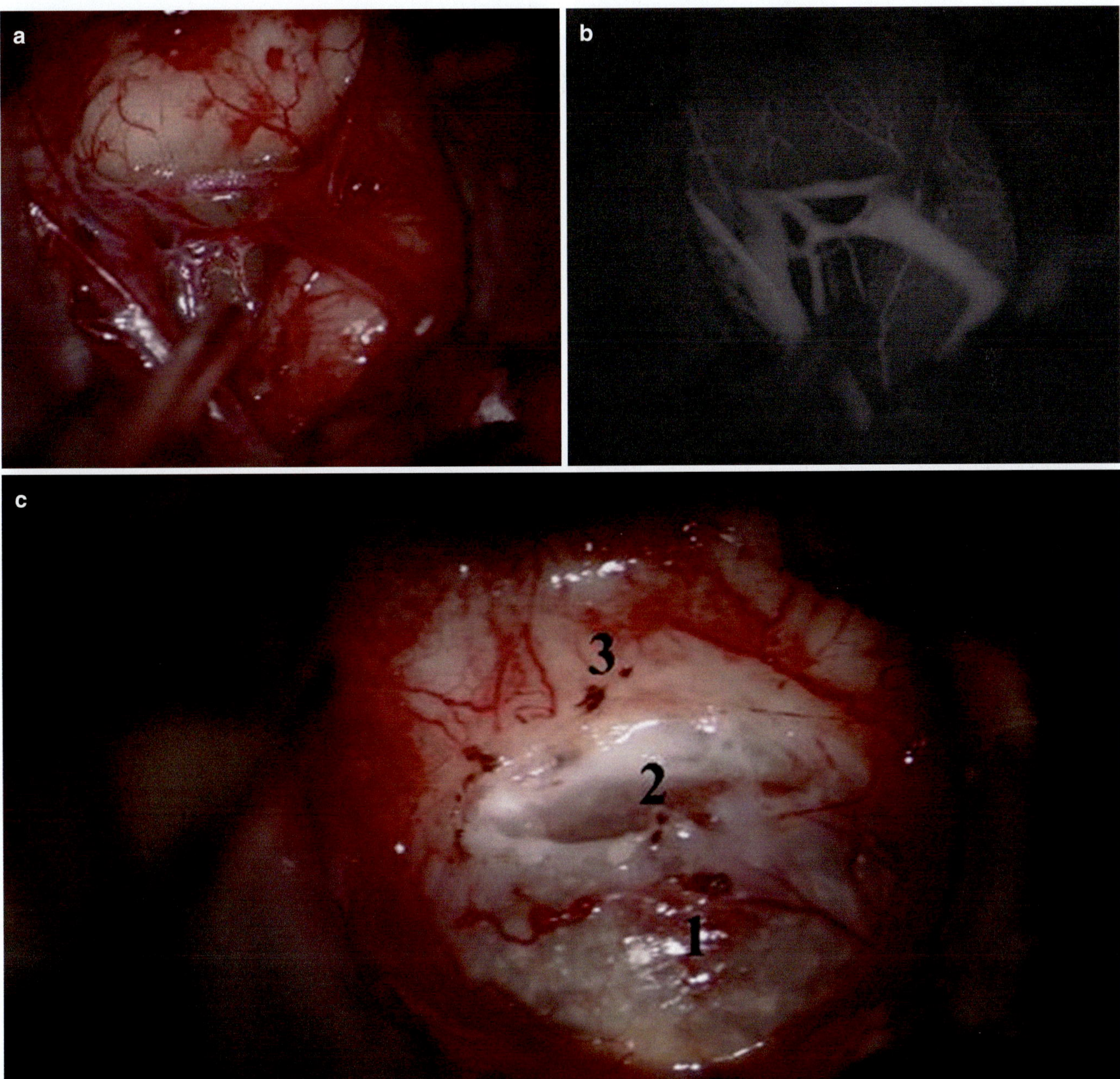

Fig. 6.49 After dissecting the anterior interhemispheric fissure, the LT space was exposed. Usually, the lamina terminalis is crowded by the anterior communicating artery complex. If split artery is required, the vascular architecture needs to be carefully evaluated. Indocyanine green angiography is a simple and easy evaluation method during the operation. After blocking the anterior communicating artery using a temporary blocking clip, if both sides A1 and A2 are well filled, it is an indicative that helps to break the vessel. In this case, the AcoA was safely divided after assessment of the angioarchitecture of the anterior communicating artery complex (com-ACA). The LT space was widely exposed facilitating dissecting the tumor. After careful dissection, the covering layers of the tumor at the LT space were illustrated. (1) Membrane layer of the LT, (2) tumor wall revealed after incision of the LT membrane, (3) optic chiasm

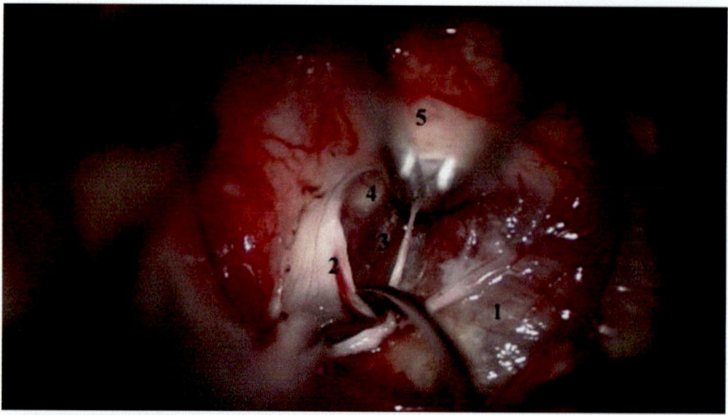

Fig. 6.50 Tracing the tumor boundary through a relatively narrow space such as the LT sometimes leads to extreme difficulties. Anatomic maintenance of the ventricular floor and walls and of the infundibulum is of paramount importance during tumor removal. (1) Membrane layer of the LT, (2) left optic tract, (3) tumor wall revealed after incision of the LT membrane, (4) neuro-layer at the hypothalamic structures, (5) optic chiasm

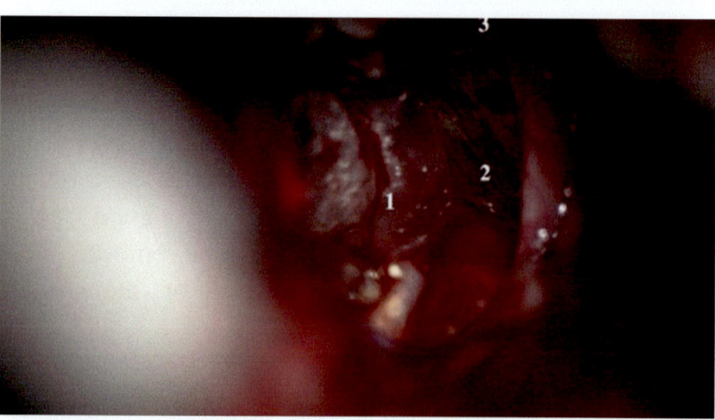

Fig. 6.52 Dissection of the tumor should be accomplished in an en bloc manner tracing along the cystic tumor wall. Piecemeal resection may cause tumor residue. Internal decompression by aspirating cystic components can help in gaining space to facilitate dissection of the tumor from the third ventricle margins. (1) Posterior tumor boundary in the third ventricle cavity, (2) tumor wall at the anterolateral portion of the third ventricle wall, (3) thin layer of the right optic tract

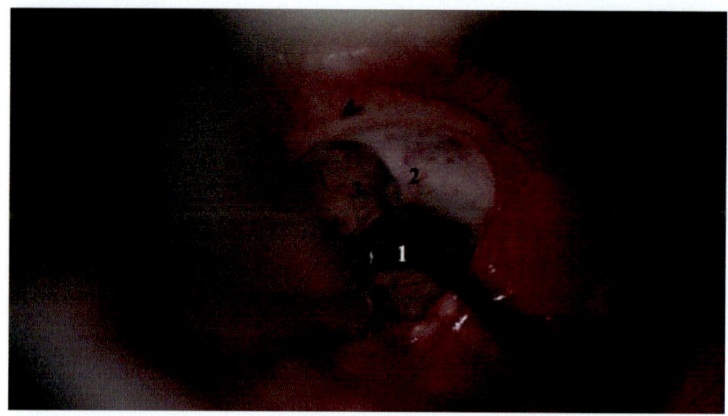

Fig. 6.51 One should always remember that the capsule of the tumor is dissected and delivered from the surrounding layer of gliosis. This neuroglial layer intervening between the tumor and viable hypothalamic nuclei may provide a safe dissecting plane. (1) Tumor wall at the posterior third ventricle cavity, (2) neuro-layer covering the tumor at the median eminence, (3) neuroglial layer between the tumor and hypothalamic nuclei, (4) optic chiasm

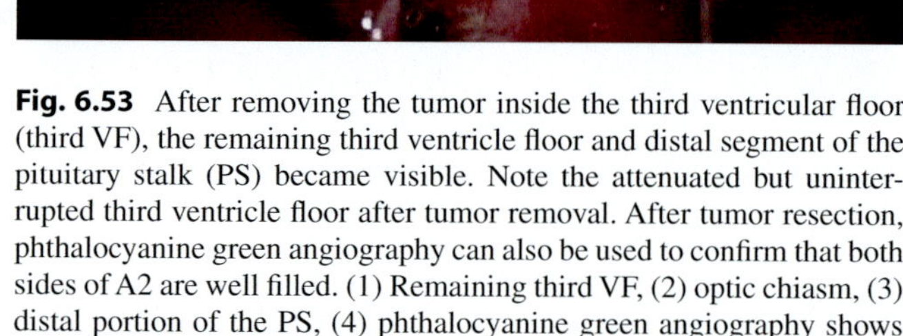

Fig. 6.53 After removing the tumor inside the third ventricular floor (third VF), the remaining third ventricle floor and distal segment of the pituitary stalk (PS) became visible. Note the attenuated but uninterrupted third ventricle floor after tumor removal. After tumor resection, phthalocyanine green angiography can also be used to confirm that both sides of A2 are well filled. (1) Remaining third VF, (2) optic chiasm, (3) distal portion of the PS, (4) phthalocyanine green angiography shows good bilateral A2 development

Perioperative Treatment The patient developed water–electrolyte imbalance that required fluid supplementation and sodium level adjustments. Otherwise, postsurgical recovery was uneventful.

Long-Term Follow-Up No tumor recurrence was detected after a 3-year follow-up study. The patient continued to require hormone substitution therapy. She also exhibited moderate weight gain, with an increase in BMI from 15.97 before surgery to 22.6 postoperatively. No significant cognitive dysfunction was noted during the follow-up period.

6.4.3.2 Case 2

Medical History This was the case of a 7-year-old male patient who presented with a 6-month history of progressively aggravated headache, dizziness, and decreased visual acuity. The boy did not exhibit significant polyuria and polydipsia. He had undergone surgery for CP resection via a right transcallosal interforniceal approach at a local hospital. A ventriculoperitoneal shunt was also used to relieve hydrocephalus. However, shunt obstruction occurred, and the patient consequently experienced severe headaches and significantly decreased visual acuity.

Physical and Experimental Examination The patient exhibited normal consciousness with significantly decreased right visual acuity (0.5) and slightly decreased left eye acuity (0.8). A surgical scar was found on his right frontal scalp. Endocrinological detection indicated slightly increased PRL levels and decreased FSH and free thyroxine (fT4) levels.

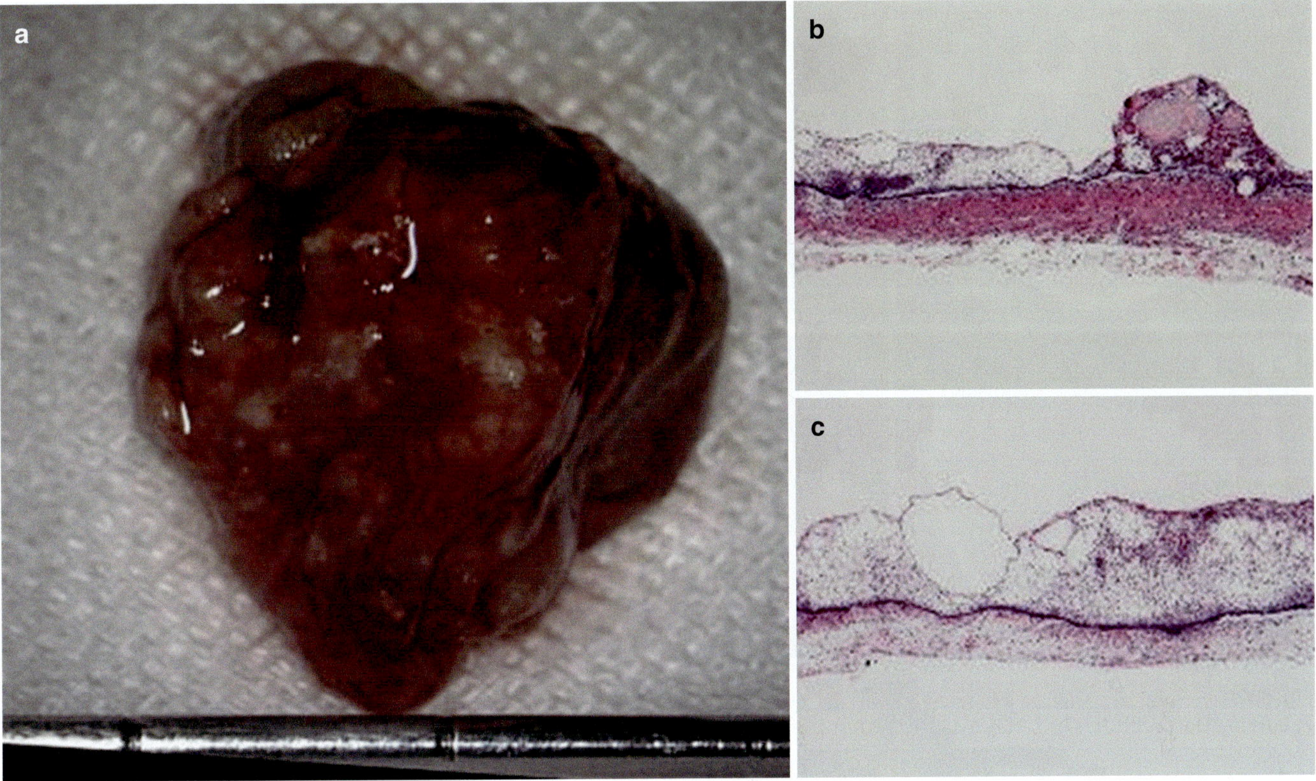

Fig. 6.54 Tumor specimen after en bloc resection. Pathological examination showed that the tumor had significant gliosis and nerve tissue structure near the infundibular tuberculum (**b**), while the tumor within third ventricle wall was similar to the ependymal membrane structure (**c**)

Radiological Images Before Surgery CT indicated a mixed cystic-solid lesion occupying the intrasellar and suprasellar region along with a large calcification mass in the suprasellar region. The cystic tumor occupied the third ventricular cavity and had caused hydrocephalus. MRI showed a lesion that had originated from the infundibulotuberum with a cyst that had extended excessively upward to the third ventricular cavity and backward to the interpeduncular cistern. According to our classification, the tumor type was T. The solid tumor had compressed the diaphragm and pituitary gland downward. The lower segment of the PS was normal, as indicated by the black arrow in Fig. 6.55 (Fig. 6.56).

Analysis Before Surgery Regarding the morphological features, the tumor was classified as type T and differed from the typical example only in terms of extension. Although two main extension directions (upward and backward) were observed on sagittal MRI, the site of origin remained at the infundibulum and under the pia mater. The tumor had remained external to the ventricular system. The third VF structure was invaginated and inflated by the tumor, but the ependymal layer remained intact. Because the posterior tumor border was located behind the AcoA complex and reached the anterior commissure, a frontobasal interhemispheric approach was suggested. However, use of the extra-axial space was suggested for removal of the tumor, which was not truly inside the third ventricular cavity. Although opening of the lamina terminalis was required to remove the upward tumor growth, the residual third VF nervous tissue should be preserved as much as possible. Conversely, the backward tumor growth had occupied the interpeduncular cistern; however, septation of the Liliequist membrane between the tumor and brain stem and the basilar artery and its branches allowed relatively safe tumor removal. Notably, several arachnoidal trabeculae connected the artery branches to the arachnoid mater. During surgery, these branches might have been dissected while pulling the tumor. Therefore, dissection of these transverse trabeculae was needed to avoid arterial injury.

Intraoperative Findings After dissecting the interhemispheric fissure, the AcoA was divided to increase exposure of the lamina terminalis space. The tumor had grown inside the nervous tissue layer of the third VF, so the lamina terminalis and third VF were spliced to dissect the tumor. The tumor was removed in a piecemeal manner, and the infundibulum and proximal segment of the PS, which were inflated by the tumor, were vertically incised to remove the tumor (Fig. 6.57).

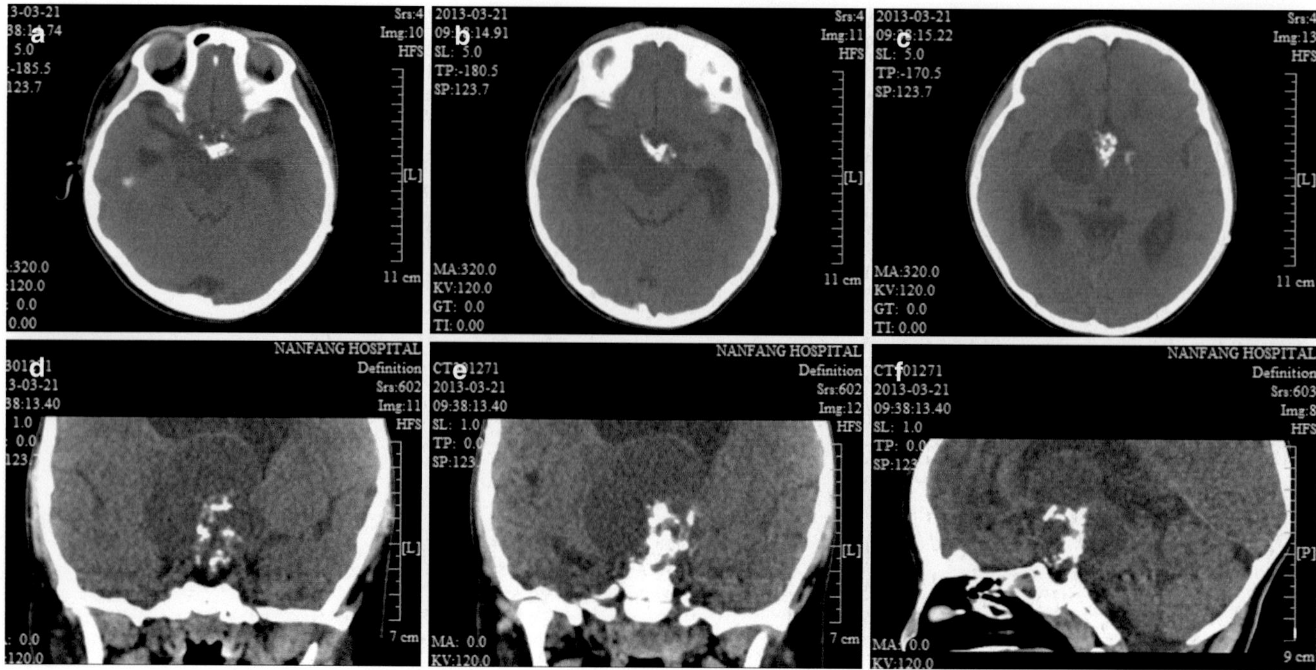

Fig. 6.55 Presurgical computed tomography scans of Case 2 (reproduced with permission from Qi (Ed.), *Craniopharyngioma*, People's Medical Publishing House, ISBN 978-7-117-26463-1, 2018)

Perioperative Treatment The patient developed water–electrolyte imbalance that required fluid supplementation and sodium level adjustments. Otherwise, postsurgical recovery was uneventful.

Long-Term Follow-Up No tumor recurrence was detected after a 3-year follow-up study. The patient continued to require hormone substitution therapy. He also exhibited moderate weight gain, with an increase in BMI from 18.5 before surgery to 24.6 postoperatively. No significant cognitive dysfunction was noted during the follow-up period.

6.4.3.3 Case 3

Medical History A 10-year-old female patient presented with a 3-month history of headache and decreased visual acuity. The patient had not undergone any surgical treatment at other hospitals.

Physical and Experimental Examination The patient exhibited normal consciousness, with visual acuity of 0.6 and 0.8 in the left and right eyes, respectively. Ophthalmoscopy indicated papilledema in both eyes. Endocrinological detection indicated near-normal status except for a slightly decreased FSH level.

Radiological Images Before Surgery MRI indicated a mixed cystic-solid tumor in the suprasellar region. The main tumor body occupied the third ventricular cavity and caused severe hydrocephalus. The solid tumor was located at the infundibulum, a possible site of origin. The posterior part of the cystic tumor occupied the interpeduncular cistern. The lower segment of the PS was normal as indicated by the red arrow in Fig. 6.58.

Analysis Before Surgery This was a case involving a third VF tumor with backward expansion to the posterior third ventricle. A clearly identifiable interface was present between the tumor and surrounding nervous tissue layer.

Membranous Structures and Hierarchical Layers See the schematic Fig. 6.59.

Intraoperative Findings (Fig. 6.60)

Perioperative Treatment The patient's postsurgical recovery was uneventful except for transient DI and minor water–electrolyte disorder.

Long-Term Follow-Up No tumor recurrence was observed after a 6-year follow-up. The patient had no significant dysfunction except for a slight weight increase. Her BMI slightly increased from 22 to 25.

6.4.3.4 Case 4

Medical History This was the case of a 7-year-old male patient who complained of "dizziness for 3 weeks and aggravated vomiting for 1 week."

Physical Examination and Laboratory Tests The patient's consciousness was normal, his visual acuity was normal, and no obvious visual field defect was observed. The size of both pupils and normal light reflection were normal. Endocrinology tests suggested that hormone levels were normal.

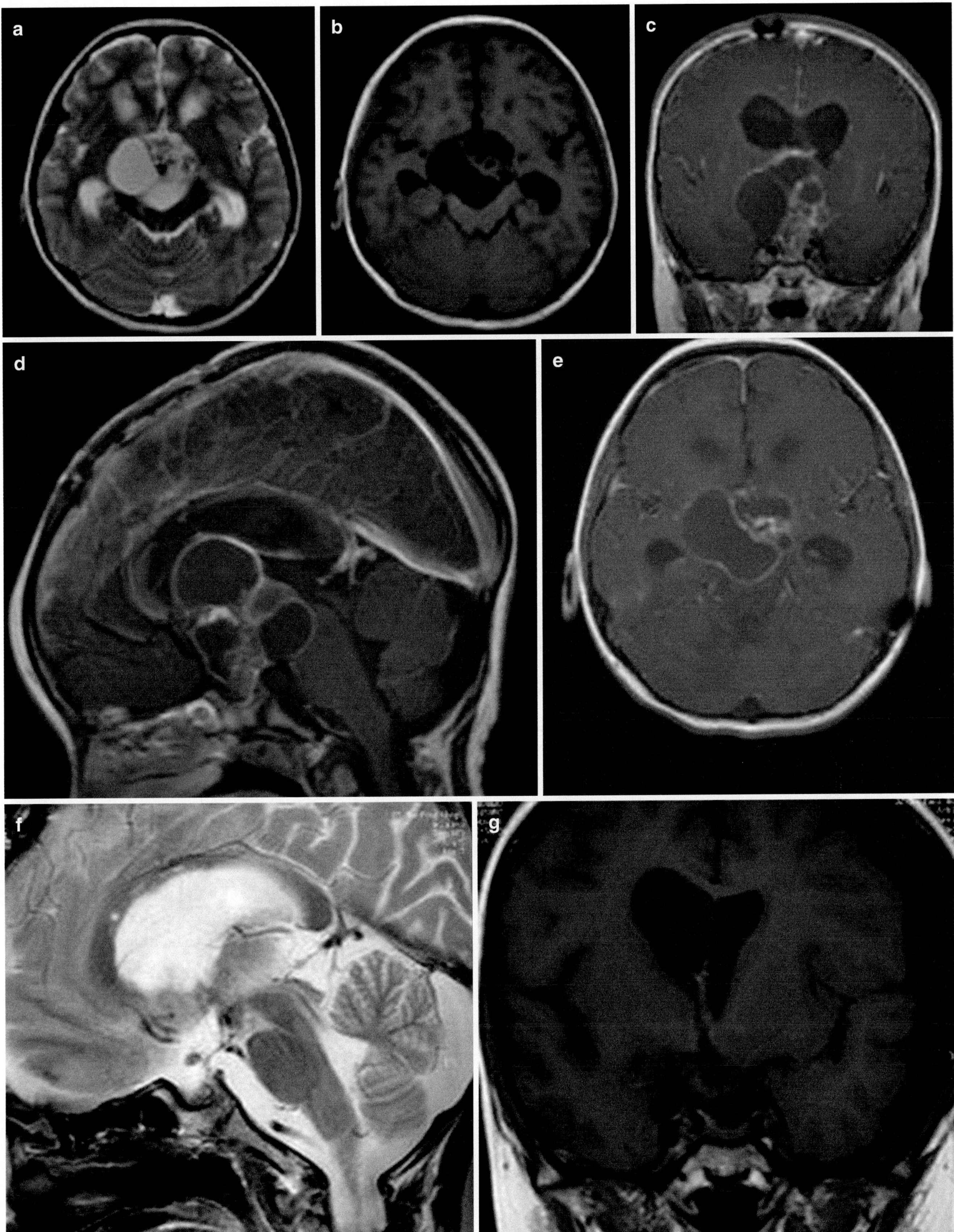

Fig. 6.56 Presurgical magnetic resonance imaging of Case 2 (reproduced with permission from Qi (Ed.), *Craniopharyngioma*, People's Medical Publishing House, ISBN 978-7-117-26463-1, 2018)

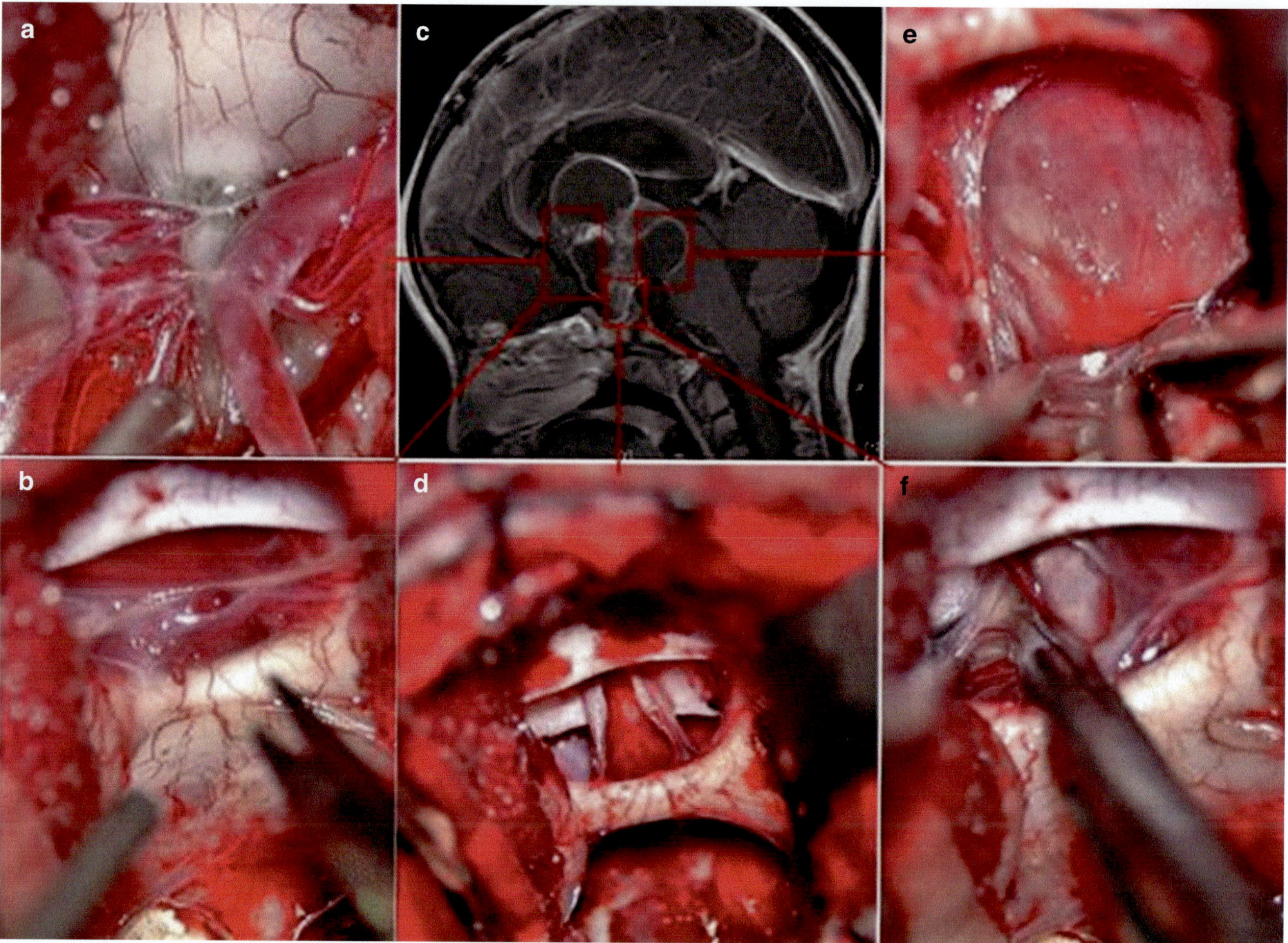

Fig. 6.57 Preoperative magnetic resonance imaging (MRI) and intraoperative images of a 7-year-old boy with a typical type T CP. Presurgical sagittal contrast-enhanced T1-weighted MRI after a flawed surgery via a trans-corpus callosum trans-fornix approach at a local hospital (**c**). Intraoperative images showing tumor removal. The anterior communicating artery was divided to enhance tumor exposure (**a**). After dissecting the arachnoid enveloping the pituitary stalk (**b**), the bulged pituitary stalk was exposed (**f**). The tumor was entirely removed using a combined trans-lamina terminalis and extra-axial route. The pituitary stalk was split vertically to expose the tumor (**d**). Note the attenuated but uninterrupted third ventricle floor after tumor removal (**e**) (reproduced with permission from Qi (Ed.), *Craniopharyngioma*, People's Medical Publishing House, ISBN 978-7-117-26463-1, 2018)

Preoperative Imaging (Fig. 6.61)

Preoperative Analysis

1. This is a typical type T craniopharyngioma with a trans-stalk growth. The tumor completely grows through the long axis of the pituitary stalk.
2. The solid part of the tumor is mainly located in the arachnoid sleeve of the pituitary stalk.
3. This type of craniopharyngioma is the best indication for the anterior interhemispheric approach. The main surgical corridor is the lamina terminalis, and the tumor can be separated by longitudinally dissecting the long axis of the pituitary stalk. If the bilateral A1 and A2 parts of the anterior cerebral arteries are well developed, the anterior communicating artery can be divided to facilitate more adequate exposure. Therefore, preoperative angiography or CTA can help with the preoperative judgment of the anterior communicating artery complex blood vessel structure.

Intraoperative Findings After interhemispheric fissure dissection, an inflated pituitary stalk became visible; the tumor originated from the pars distal tuberoinfundibular part of pituitary stalk and grew longitudinally along the long axis of the pituitary stalk. The posterior tumor occupied the space

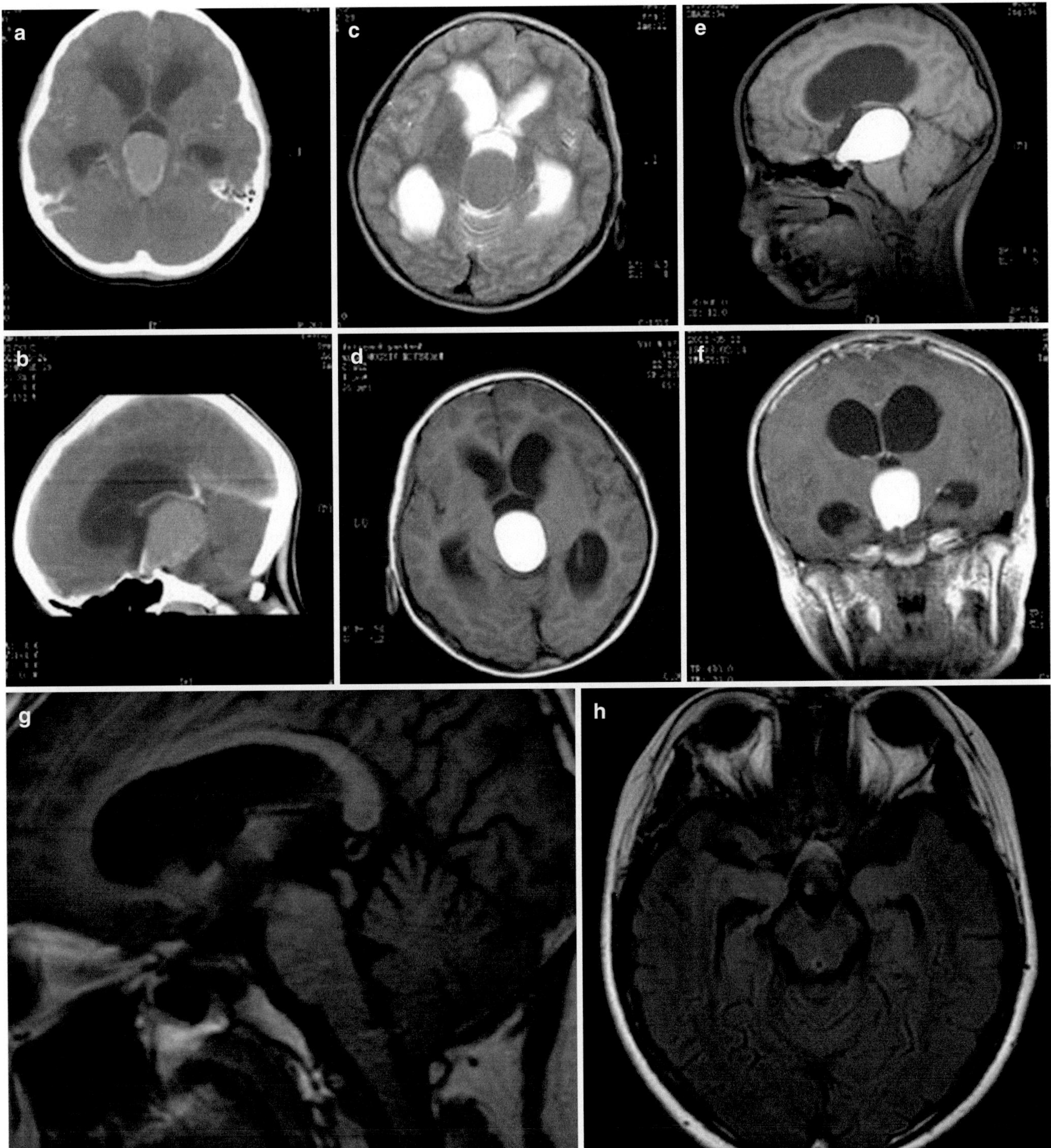

Fig. 6.58 Presurgical and postsurgical radiological images. (**a**–**f**) Presurgical computed tomography and magnetic resonance imaging (MRI). (**g**, **h**) Postsurgical MRI

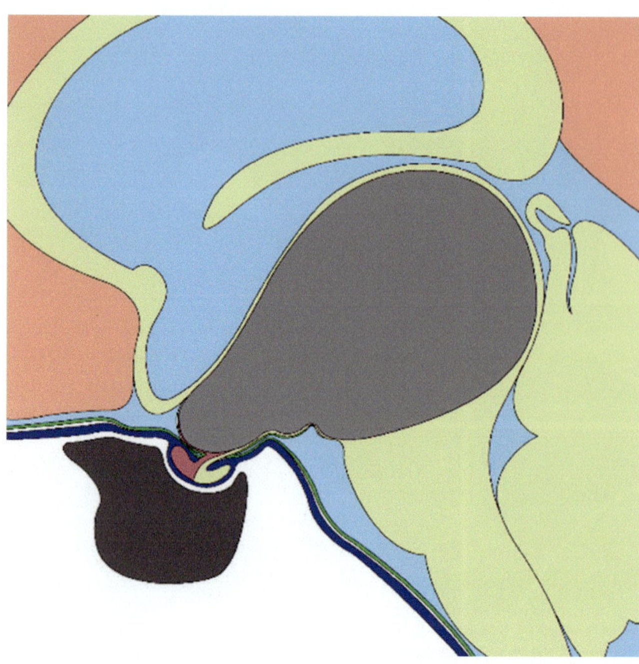

Fig. 6.59 Schematic figure showing the tumor morphology and relationships with the surrounding structures

of the third ventricle by invaginating the basal nerve tissue of the third ventricle floor (Fig. 6.62).

Postoperative Treatment Postoperative recovery was successful, perioperative period was characterized by mild diabetes insipidus, water and electrolyte disorders, and partial pituitary dysfunction.

During the perioperative period, the patient's fluid intake and blood sodium levels required measurement.

Long-Term Follow-Up After 1 year of follow-up, the patient's pituitary function was completely restored, and hormone replacement was gradually stopped. The patient's general condition was good, with normal schooling and excellent academic performance. The patient slightly increased in weight within 6 months after surgery, and then gradually returned to normal, and the BMI was normal.

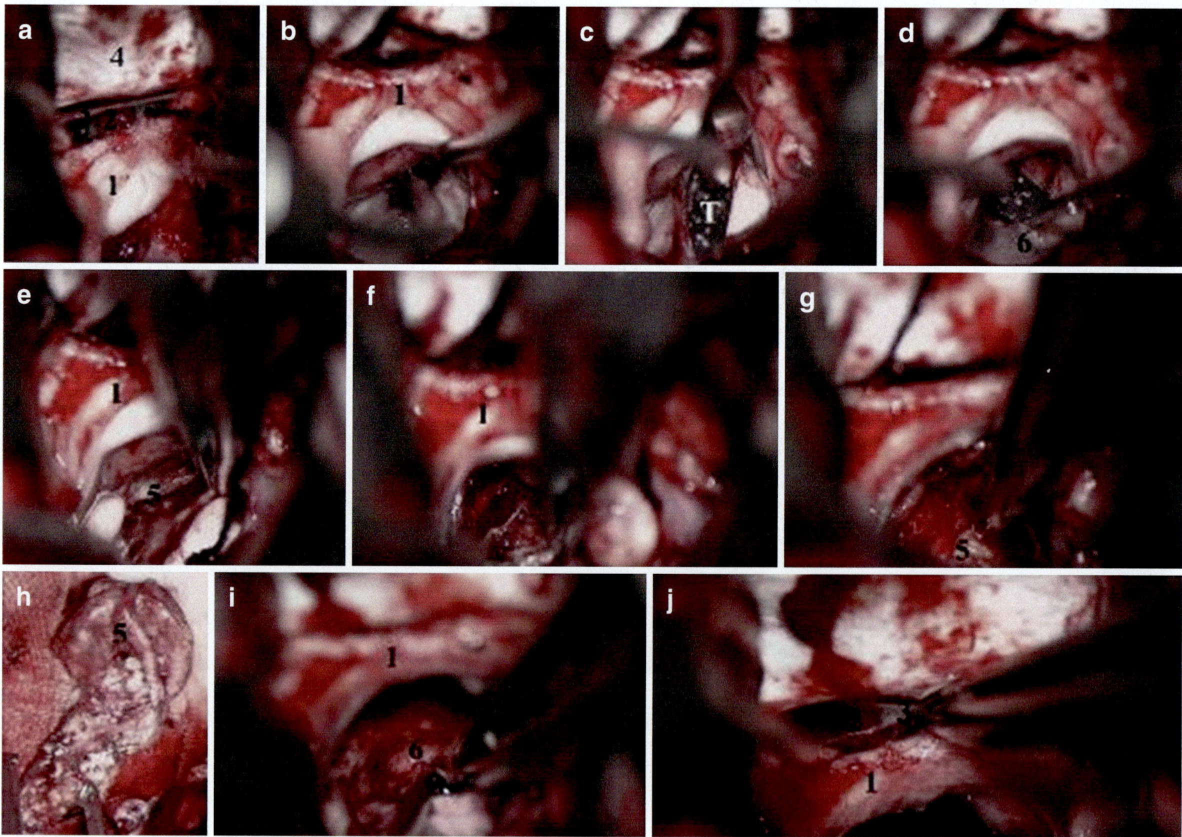

Fig. 6.60 Intraoperative findings. (**a**) After interhemispheric fissure dissection, the prefixed optic chiasm was observed. The intact arachnoid sleeve-covered pituitary stalk was observed through the small prechiasmatic space. (**b–d**) The lamina terminalis was opened to identify the intact third ventricular floor (third VF). The third VF nervous tissue layer was opened to expose the true tumor. (**e**, **f**) The tumor was separated along its interface with the third VF nervous tissue layer. (**g**) The site of tumor origin remained at the tuberoinfundibular part of the pituitary stalk. (**h**) The tumor was totally removed. (**i**, **j**) After tumor removal, the third VP was preserved and the pituitary stalk was maintained. (1) Optic chiasm, (2) pituitary stalk, (3) arachnoidal sleeve of the pituitary stalk, (4) planum sphenoidale, (5) tumor, (6) remaining third ventricle floor

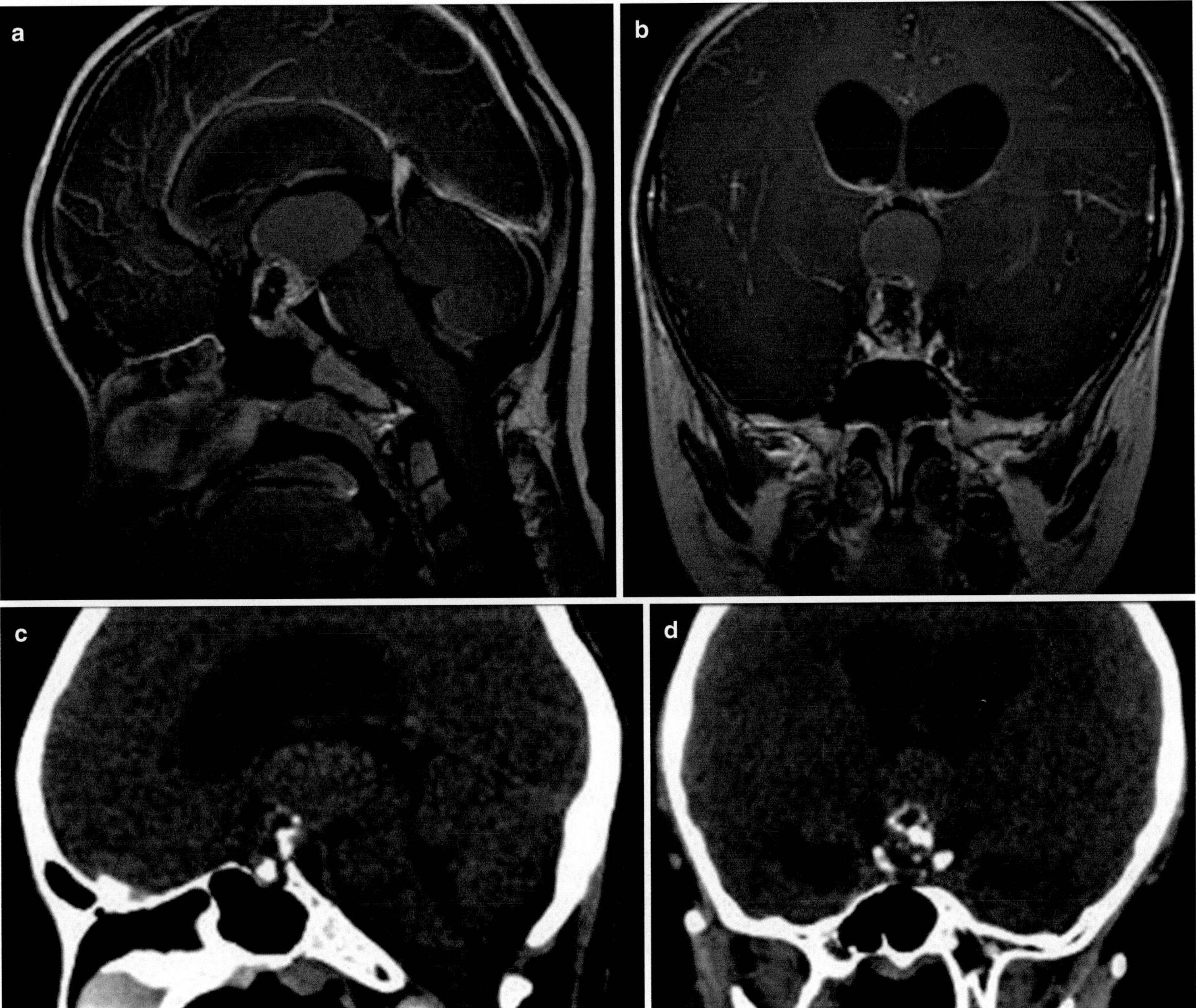

Fig. 6.61 Preoperative imaging of a typical type T craniopharyngioma. Preoperative MR images (**a**, **b**) showing the mixed cystic-solid tumor in the sellar region; the solid part of the tumor is located in the tuberculum of the pituitary stalk behind the optic chiasm, and the cystic part is involved in the floor of the third ventricle and occupies the chamber of the third ventricle, leading to obstructive hydrocephalus. CT scans (**c**, **d**) showed calculus-like calcification within the parenchymal part of the tumor. According to our classification, the tumor belongs to the "T" type with subarachnoid expansion (traditional ventricular trans-talk craniopharyngioma). In this case, the extraventricular part of the tumor grew through the arachnoid sleeve of the pituitary stalk and involved the pituitary fossa from above. The distal end of the pituitary stalk into the diaphragm opening was retained, and the shape of the pituitary gland was normal

However, in the routine follow-up at 2.5 years after surgery, the tuberoinfundibular tumor recurred, although the patient had no symptoms (Fig. 6.63).

Treatment of Recurrent Tumor The patient's tumor enlarged during close follow-up, and a second surgery was performed. Through the same anterior interhemispheric approach, we successfully exposed and separated the tumor. This time, the management of the infundibular stalk was more aggressive, but the continuity of the pituitary stalk was still preserved, and the tumor was completely resected under the microscope. The quality of life of the patient after the follow-up period remains good, with normal schooling and excellent academic performance (Fig. 6.64).

Postoperative Neuroimaging (Fig. 6.65)

Postoperative Course The patient's postoperative course was uneventful; the water sodium disorder and the urine collapse gradually recovered after treatment. The patient returned to normal learning and living conditions after surgery, and the academic performance was excellent. Routine follow-up.

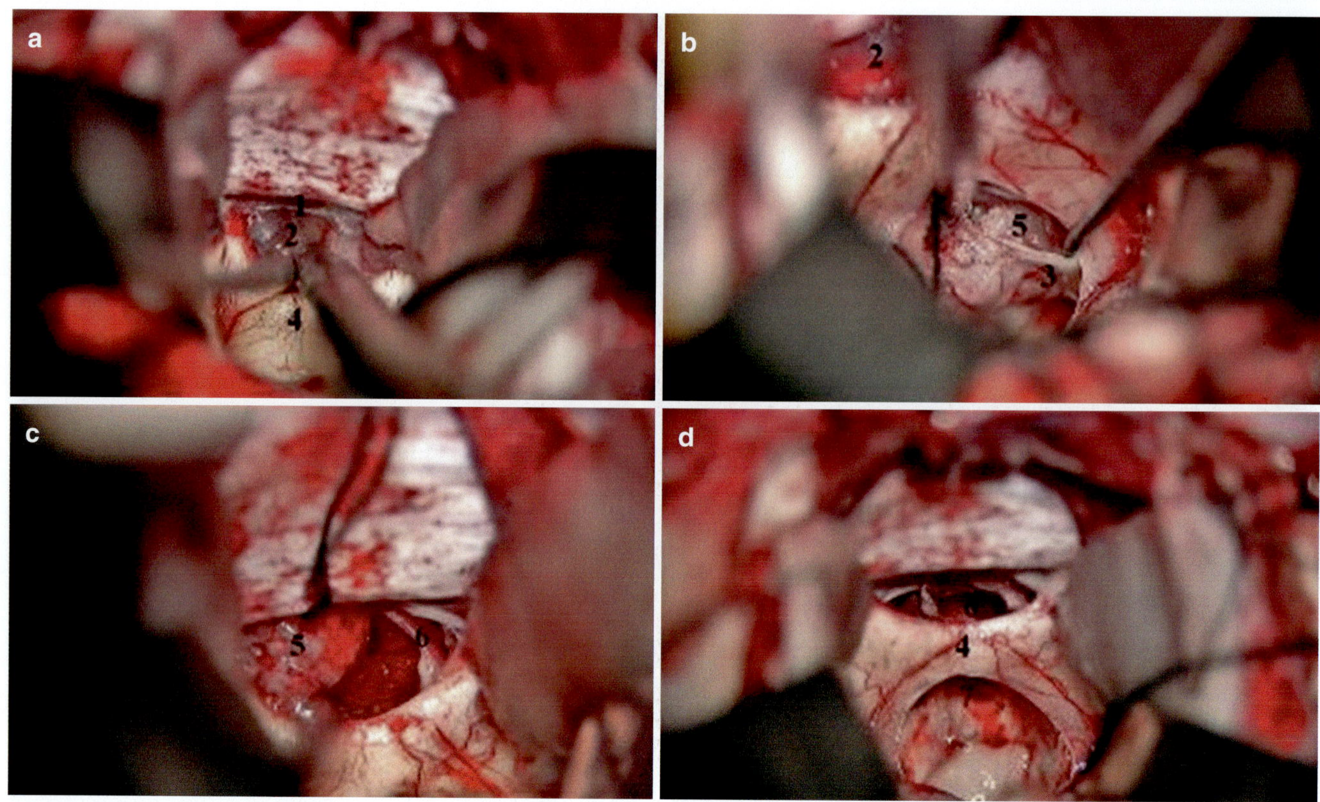

Fig. 6.62 Intraoperative images showing the morphological relationship between the tumor and the long axis of hypothalamic-pituitary stalk-pituitary. (**a**) Revealing the dilated pituitary stalk fiber in the pre-optic chiasmatic space, the superior pituitary arteries distribute on the surface. The parenchymal part of the tumor located within the dilated pituitary stalk. (**b**) The tumor was dissected and delivered from the surrounding layer of gliosis. This neuroglial layer intervening between the tumor and viable hypothalamic nuclei may provide a safe dissecting plane. (**c**) A longitudinal incision was made on the pituitary stalk to separate the tumor, and the interface between the tumor and the pituitary stalk is visible behind the tumor; usually the interface is not smooth, which can easily cause residual tumor, especially when attempting to retain the structure of the pituitary stalk. (**d**) Residual flaky bulging fibers of the pituitary stalk at the base of the third ventricle after tumor resection. (1) Arachnoidal sleeve of the pituitary stalk, (2) dilated pituitary stalk containing tumor revealed from the optic-chiasm space, (3) neuro-layer at the hypothalamic structures, (4) optic chiasm, (5) tumor, (6) retained lamellar stalk, (7) remaining third ventricle floor after tumor removal

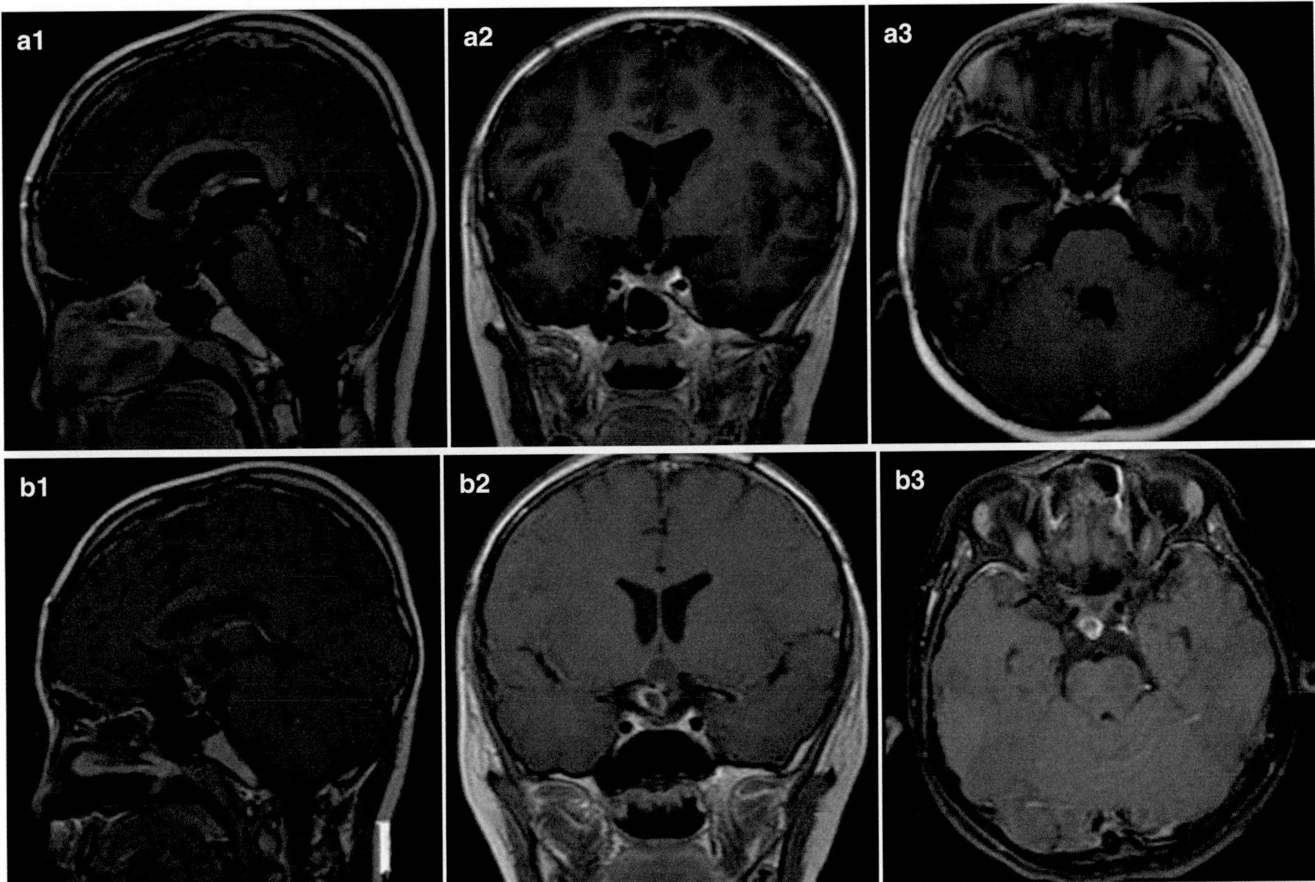

Fig. 6.63 Two-year postoperative MRI showing satisfactory tumor resection; the structure of the stalk axis of the third ventricle was well preserved (**a**1–3) and only suspicious point shadows were seen in the funnel, as well as mild enhancement. However, during follow-up MR study 2.5 years after the operation, the tumor was found to have recurred asymptomatically, suggesting the importance of regular follow-up and the need to reflect on the dispose of the pituitary stalk during surgery (reproduced with permission from Qi (Ed.), *Craniopharyngioma*, People's Medical Publishing House, ISBN 978-7-117-26463-1, 2018)

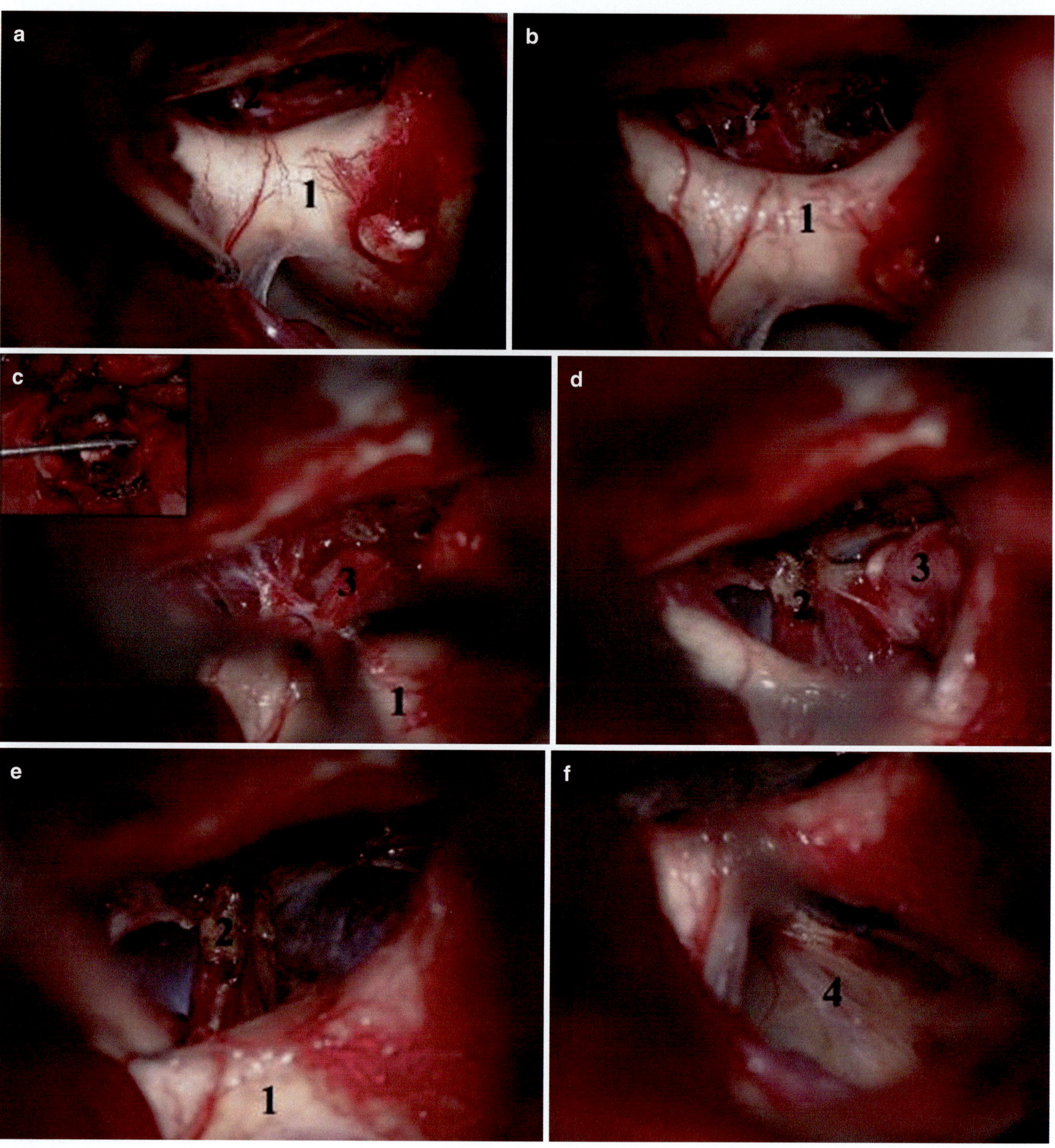

Fig. 6.64 A more adequate arachnoid dissection is needed for reoperation. In this case, the anterior interhemispheric fissure is fully dissected to expose the tumor. (**a**) The tumor mainly grows at the pituitary stalk entering the diaphragm opening. It is also considered to be the origin site of the tumor. The nerve tissue layer is lifted from below, dissecting and separating the boundary between the tumor and the pituitary stalk, and retaining part of the pituitary stalk becomes a key point of surgery. (**b**) The boundary between the origin of the tumor and the pituitary stalk fiber is unclear. (**c**) Attempt to separate the tumor interface on the premise of retaining part of the pituitary stalk and pursue total resection. (**d**) The posterior portion of the tumor, the dissecting plane between the tumor and pituitary stalk, and the infundibular part of the third ventricle are clear. (**e**) After the tumor was completely resected, the pituitary stalk was partially preserved and the right part of the pituitary stalk fiber was removed. (**f**) A fissure-like defect in the infundibular part of the third ventricle was retained after tumor removal. In this recurrent tumor, a dural window of approximately 2 cm in diameter was sufficient to complete the surgery (black frame on **c**). (1) Optic chiasm, (2) pituitary stalk containing tumor revealed from the optic-chiasm space, (3) tumor, (4) remaining third ventricle floor after tumor removal (reproduced with permission from Qi (Ed.), *Craniopharyngioma*, People's Medical Publishing House, ISBN 978-7-117-26463-1, 2018)

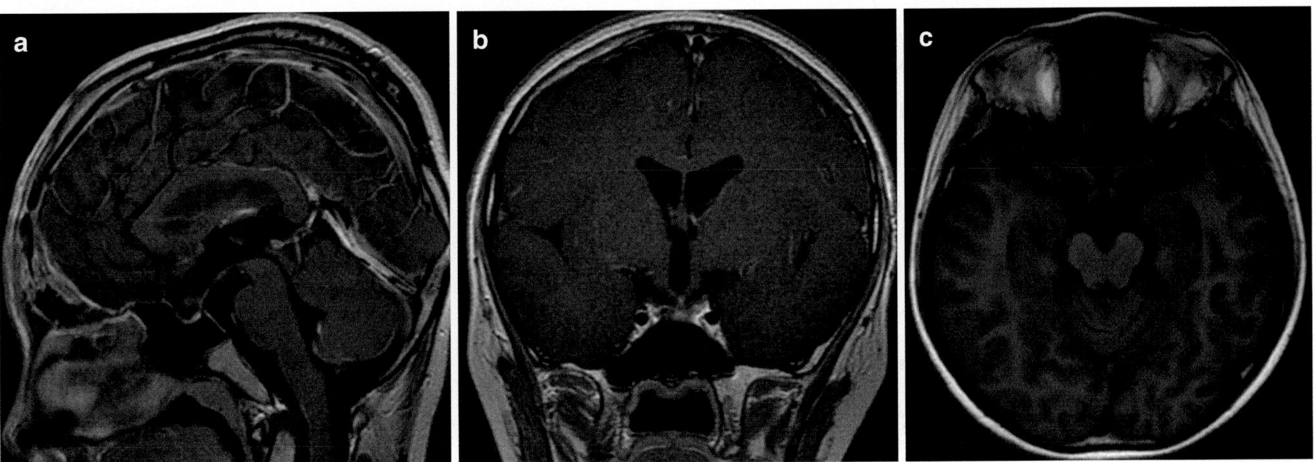

Fig. 6.65 Postoperative MRI showing satisfactory tumor resection and normal structural protection (reproduced with permission from Qi (Ed.), *Craniopharyngioma*, People's Medical Publishing House, ISBN 978-7-117-26463-1, 2018)

References

1. Pan J, Qi S, Liu Y, Lu Y, Peng J, Zhang X, et al. Growth patterns of craniopharyngiomas: clinical analysis of 226 patients. J Neurosurg Pediatr. 2016;17(4):418–33.
2. Van Effenterre R, Boch AL. Craniopharyngioma in adults and children: a study of 122 surgical cases. J Neurosurg. 2002;97:3–11.
3. Yasargil MG, Curcic M, Kis M, Siegenthaler G, Teddy PJ, Roth P. Total removal of craniopharyngiomas. Approaches and long-term results in 144 patients. J Neurosurg. 1990;73:3–11.
4. Hoffman HJ. Surgical management of craniopharyngioma. Pediatr Neurosurg. 1994;21(Suppl 1):44–9.
5. Kassam AB, Gardner PA, Snyderman CH, Carrau RL, Mintz AH, Prevedello DM. Expanded endonasal approach, a fully endoscopic transnasal approach for the resection of midline suprasellar craniopharyngiomas: a new classification based on the infundibulum. J Neurosurg. 2008;108:715–28.
6. Qi S, Lu Y, Pan J, Zhang X, Long H, Fan J. Anatomic relations of the arachnoidea around the pituitary stalk: relevance for surgical removal of craniopharyngiomas. Acta Neurochir. 2011;153:785–96.
7. Qi S, Pan J, Lu Y, Gao F, Cao Y, Peng J, et al. The impact of the site of origin and rate of tumour growth on clinical outcome in children with craniopharyngiomas. Clin Endocrinol. 2012;76:103–10.
8. Pascual JM, Carrasco R, Prieto R, Gonzalez-Llanos F, Alvarez F, Roda JM. Craniopharyngioma classification. J Neurosurg. 2008;109:1180–2; author reply 1182–3.

Part III

Recurrent Craniopharyngioma

7 Treatment of Recurrent Craniopharyngioma

Jing Nie

7.1 Introduction

Recurrence is a thorny problem in the treatment of craniopharyngioma. Recurrence is inevitable in patient with subtotal resection and postoperative radiotherapy and chemotherapy, especially in children. It has been reported that the recurrence incidence was 10–30% in cases of total resection. Reoperation is the last option for recurrent craniopharyngioma.

Both transcranial approach and transsphenoidal approach was suitable for recurrent type Q cases. The transcranial approach is mainly suitable for patients with damaged intracranial membranous structures during the first operation. Those who have undergone omaya capsule insertion or radiotherapy were also suitable for transcranial approach when they suffer tumor recurrence. The reason for this is that tumor was usually severely adherent to peripheral neurovascular during the second operation which bring much difficulty in transsphenoidal approach. Transsphenoidal approach is suitable for smaller tumors, especially in the first operation, the diaphragma sellae is not damaged, and there is no obvious adherence between tumor and supsellar structures of the saddle.

Except for rare cases where there was ectopic implantation of tumors in previous surgery, the surgical classification of recurrent craniopharyngioma is consistent with the preoperative classification.

The operation of recurrent craniopharyngioma is more difficult, but the prognosis is not necessarily worse. This depends mainly on the quality of the surgery and the extent to which the hypothalamic endocrine disorders caused by radiotherapy are harmful to the body.

The authors have a clear view that craniopharyngioma is a surgical disease and that radical surgical resection is the only possible cure for patients. Although subtotal resection and adjuvant radiotherapy and chemotherapy can delay the recurrence of tumors, recurrence is inevitable for patients with long-term survival. In addition to the difficulty of reoperation, even endocrine function is low (Q type), and hypothalamic function disorder (S and T type) is a problem that every neurosurgeon must face. Neurosurgeons need to understand that once a patient receives radiotherapy and chemotherapy and cystic fluid aspiration and intracapsular chemoradiotherapy, it signifies that the patient has lost the possibility of a true cure and high-quality survival.

At any age, radical resection is usually performed as the primary treatment for craniopharyngioma. The best outcomes can be achieved through radical resection. Nevertheless, the tumor type based on the location, size, and calcifications, frequent involvement of critical neurovascular structures, patient's age at presentation, and the surgeon's experience usually limits resection extent. However, many surgeons prefer a less radical surgical treatment followed by radiation therapy, and craniopharyngioma can also recur following total resection, despite confirmation via negative postoperative brain imaging. Craniopharyngiomas are more likely to recur during the first 3 years after primary resection, after which the recurrence incidence plateaus. The presence of tumor remnants after surgery is the strongest predictor of tumor recurrence. The 5-year RFS in patients without residual tumor was 84.9% versus 48.3% in patients with residual tumor. Large calcified lesions have been associated with an increased risk of recurrence. Third ventricular floor (VF)

J. Nie (✉)
Department of Neurosurgery, Nanfang Hospital of Southern Medical University, Guangzhou, Guangdong, China

© Springer Nature Singapore Pte Ltd. 2020
S. Qi (ed.), *Atlas of Craniopharyngioma*, https://doi.org/10.1007/978-981-13-7322-0_7

involvement is another risk factor for recurrence. Our data shows that the pathological subtype was a predictor of prognosis. The recurrence incidence of adamantinomatous craniopharyngioma (ACP) is higher.

The optimal treatment for recurrent craniopharyngioma remains controversial and under debate. The risk of significant morbidity in visual and hypothalamic functions and endocrinological disturbances could follow radical resection in recurrent craniopharyngioma, which may lead to a poor life quality. This section mainly discusses the various surgical modalities for recurrent craniopharyngiomas.

There are two main surgical modalities for recurrent craniopharyngiomas: the transcranial and transsphenoidal approaches. For various reasons, the former is more widely applied: first, most craniopharyngiomas are of suprasellar origin and rarely exhibit intrasellar invasion, thus restricting the application of a transsphenoidal approach. Second, a suitable transcranial approach can provide a wide view of the tumor, especially in some critical areas such as the pituitary stalk (PS), optic nerve, anterior cerebral artery (ACA), and the third ventricular floor. Third, only some tumors of entirely intrasellar origin, known as Q type, may be completely resected via a transsphenoidal approach.

In this section, we have provided clinical data of twelve cases of recurrent craniopharyngioma. Emphasis has been placed on performance of the selection of a proper approach to achieve satisfactory exposure for tumor removal.

7.2 Case 1: Radical Gross Tumor Resection Was Performed on the Type Q Recurrent Craniopharyngioma by Enlarging the Exposure of Pituitary Fossa Through Drilling the Tuberculum Sellae (Figs. 7.1, 7.2, 7.3, 7.4, 7.5, 7.6, 7.7, 7.8, 7.9, 7.10, and 7.11)

Although subtotal resection can temporarily alleviate the clinical symptoms, the recurrence is inevitable for patients with long-term survival. Some patients relapse very quickly. This patient has a tumor recurrence less than half a year after the first operation. Tumor recurrence of this patient caused a sharp decline in vision. The authors have a clear view that craniopharyngioma is a surgical disease. We recommend that recurrent craniopharyngioma should receive reoperation as soon as possible. The first operation was performed via the right-side pterional approach. Radical gross tumor removal via the fronto-basal interhemispheric approach was performed in order to avoid adhesion of the surrounding structure caused by the first operation. Due to the diaphragma sellae structural destruction in the first operation, the recurrent craniopharyngioma had direct contact with pituitary stalk, the pituitary stalk exhibited severe tumor involvement in recurrent tumor, and it was sacrificed to avoid tumor recurrence. The vision of the patient was significantly

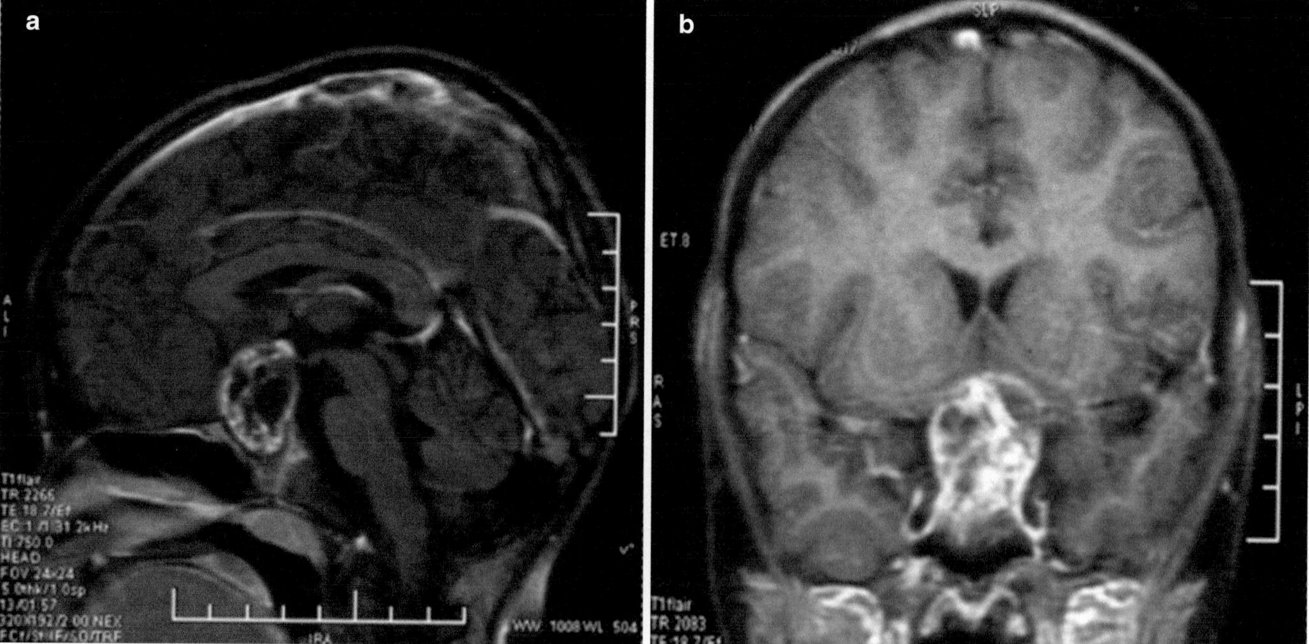

Fig. 7.1 Female, 6 years old. A type Q-CP case. Pre-surgical radiological images. (**a**, **b**) MRI revealed that a tumor in the intrasellar and suprasellar region. Partially tumor resection via the right-side pterional approach was performed in October 2013 in another hospital

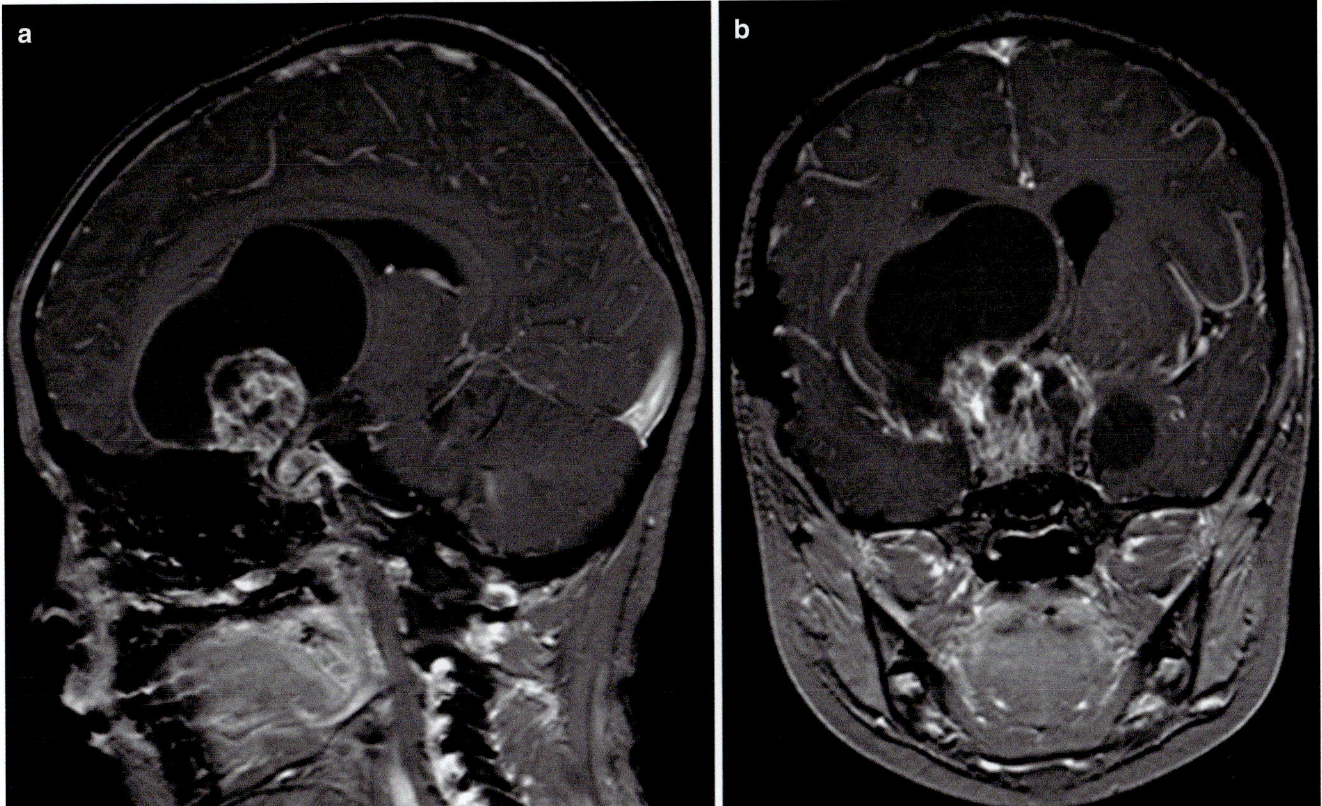

Fig. 7.2 In March 2013 (half a year after the first operation), the vision sharply declined. (**a**, **b**) MRI revealed the recurrence of the tumor in the intrasellar and suprasellar regions. Due to the diaphragma sellae structural destruction in the first operation, the recurrent craniopharyngioma could have involved several subarachnoid spaces

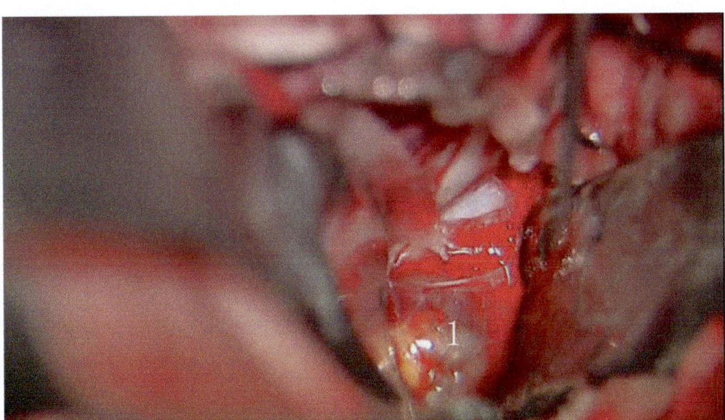

Fig. 7.3 Radical gross tumor removal (GTR) via the fronto-basal interhemispheric approach was performed in our hospital in March 2013. Intrasurgical findings. Dissect the arachnoidal trabecula and membrane between the two lobes to expose of the sellar region. (1) Tumor

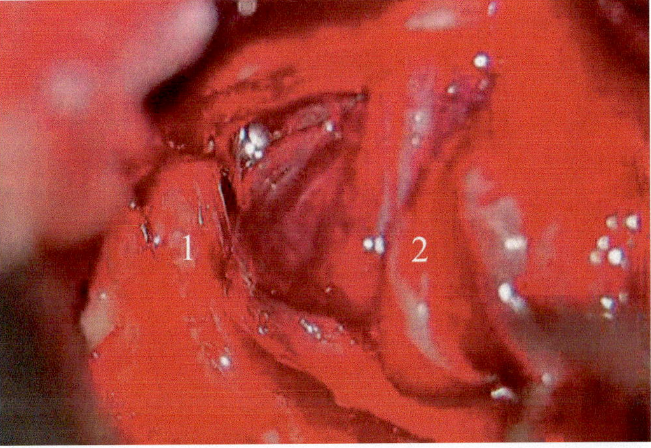

Fig. 7.4 The tumor was separated from the left-side optic nerve. (1) Left-side optic nerve, (2) tumor

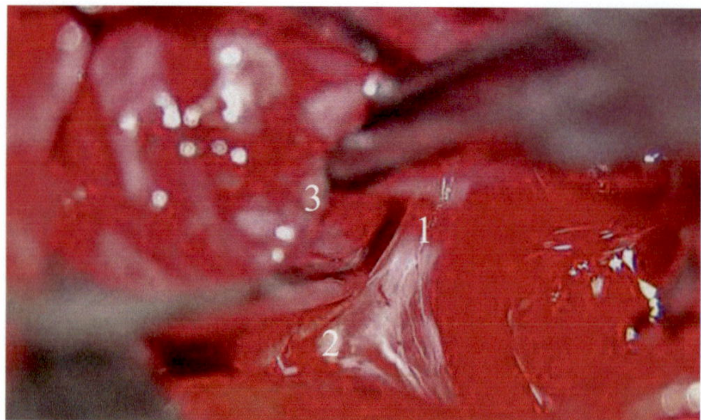

Fig. 7.5 The morphologically thin optic chiasm and right-side optic nerve were pushed by the tumor. (1) Left-side optic nerve, (2) optic chiasm, (3) tumor

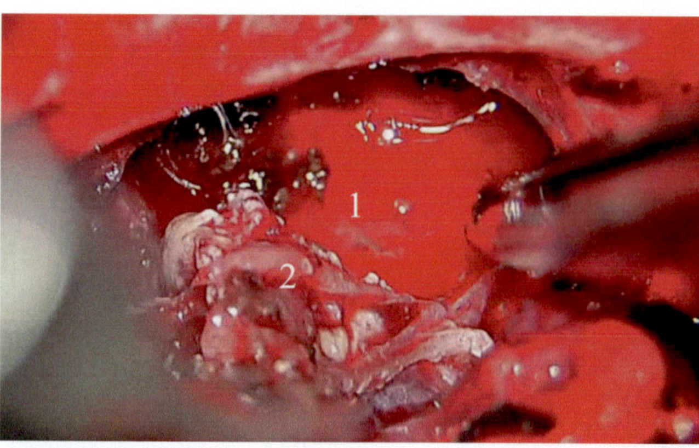

Fig. 7.8 Resection of the tumor in the intrasellar region, the pituitary stalk was located behind the tumor, expanding like a funnel, and the origin site of the tumor was located in the intrasellar region. (1) Pituitary stalk, (2) tumor

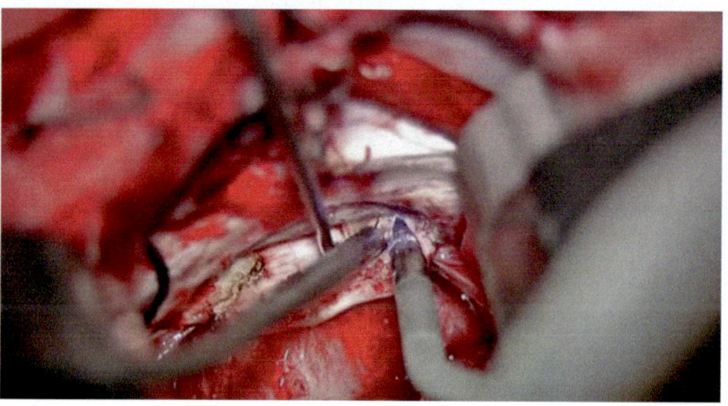

Fig. 7.6 The origin site of the tumor is located in the intrasellar region. The intrasellar tumor could be extensively exposed after drilling the tuberculum sellae. The laser knife was used to open the dura mater of the tuberculum sellae

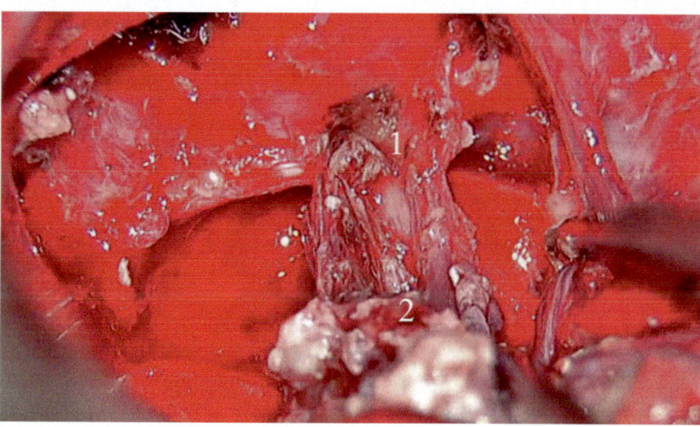

Fig. 7.9 Resection of intrasellar tumor along the pituitary capsule. The tumor grew throughout the arachnoidal sleeve segment of pituitary stalk. Due to the diaphragma sellae structural destruction in the first operation, the recurrent craniopharyngioma had direct contact with pituitary stalk. The pituitary stalk exhibited severe tumor involvement, and it was sacrificed to avoid tumor recurrence. (1) Pituitary stalk, (2) tumor

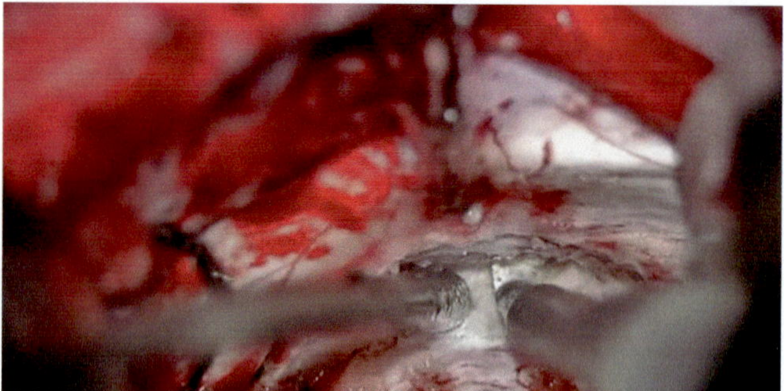

Fig. 7.7 The ultrasonic bone scalpel was used to drill the tuberculum sellae to expose the intrasellar tumor

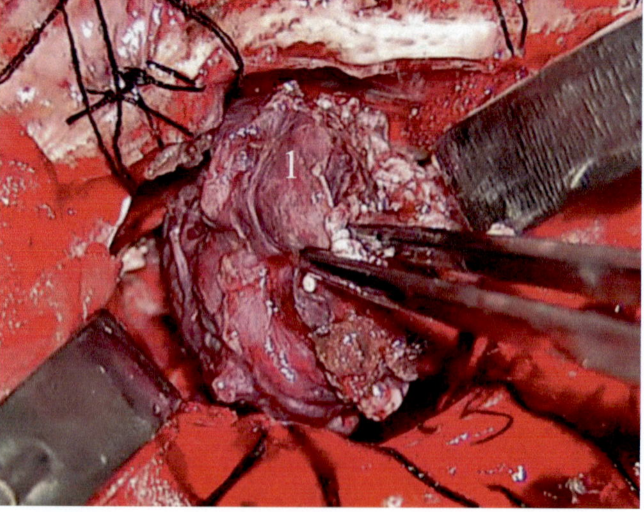

Fig. 7.10 The tumor was en bloc removed. (1) Tumor

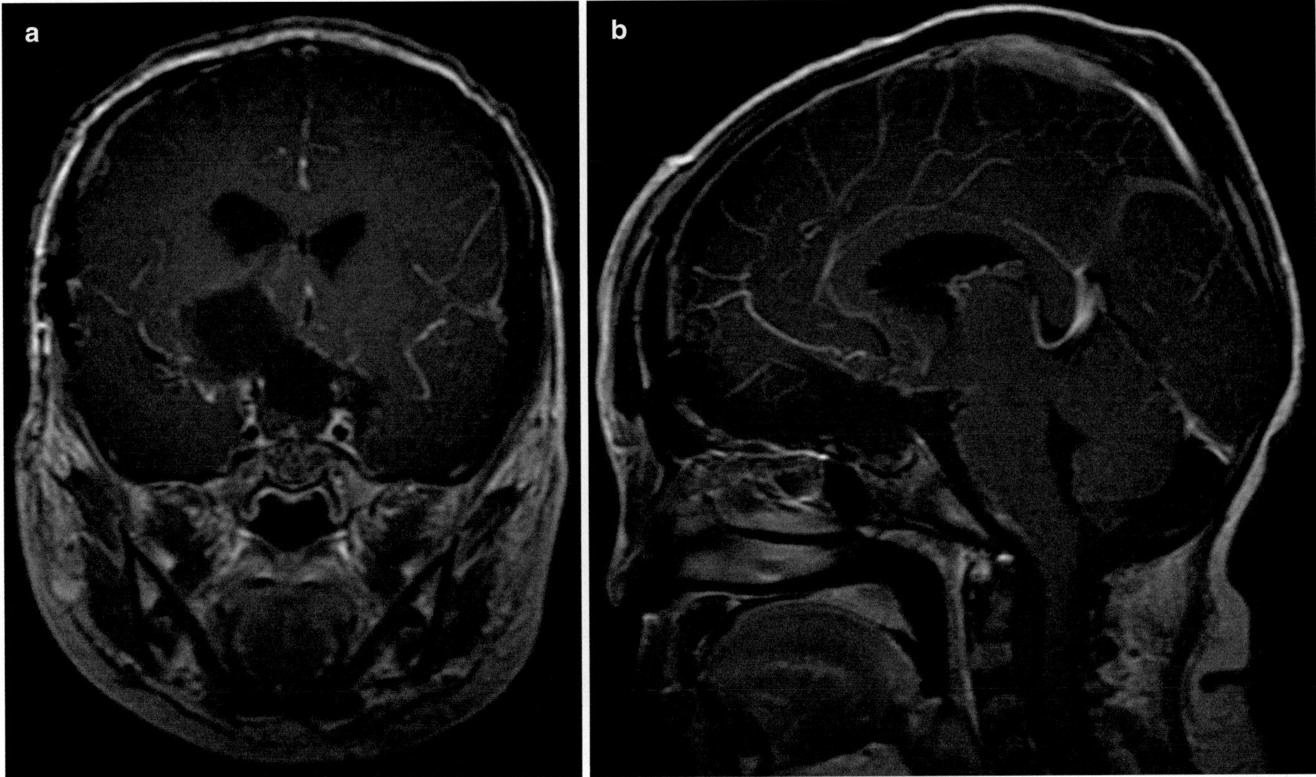

Fig. 7.11 (**a**, **b**) MRI postsurgery showed no residual tumor, and the neurohypophysis was preserved. The vision of the patient was significantly improved

improved after the operation. We believe that radical surgical resection is the only possible cure for patients. The intrasellar tumor could be extensively exposed after drilling the tuberculum sellae.

7.3 Case 2: The Preservation of Pituitary Stalk and Pituitary Capsule May Lead to Recurrence of the Type Q Tumor (Figs. 7.12, 7.13, 7.14, 7.15, 7.16, 7.17, and 7.18)

In this case, pre-surgical radiological images revealed a tumor in the intrasellar and suprasellar regions; the surgical classification of the craniopharyngioma was Q type. The first operation was performed through fronto-basal interhemispheric approach; the tumor in the intrasellar and suprasellar regions was totally removed. For the postoperative endocrine function retention, the pituitary stalk and pituitary capsule were preserved during the first operation, resulting in postoperative tumor recurrence. The surgical classification of recurrent craniopharyngioma is consistent with preoperative classification. Most recurrent craniopharyngioma still retains the initial growth pattern. The recurrent tumor of Q type might be completely restrained in the intrasellar region when the diaphragma sellae was reconstructed. The recurrent tumor may be completely resected via a transsphenoidal approach.

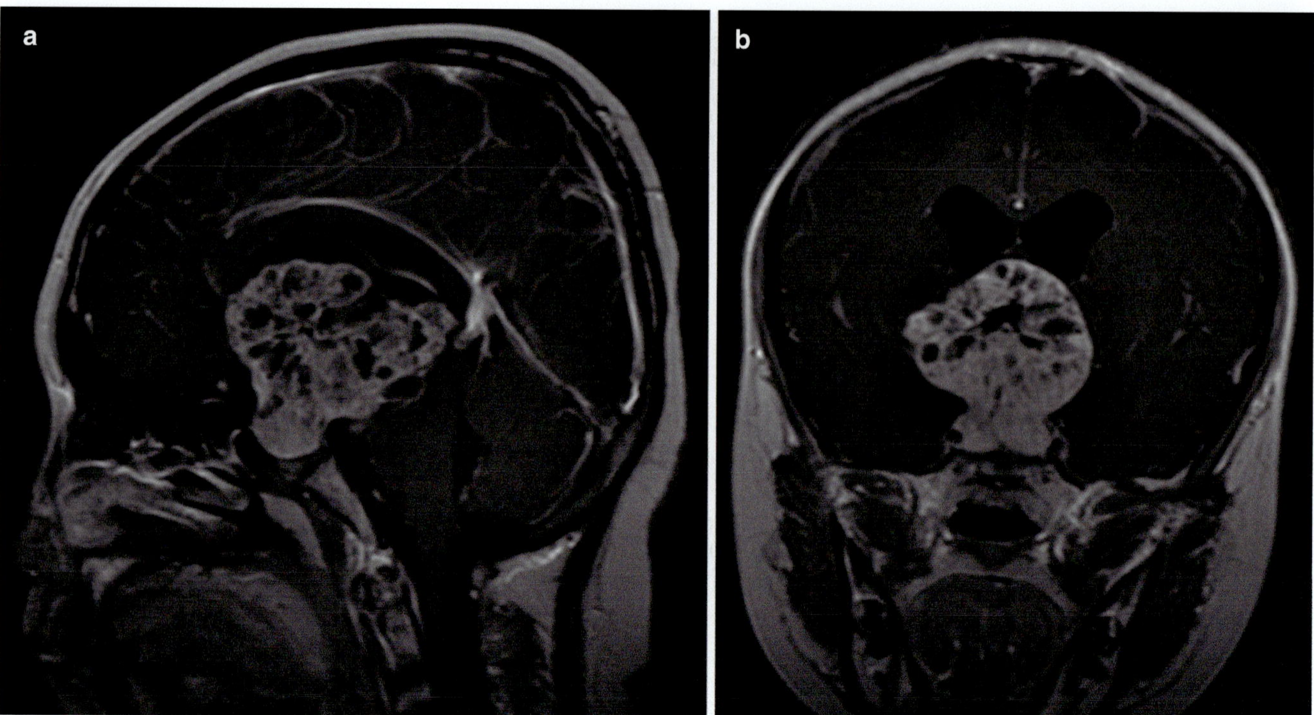

Fig. 7.12 Female, 14 years old. A type Q-CP case. Preoperative radiological images. (**a**, **b**) MRI revealed a tumor in the intrasellar and suprasellar regions

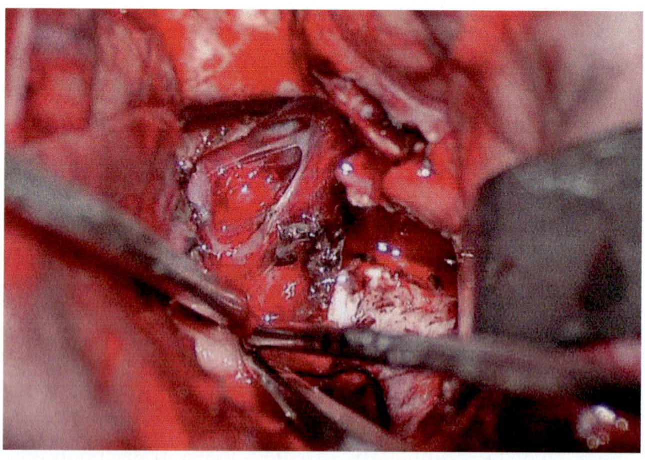

Fig. 7.13 Radical gross tumor removal (GTR) by the fronto-basal interhemispheric approach was performed in our hospital in May 2014. After total tumor removal, the diaphragma sellae was reconstructed with artificial dura mater, and the neurovascular structures of the sellar region were preserved. (1) Artificial dura mater

7.4 Case 3: Repeated Resection and Radiotherapy May Lead to Malignant Transformation of the Tumor (Figs. 7.19., 7.20, 7.21, 7.22, 7.23, 7.24, 7.25, 7.26, 7.27, 7.28, 7.29, 7.30, 7.31, 7.32, 7.33, 7.34, and 7.35)

In this case, the patient had several tumor recurrences. In 2009, intrasellar tumor resection combined with the removal of the pituitary capsule was performed, and the diaphragma sellae was reconstructed with artificial dura mater, which limited the tumor to suprasellar invasion, but the intrasellar tumor still recurred. The pathological findings indicated that the tumor had more invasive features and hinted at malignant transformation. The tumor cells were positive for Ki-67 (++, 18%). We believe that pathological malignancy may be one of the causes of tumor recurrence. The most recurrent craniopharyngioma still retains the initial growth pattern.

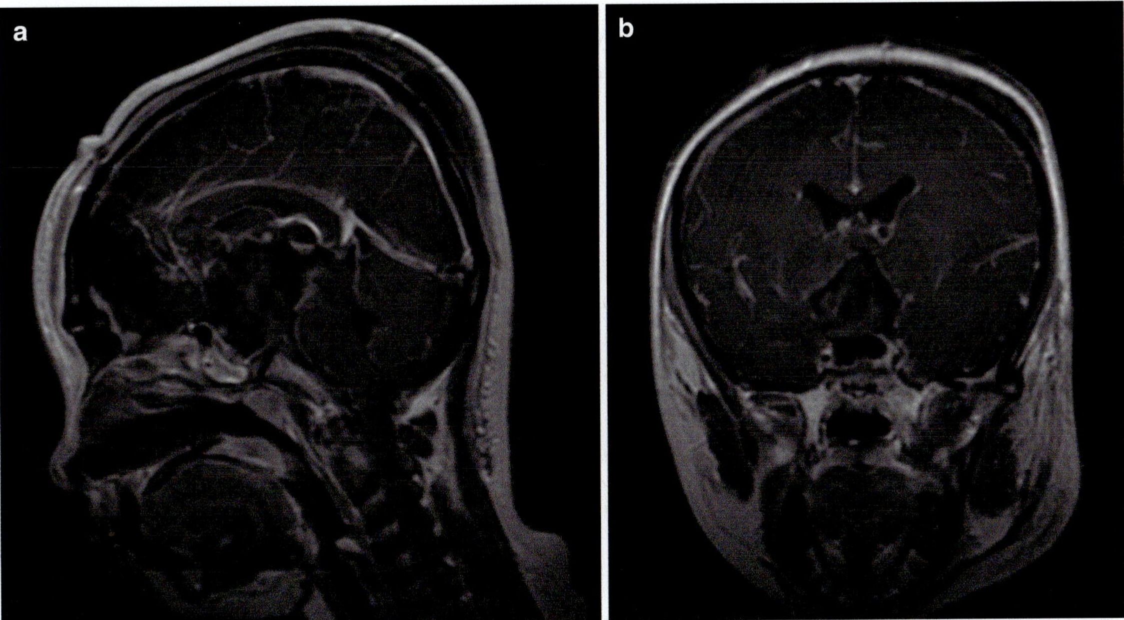

Fig. 7.14 Postoperative radiological images. (**a**, **b**) MRI indicated no residual tumor. The neurohypophysis and partial adenohypophysis were preserved

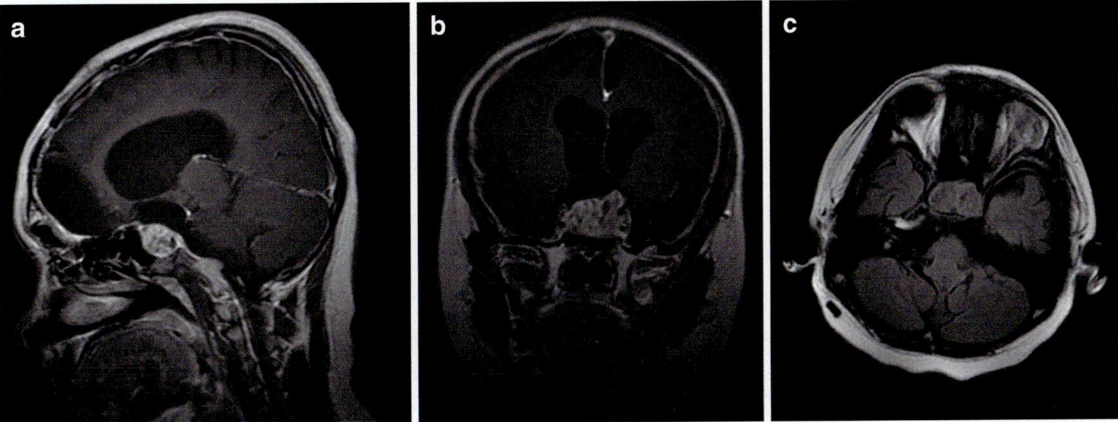

Fig. 7.15 In October 2014, (**a**–**c**) MRI revealed the recurrence of the tumor in the intrasellar region. The diaphragma sellae was reconstructed with an artificial dura mater in the first operation, which limited the recurrent tumor to suprasellar invasion

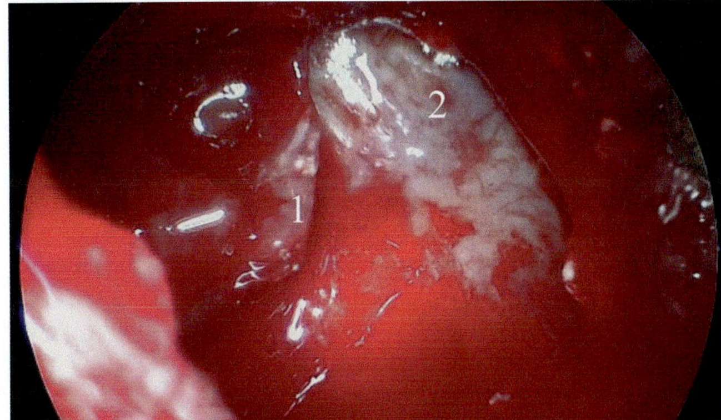

Fig. 7.16 Radical gross tumor removal by the transsphenoidal approach was performed in our hospital in October 2014. Intrasurgical findings. After drilling the sellar floor bone, and opening the dura, the intrasellar tumor was exposed. (1) Tumor, (2) artificial dura mater

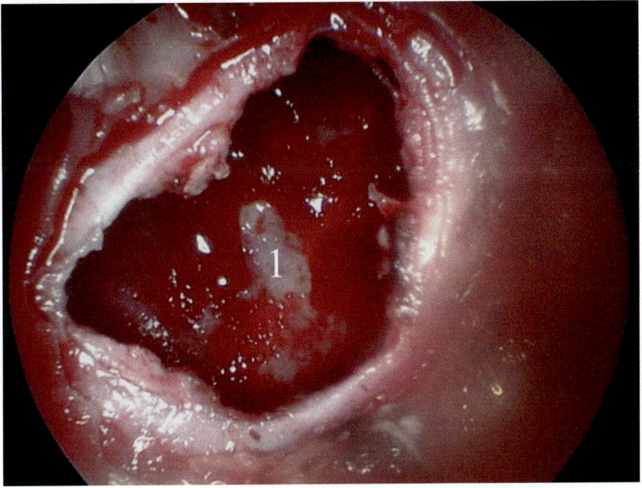

Fig. 7.17 The artificial dura mater which was used to reconstruct the diaphragma sellae in the first operation was exposed after the total intrasellar tumor removal. (1) Artificial dura mater

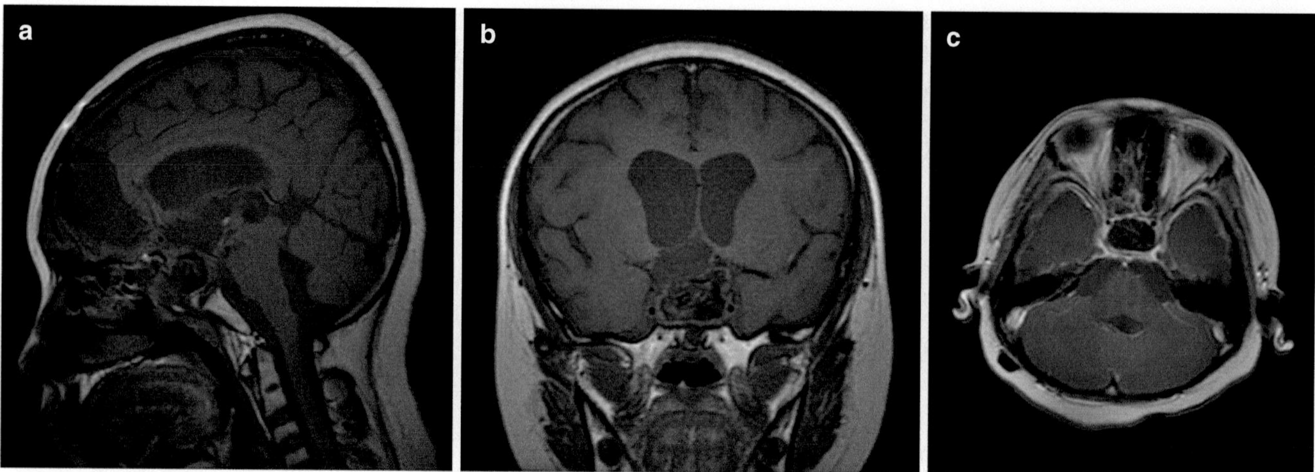

Fig. 7.18 In 2016 (2 years after the last operation), postsurgical radiological images. (**a**–**c**) MRI indicated total tumor removal and proved that the tumor had not recurred

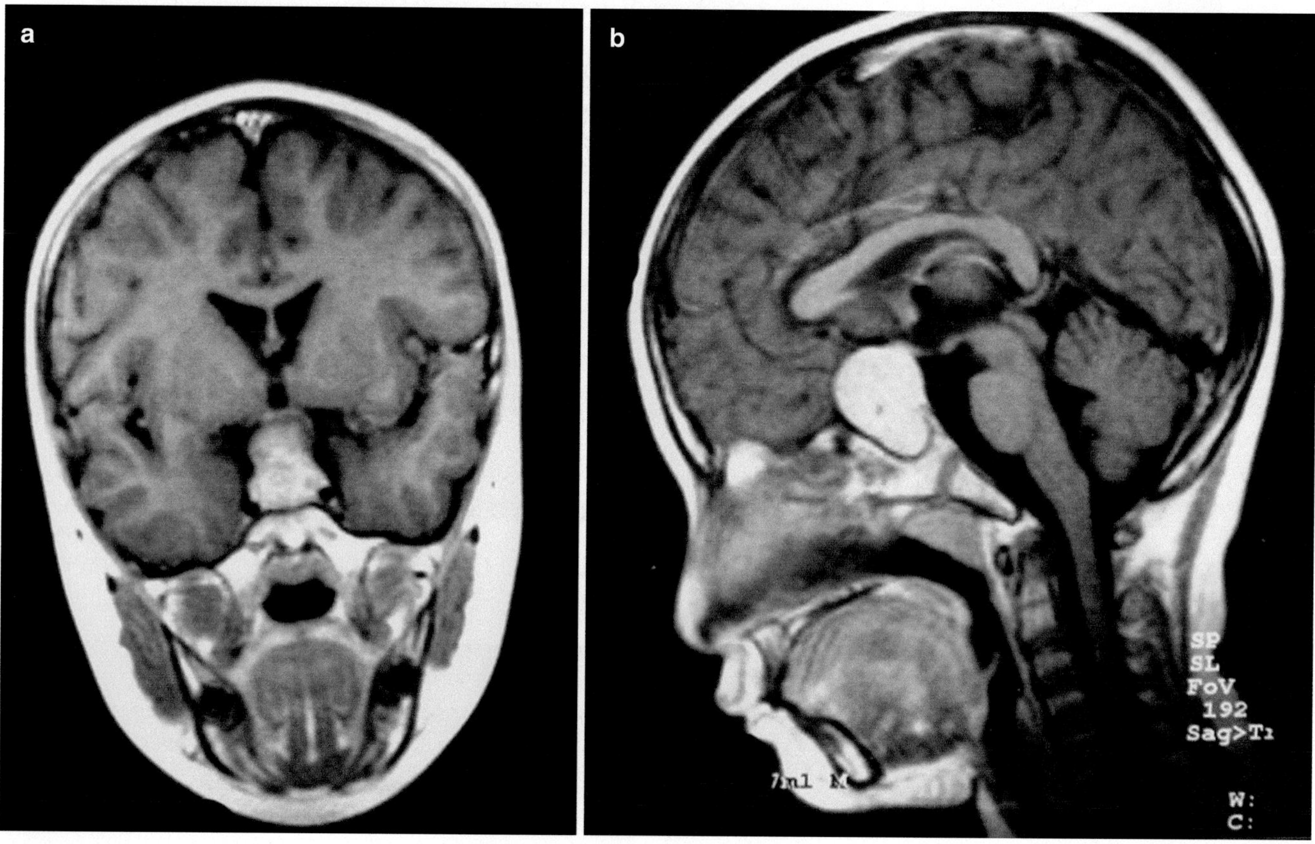

Fig. 7.19. Male, 9 years old. A type Q-CP case. Pre-surgical radiological images. (**a**, **b**) Magnetic resonance imaging revealed a cystic predominantly tumor in the sellar region

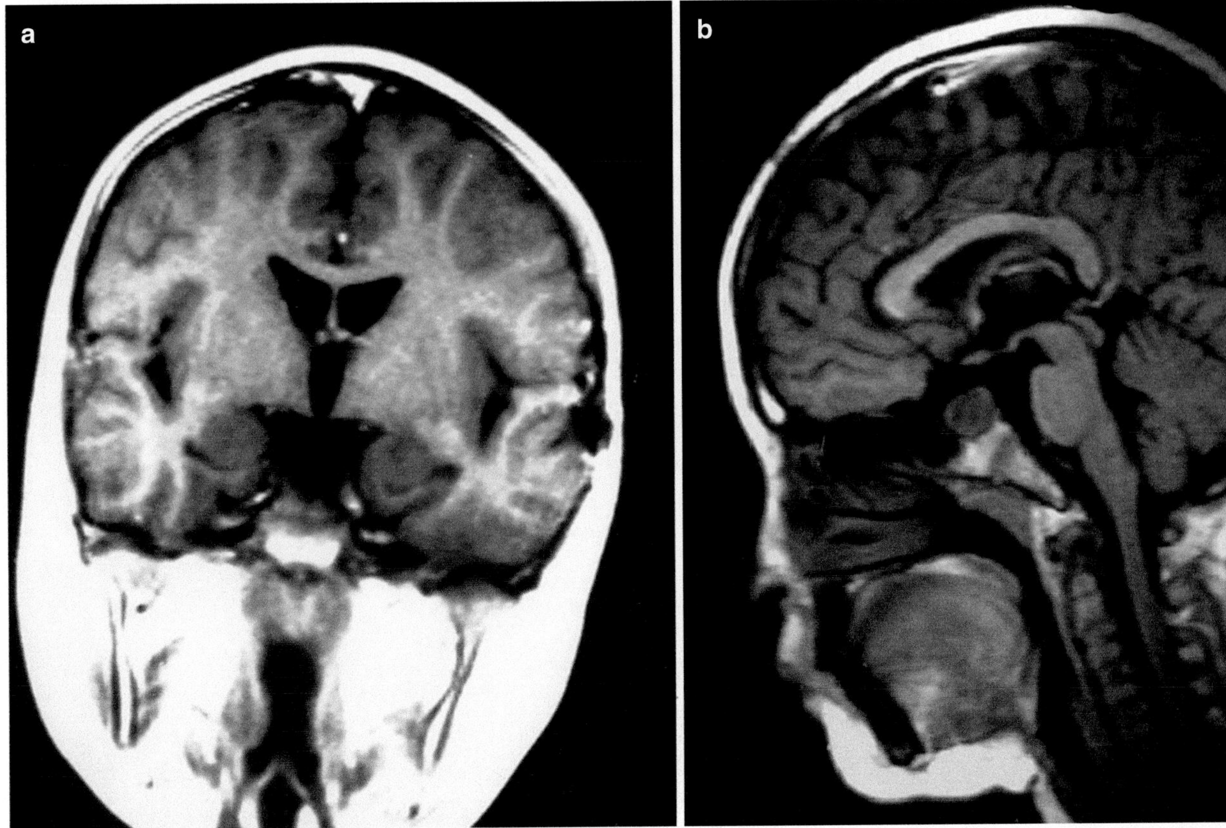

Fig. 7.20 In 1998, subtotal tumor resection via the left-side pterional with lateral frontal expanding approach was performed in another hospital. Postsurgical radiological images. (**a**, **b**) MRI revealed the patient with residual tumor in the sellar region. There was visual improvement in the left eye, but there was complete loss of vision in the right eye after surgery

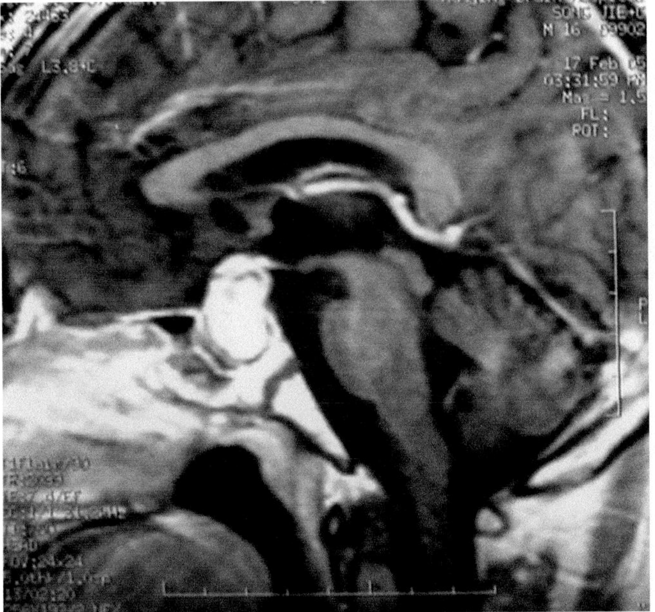

Fig. 7.21 The first recurrence of the type Q-CP case. In 2004, the vision in the left eye decreased. MRI showed the recurrence of the tumor; irradiation with gamma knife was performed in another hospital

We emphasized that the origin site is the source of tumor recurrence. Some type Q craniopharyngiomas may originate from intrasellar residues. The removal of intrasellar residues may explain why the recurring Q-type tumor may be completely resected via a transsphenoidal approach. We suggest to reconstruct the diaphragma sellae which might limit the tumor to suprasellar invasion in Q-type tumor. Incomplete tumor resection can lead to tumor recurrence. Repeated resection and repeated radiotherapy may lead to malignant changes of the tumor, but even if it is malignant, it can still not relapse if the total resection is performed. This patient has no recurrence for 5 years. This patient returned to normal work and life through endocrine therapy after operation.

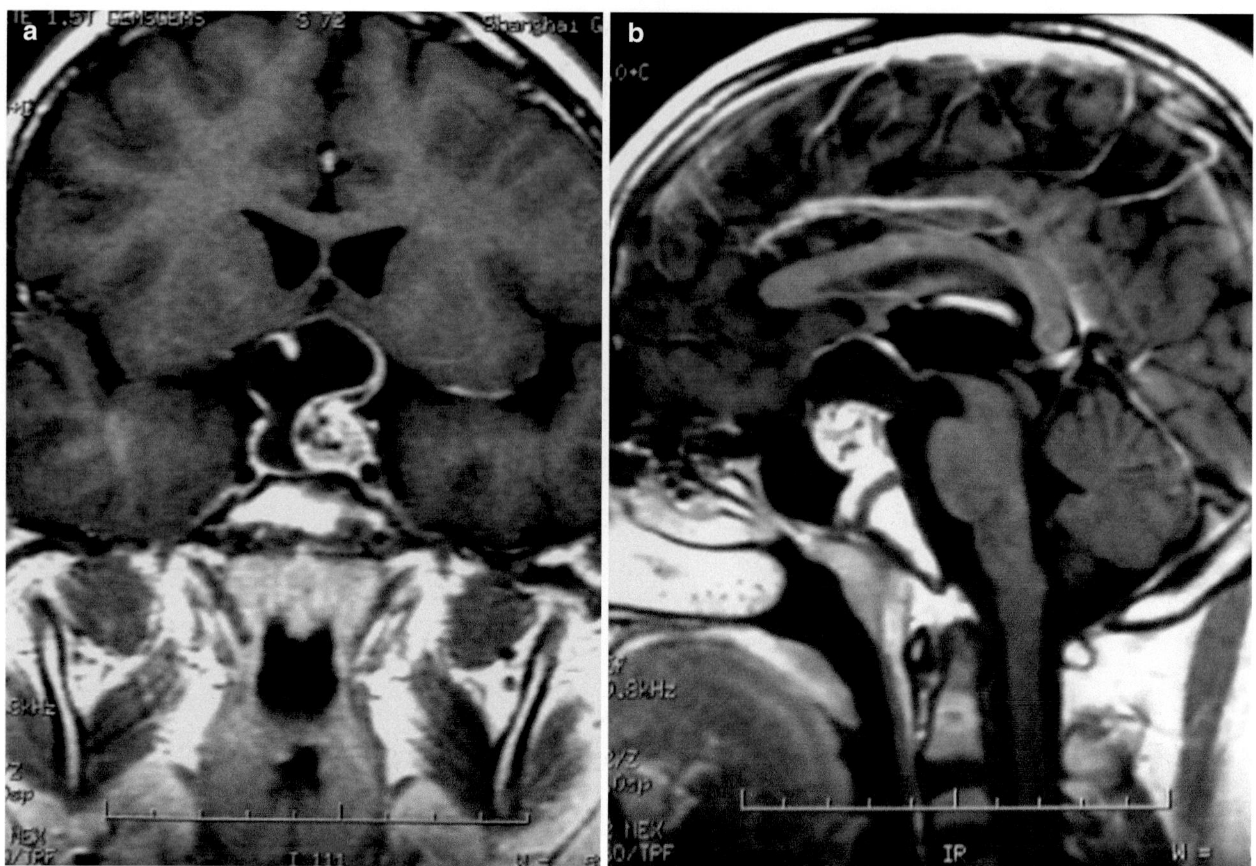

Fig. 7.22 The second recurrence of the type Q-CP case. Early in 2006, the vision in the left eye began to decline. The tumor recurred, predominantly growing through cysts

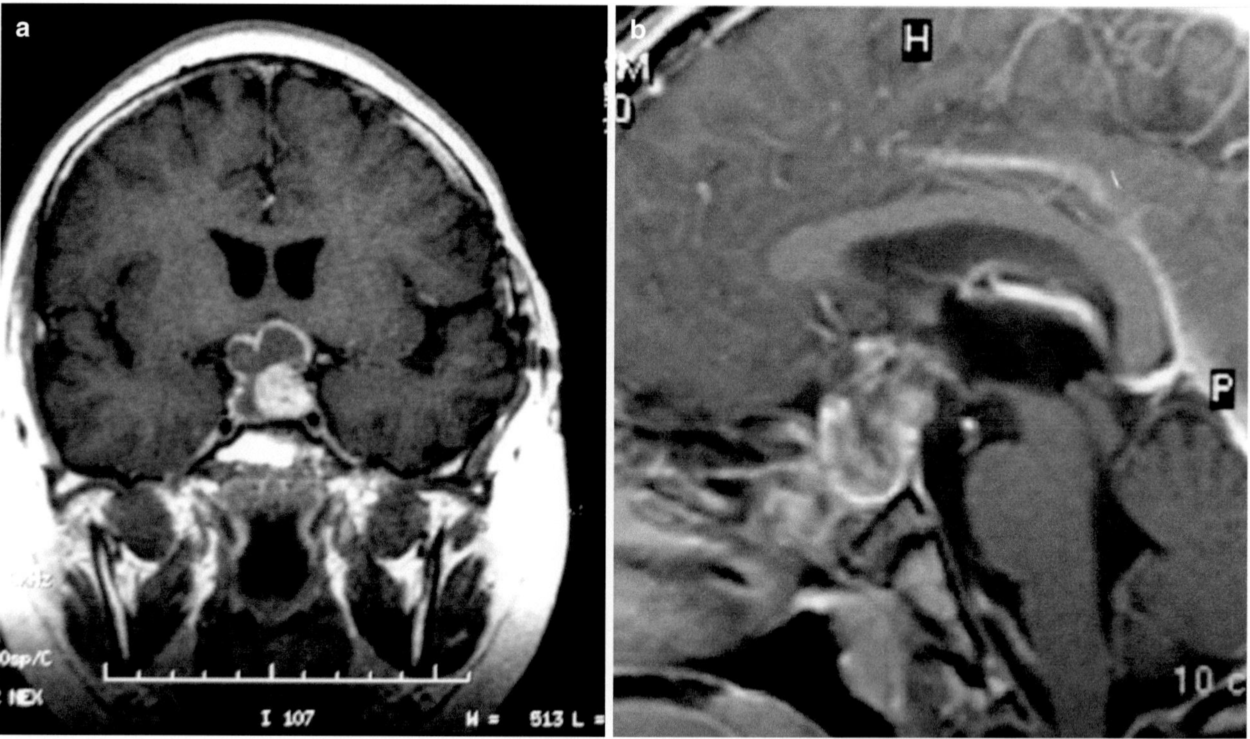

Fig. 7.23 Cystic fluid drainage followed by P32 intra-cystic irradiation was used to treat the recurrent tumor. However, the patient's vision had no improvement; MRI showed no significant shrink of the tumor

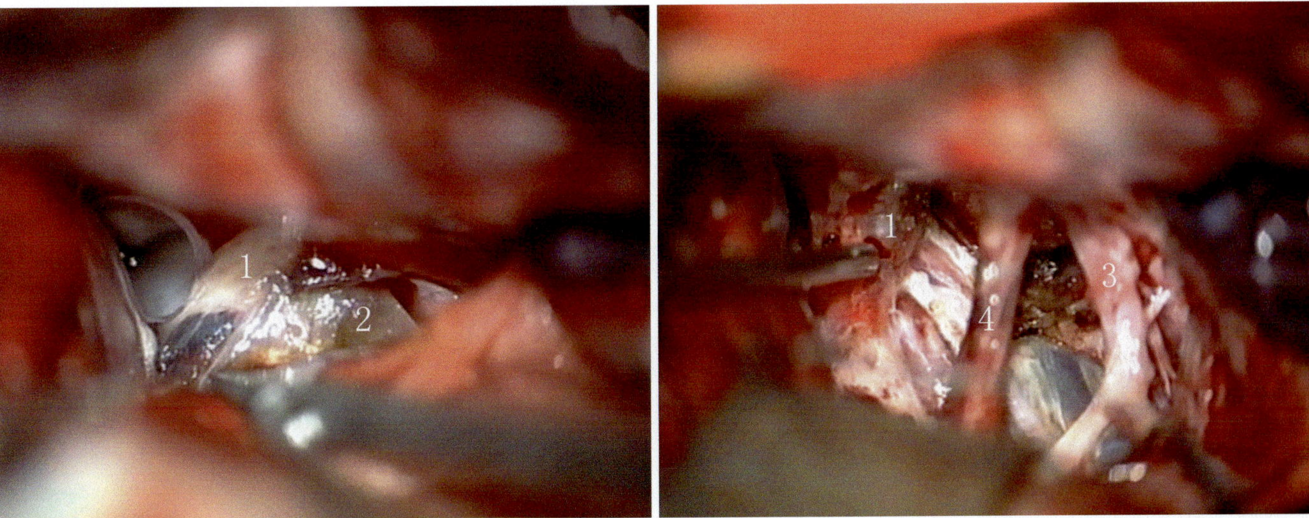

Fig. 7.24 Radical gross tumor removal (GTR) by the fronto-basal interhemispheric approach was performed in our hospital in October 2007. The purpose of the operation was to save the vison. (**a**, **b**) Intrasurgical findings. (1) Degenerative optic nerve (left side), (2) tumor, (3) optic nerve (right side), (4) internal carotid artery

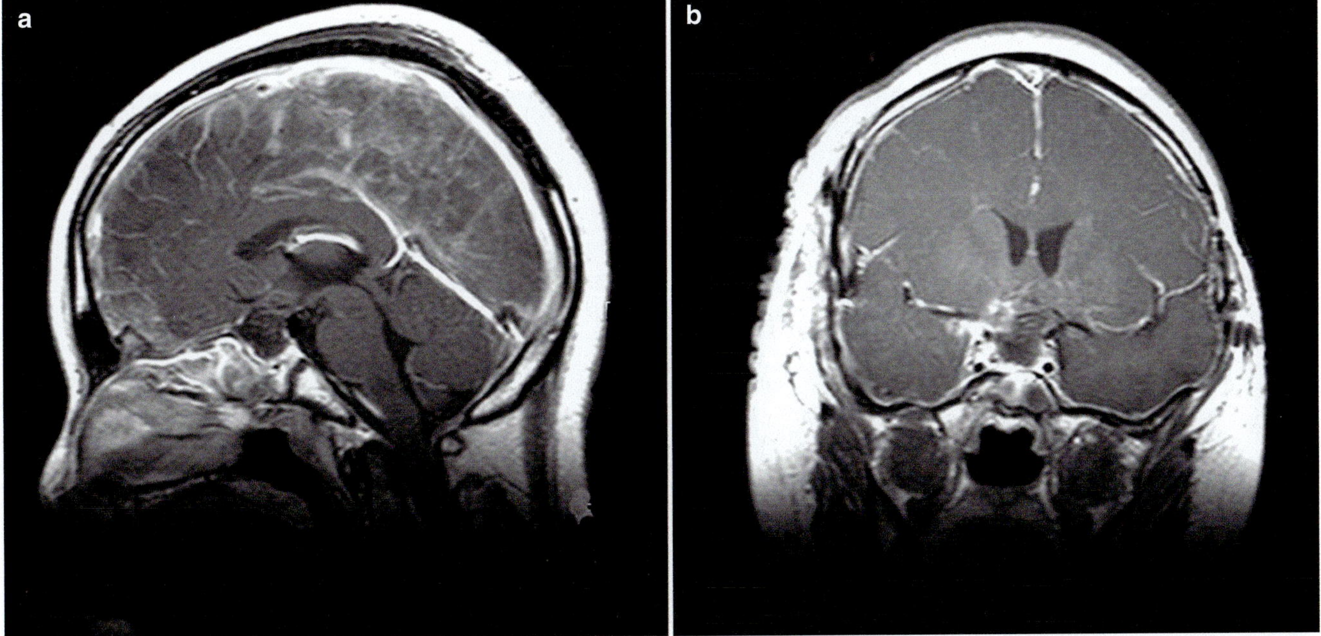

Fig. 7.25 Radical gross tumor removal (GTR) was performed in our hospital in 2007, and the postoperative MRI showed no visibly residual tumor. The neurovascular structures of the sellar region were preserved. The vision in the left eye of the patient was significantly improved

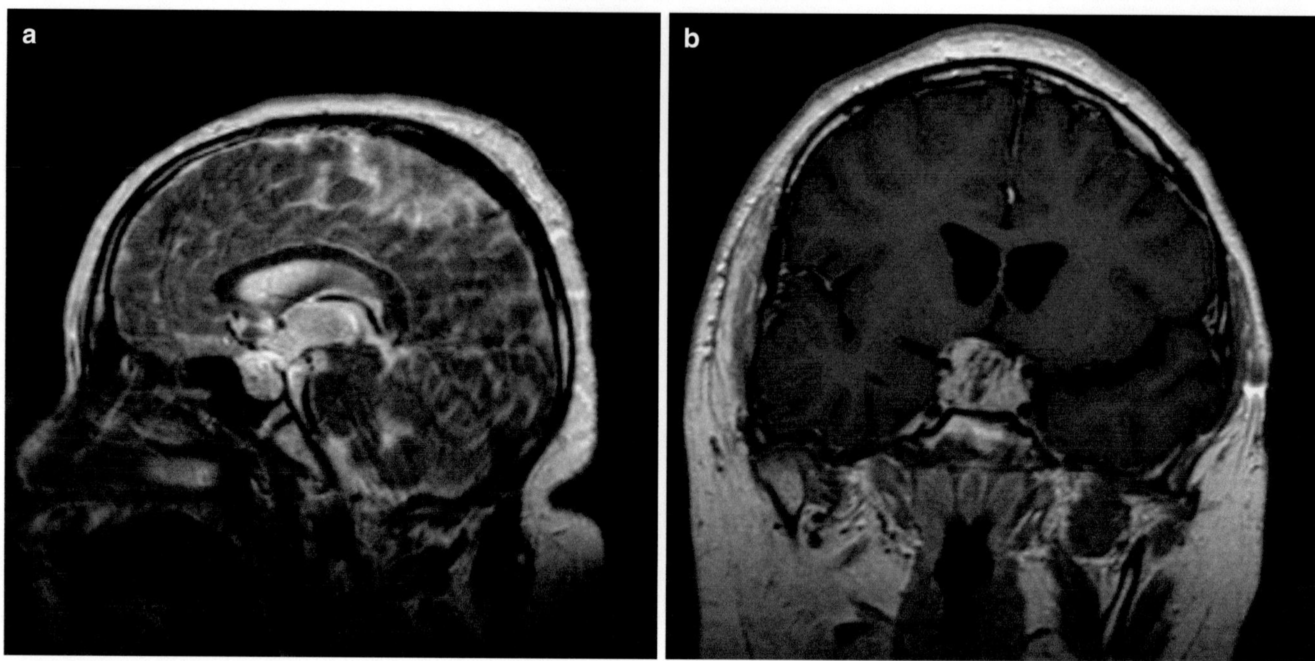

Fig. 7.26 In March 2008, there was intrasellar tumor recurrence in postoperative MRI (**a**, **b**)

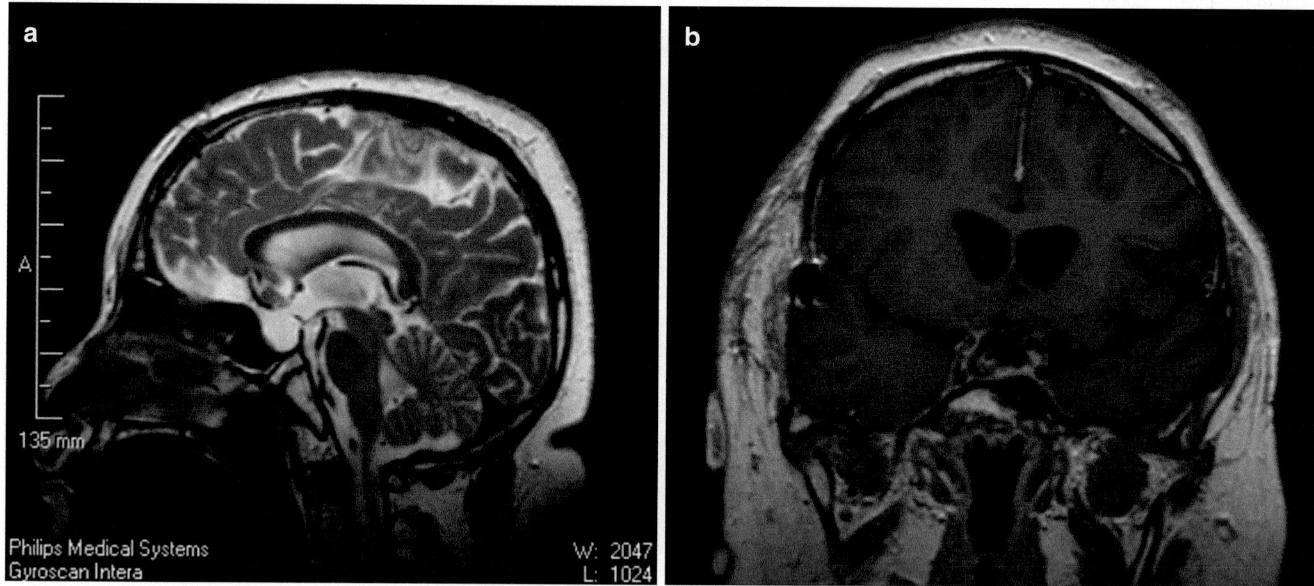

Fig. 7.27 In April 2008, radical gross tumor removal was performed. in postoperative MRI (**a**, **b**)

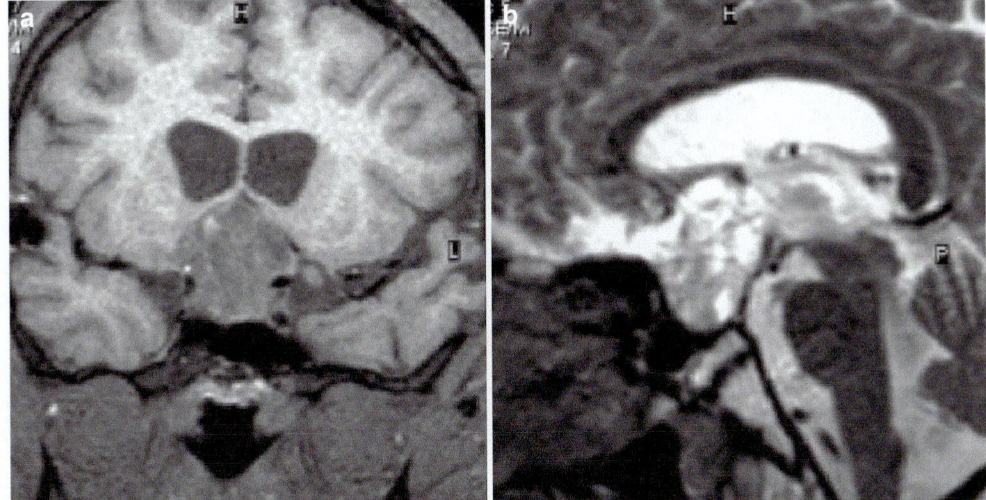

Fig. 7.28 In March 2009, the tumor recurred again in postoperative MRI (**a**, **b**)

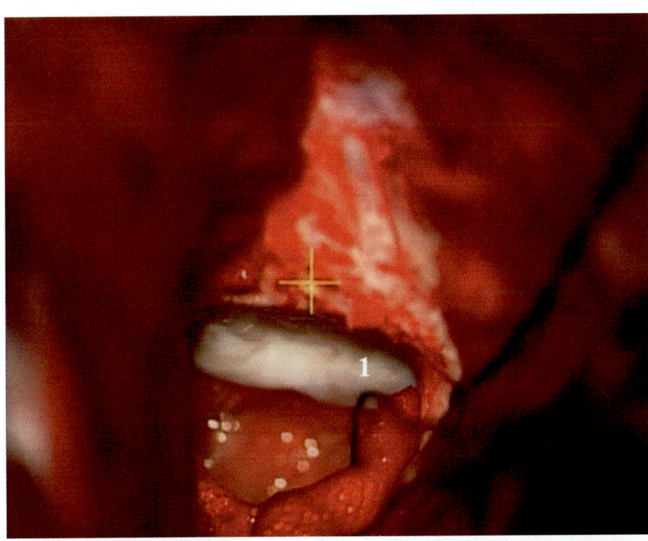

Fig. 7.29 In April 2009, radical gross tumor removal was performed. The tumor was separated from the surrounding neurovascular structures along the suprasellar arachnoid interface. The diaphragma sellae was reconstructed with artificial dura mater. (1) Artificial dura mater

7.5 Case 4: Inappropriate Preservation of the Pituitary Stalk Retention May Lead to Tumor Recurrence (Figs. 7.36, 7.37, 7.38, 7.39, 7.40, 7.41, 7.42, 7.43, 7.44, 7.45, 7.46, 7.47, 7.48, 7.49, 7.50, and 7.51)

In this case, the patient had only mild hypothalamic-pituitary dysfunction before surgery, and the clinical symptoms were mild. The pituitary stalk was clearly identifiable during the operation. For postoperative endocrine function retention, the pituitary stalk was preserved during the first operation, resulting in postoperative tumor recurrence. Once the tumor recurs, it is recommended to perform surgery as soon as possible. The origin site of recurrent craniopharyngioma was consistent with the first operation. Due to the destruction of the diencephalon lobe and mesencephalic lobe of Liliequist membrane in the first operation, the recurrent tumor could have serious adhesion to the peripheral blood vessels, nerves, and third VF, which increases the difficulty of surgery, and

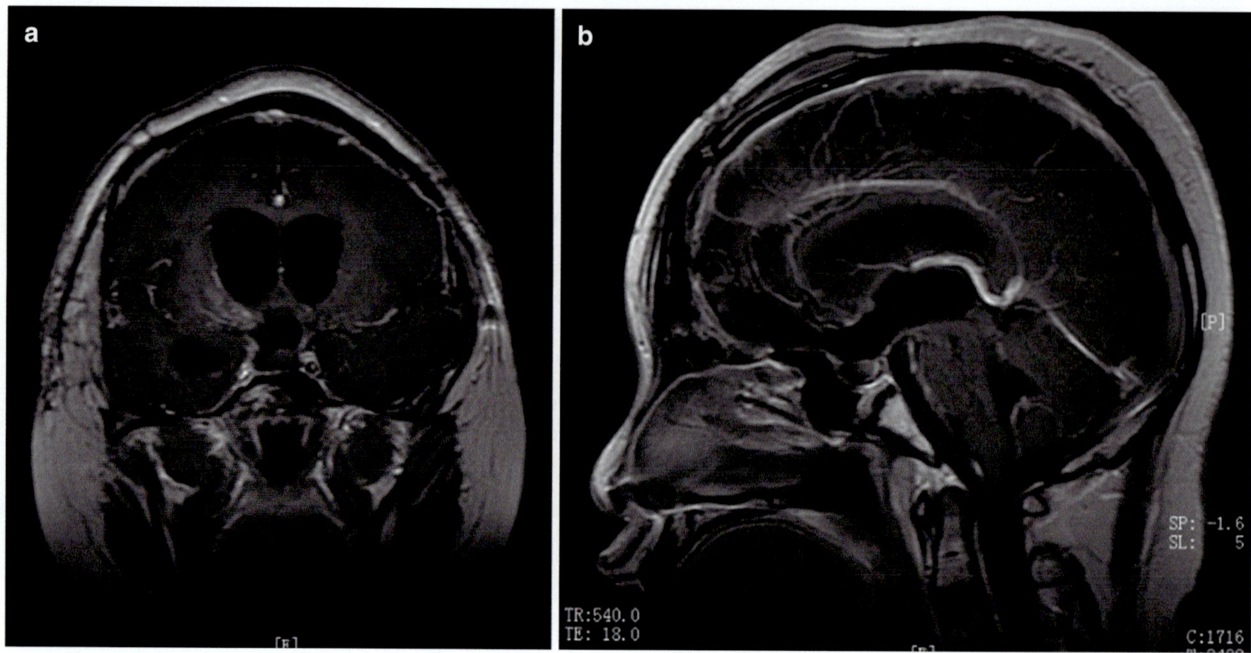

Fig. 7.30 Postoperative radiological images. (**a**, **b**) MRI indicated no residual tumor. The reconstructed diaphragma sellae remained intact

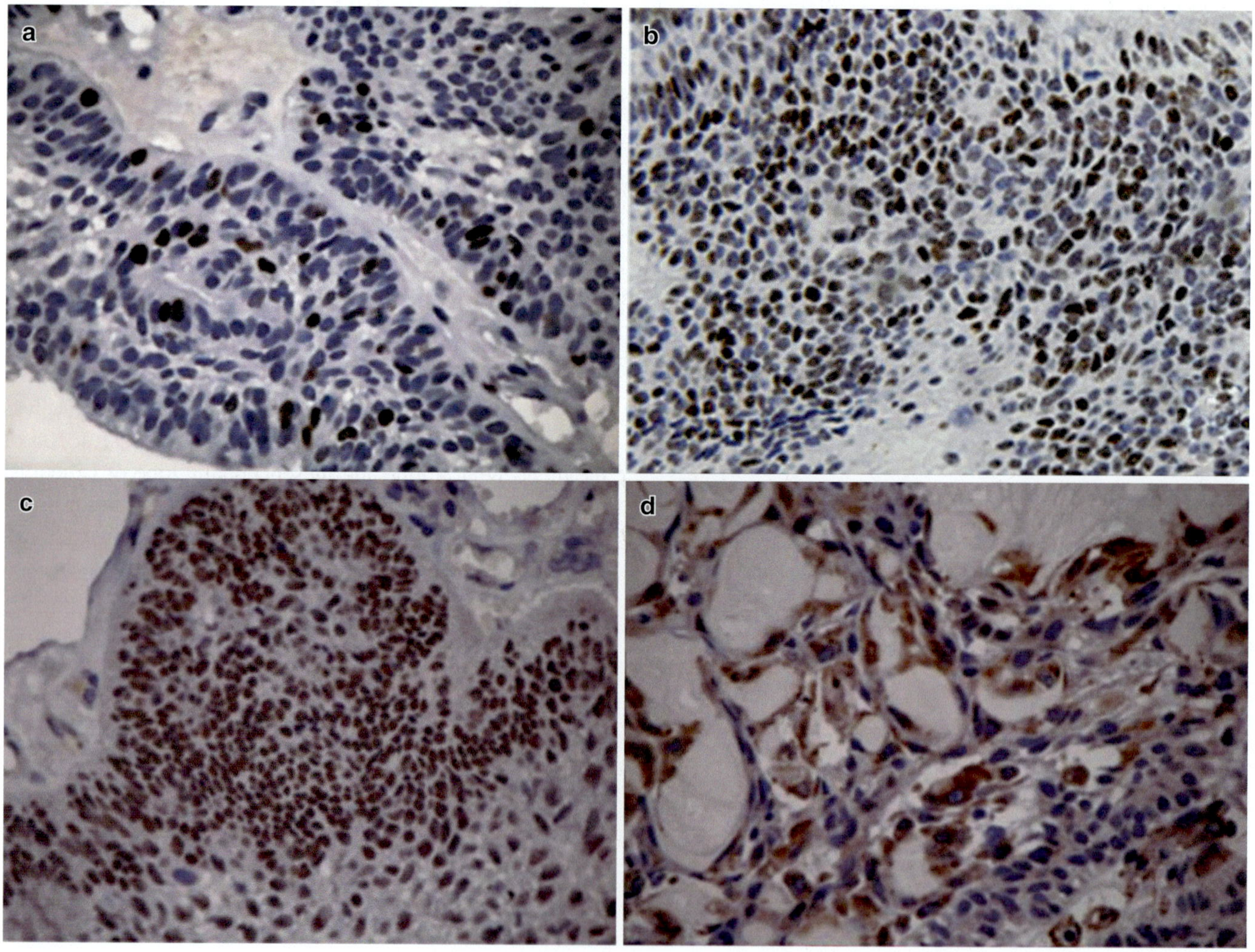

Fig. 7.31 The pathological findings indicated that the tumor had more invasive features and hinted at malignant transformation. Immunohistochemically, the tumor cells were positive for Ki-67 (++, 18%) (**a**), p53 (++) (**b**), p63 (+) (**c**), and VEGF (+) (**d**). And HE staining showed malignant transformation including increased cell density (**e**) and pathologic mitosi (**f**).

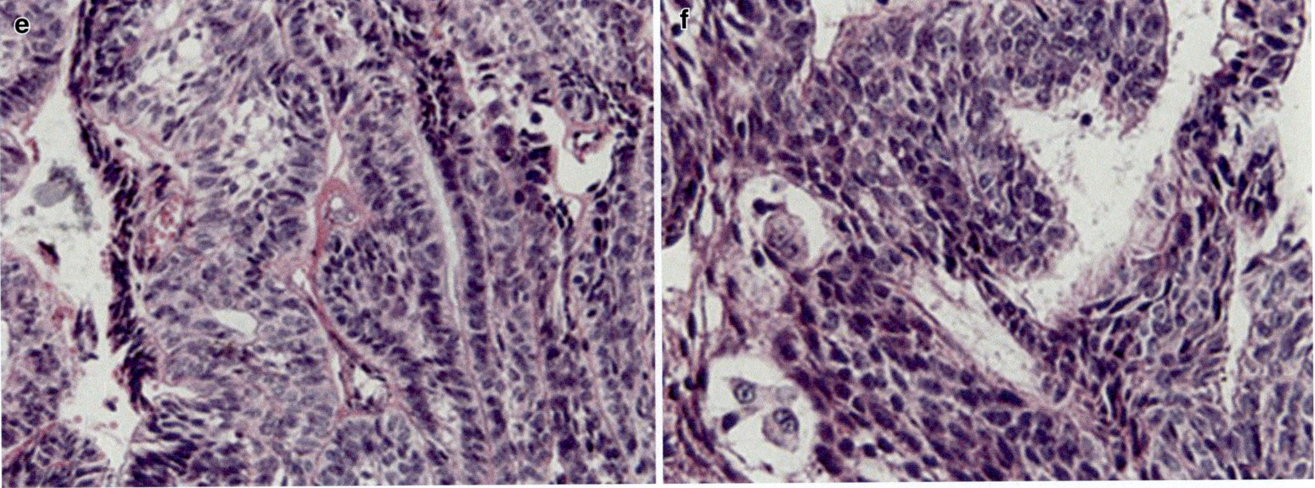

Fig. 7.31 (continued)

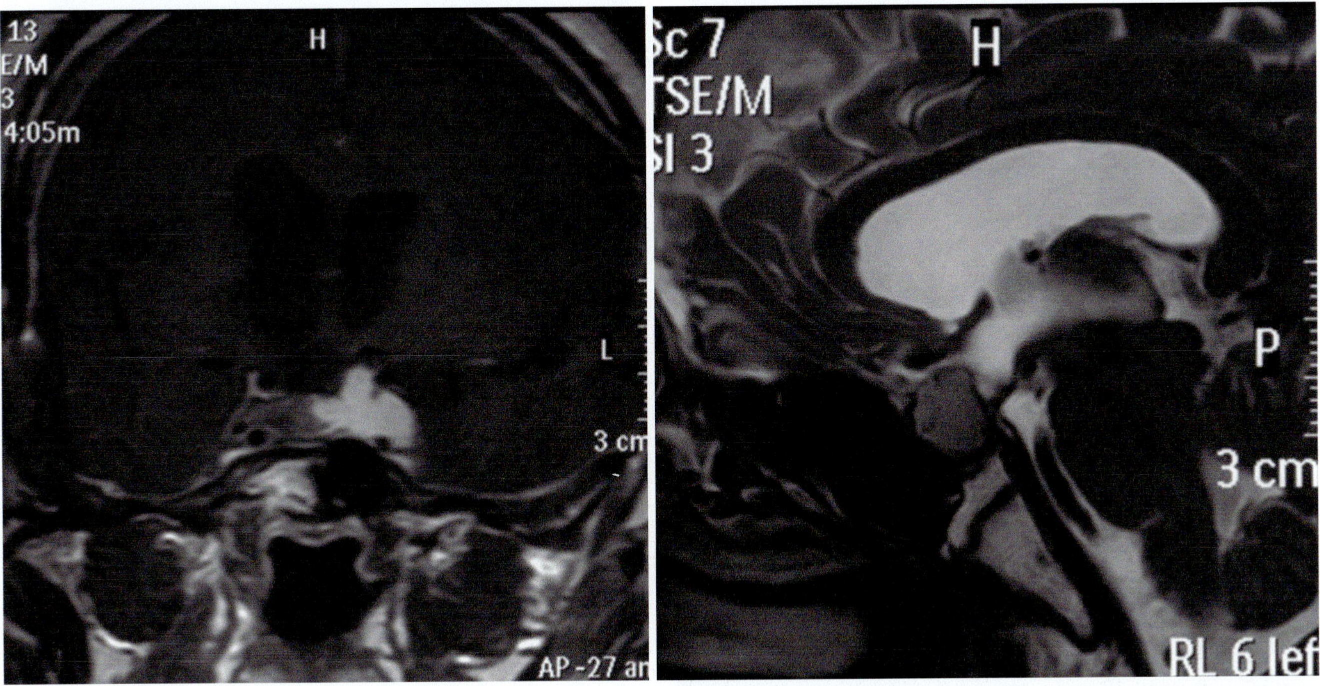

Fig. 7.32 In 2010, there was intrasellar tumor recurrence and the tumor was intrasellarly restricted

sometimes, even smaller recurrent tumors require complex procedures. Due to the peripheral arachnoid membrane structural destruction in the first operation, the resulting recurrent craniopharyngioma could have involved several subarachnoid spaces, including the posterior cranial fossa, which restricts the application of transsphenoidal surgery in recurrent tumors. Therefore, in our opinion, for type S recurrent CP, especially several subarachnoid spaces expanding the tumor, the transcranial approach is preferred.

It can be seen from this example that the patient of S-type craniopharyngioma has mild symptoms, mild postoperative reaction, and good endocrine function after the operation. Even with such a huge tumor, the postoperative response is not serious. Retention of pituitary stalk may lead to tumor recurrence.

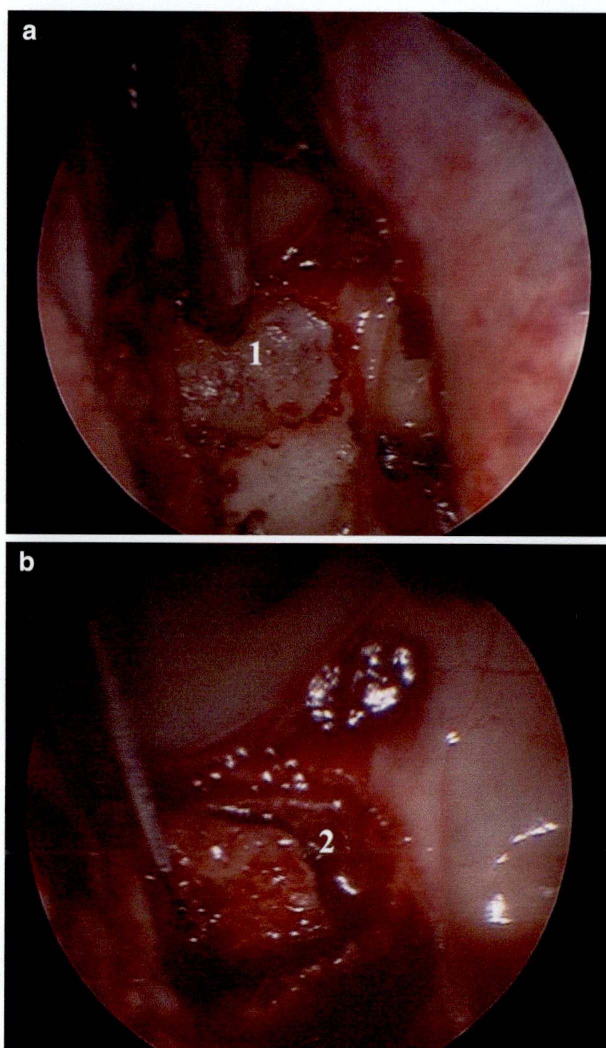

Fig. 7.33 After drilling the sellar floor bone and opening the dura, (**a**, **b**) the intrasellar tumor was exposed. The tumor grew from the intrasellar residues to intrasellar region, and the intrasellar tumor was removed together with the dura mater. (1) Dura, (2) tumor

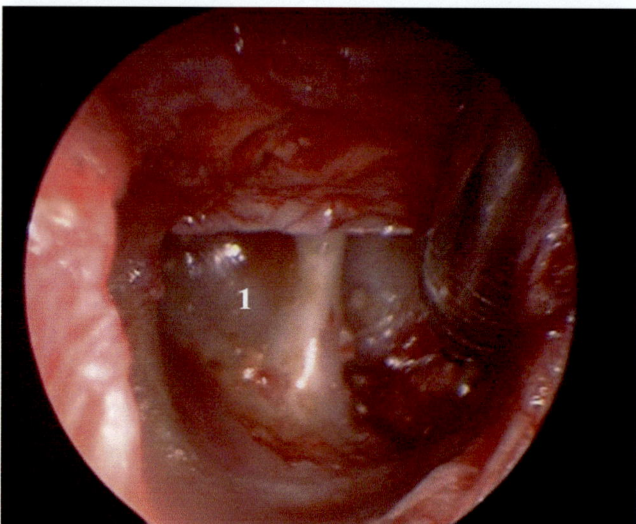

Fig. 7.34 The artificial dura mater which was used to reconstruct the diaphragma sellae was exposed after the total intrasellar tumor removal. (1) Artificial dura mater

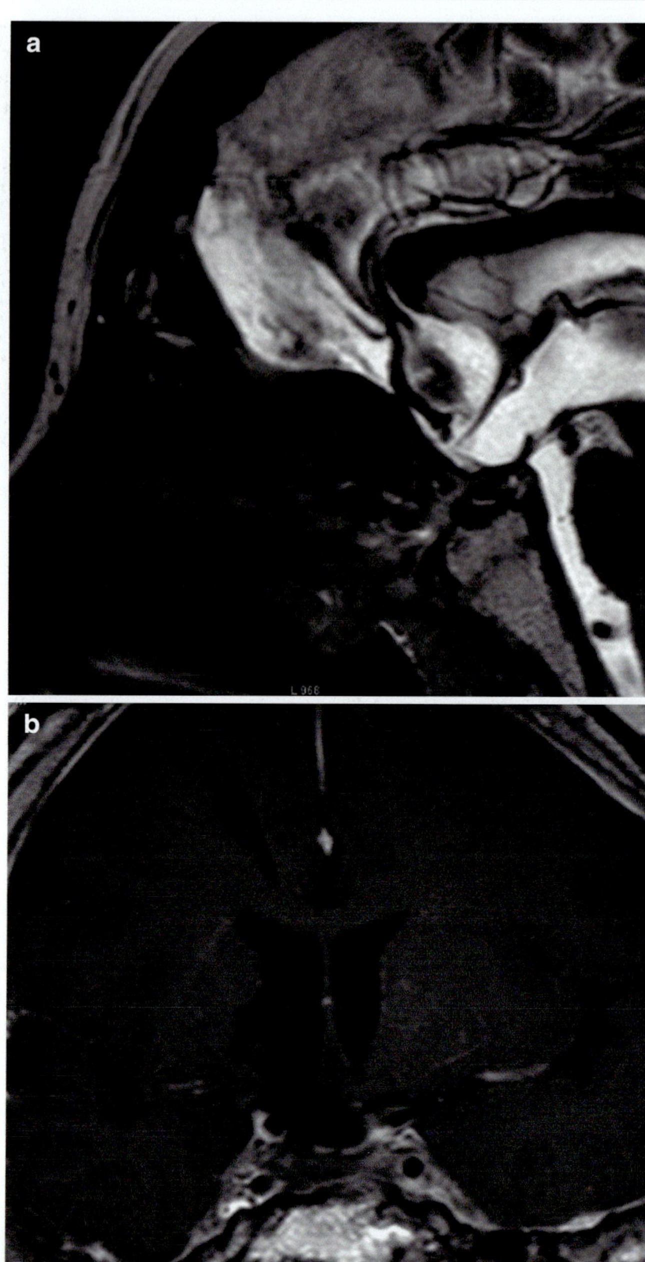

Fig. 7.35 In 2013 (3 years after the last operation), postoperative radiological images. (**a**, **b**) MRI indicated total tumor removal and proved that the tumor had not recurred

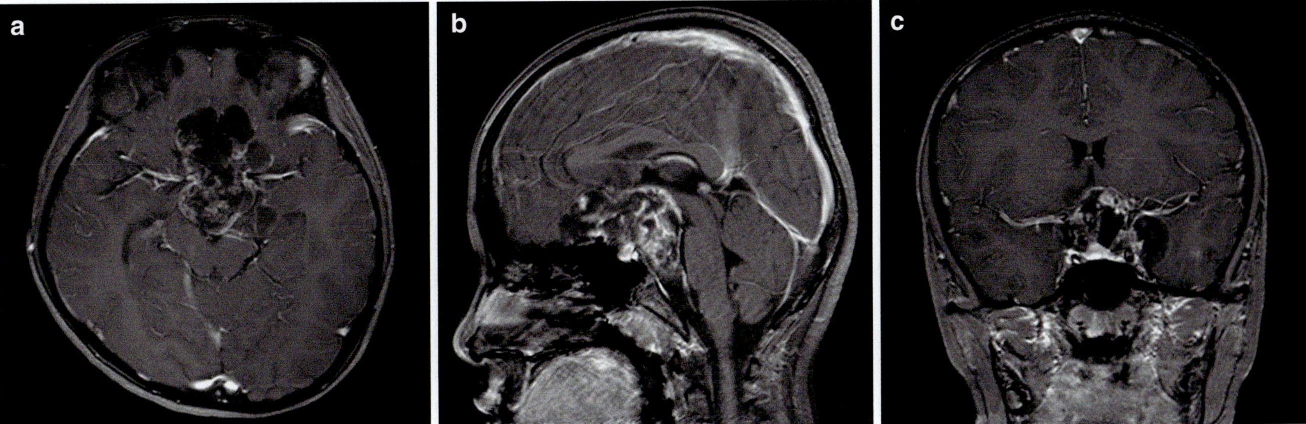

Fig. 7.36 A type S-CP case. Preoperative radiological images obtained in November 2016. (**a–c**) MRI revealed a cystic-solid tumor in the suprasellar region. The tumor arose from the arachnoidal sleeve segment of the pituitary stalk and mainly spread forward through the prechiasmatic cistern into the anterior fossa, lateral fissure cistern, and frontotemporal lobe

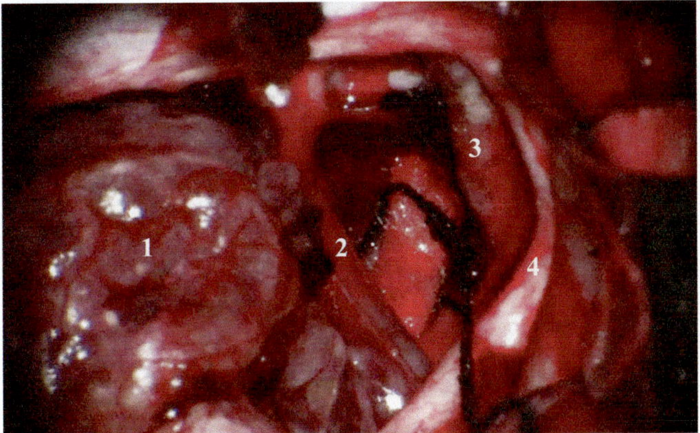

Fig. 7.37 Radical gross tumor removal (GTR) via the fronto-basal interhemispheric approach was performed in our hospital in December 2016. Intraoperative findings. The tumor arose from the arachnoidal sleeve segment of the pituitary stalk; the lower segment of the pituitary stalk remained intact. The tumor was mainly dissected through the prechiasmatic space and optic-internal carotid artery space. The pituitary stalk was pushed back to the right by the tumor. (1) Tumor, (2) pituitary stalk, (3) internal carotid artery, (4) optic nerve

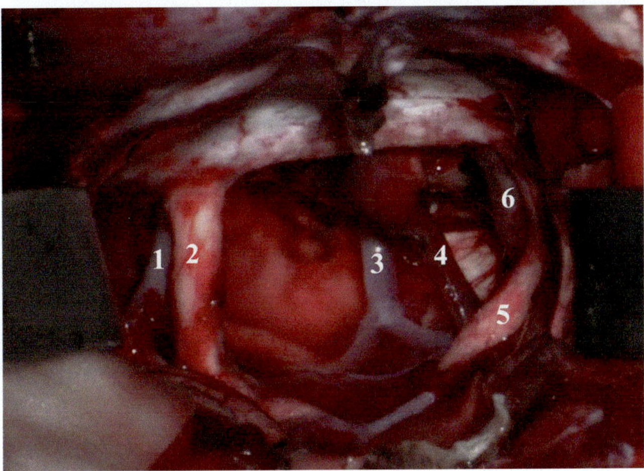

Fig. 7.39 After total tumor removal, the neurovascular structures of the sellar region were preserved. In addition to the origin site, the pituitary stalk remained intact. The origin site of the tumor was clearly visible. (1) internal carotid artery (left), (2) optic nerve (left), (3) basilar artery and its branches, (4) the origin site of the tumor in pituitary stalk, (5) optic nerve (right), (6) internal carotid artery (right)

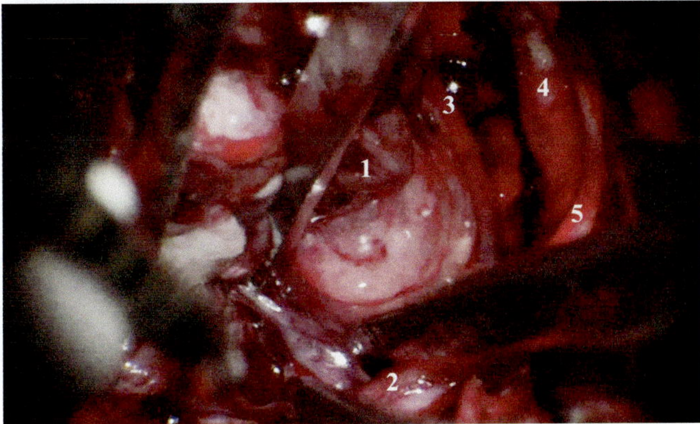

Fig. 7.38 The tumor tightly adhered to the third VF and was separated from the floor of the third VF. (1) Tumor, (2) third VF, (3) pituitary stalk, (4) internal carotid artery, (5) optic nerve

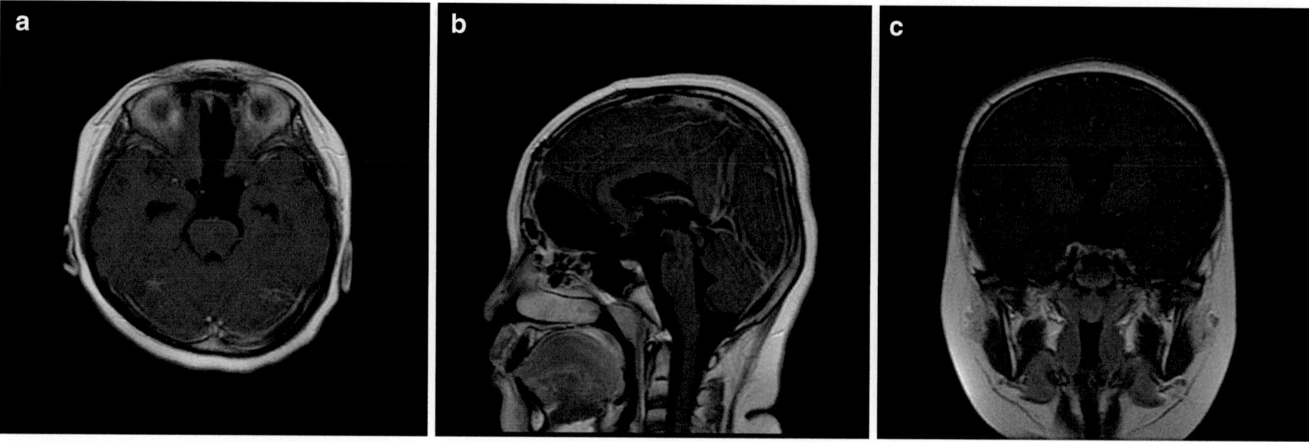

Fig. 7.40 Postoperative radiological images. (**a**–**c**) MRI indicated no residual tumor

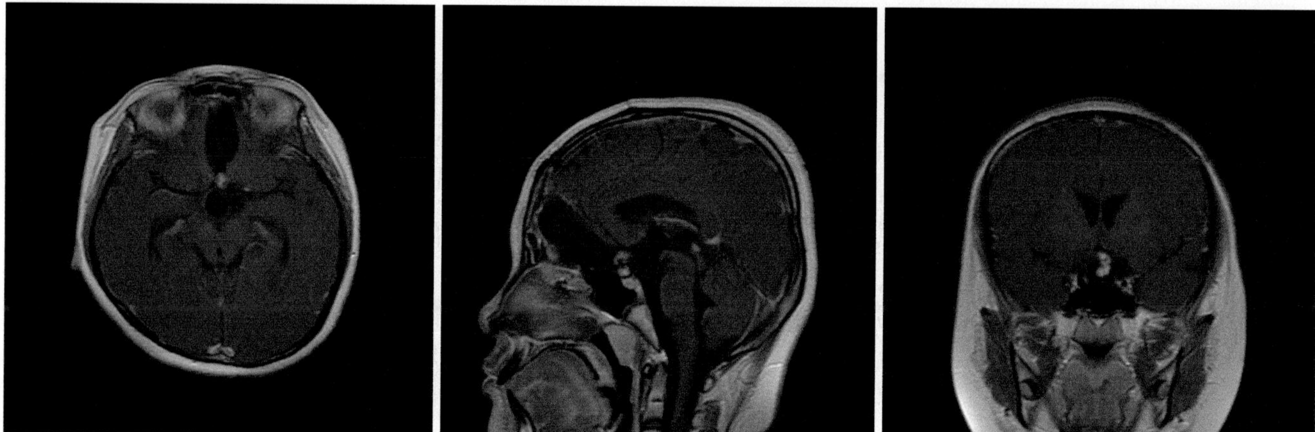

Fig. 7.41 In November 2017, postoperative MRI (**a**–**c**) showed the recurrence of the tumor and the recurrent tumor was closely related to pituitary stalk

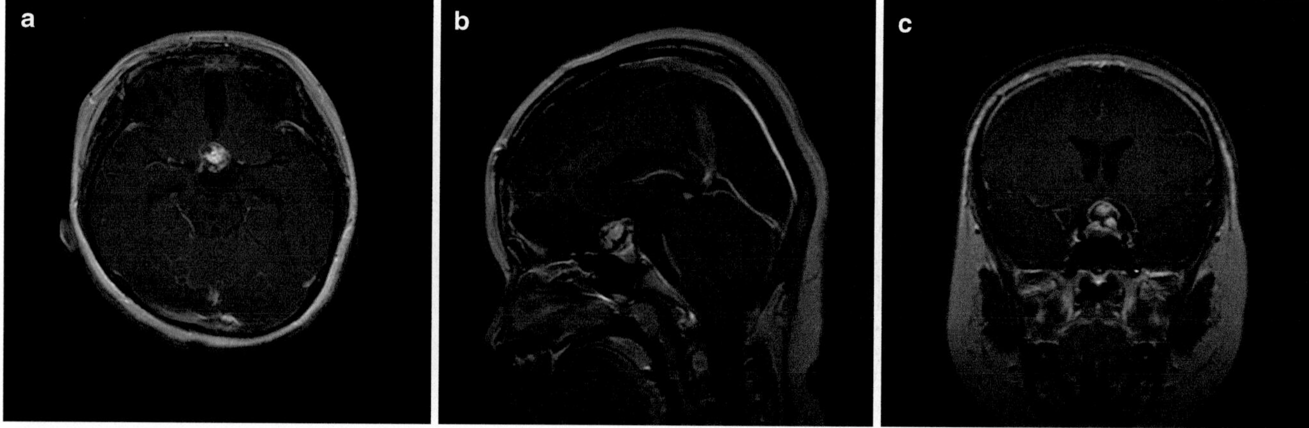

Fig. 7.42 In March 2018, postoperative MRI (**a**–**c**) showed that the recurrent tumor was larger

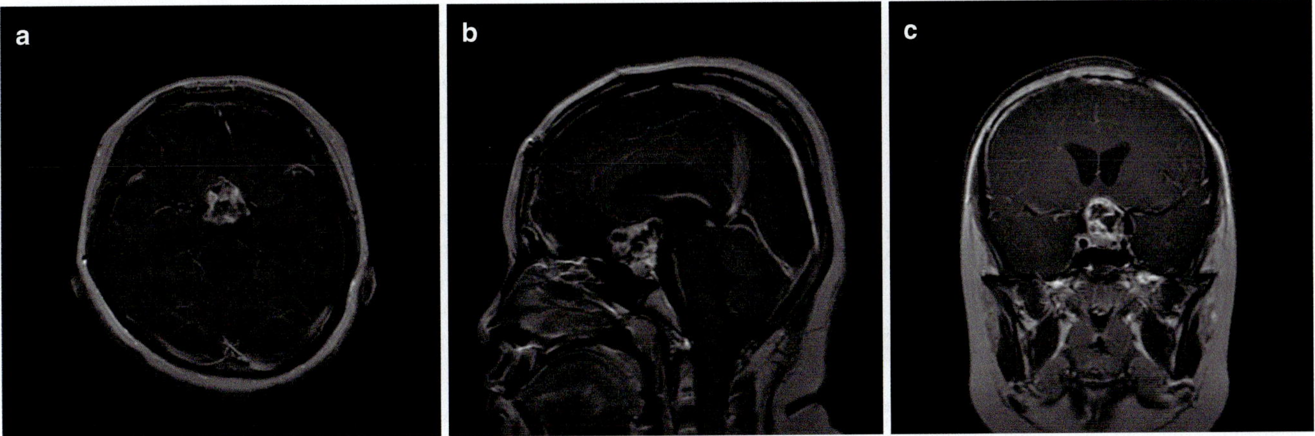

Fig. 7.43 Pre-surgical radiological images (**a–c**) obtained in June 2018

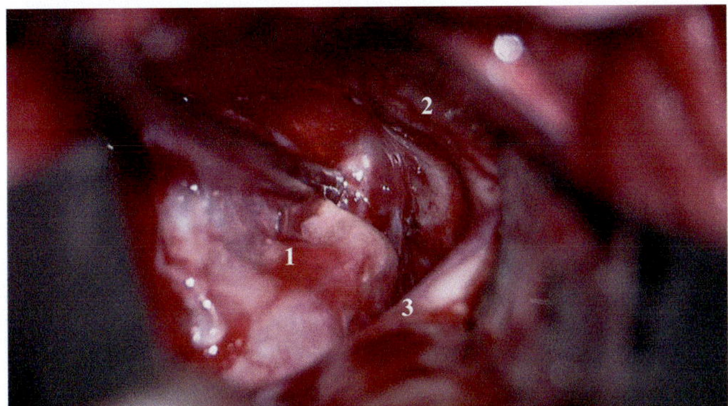

Fig. 7.44 Radical gross tumor removal (GTR) via the fronto-basal interhemispheric approach was performed in our hospital in May 2018. Intraoperative findings. The tumor was dissected through the pre-chiasmatic space. (1) Tumor, (2) optic nerve, (3) optic chiasm

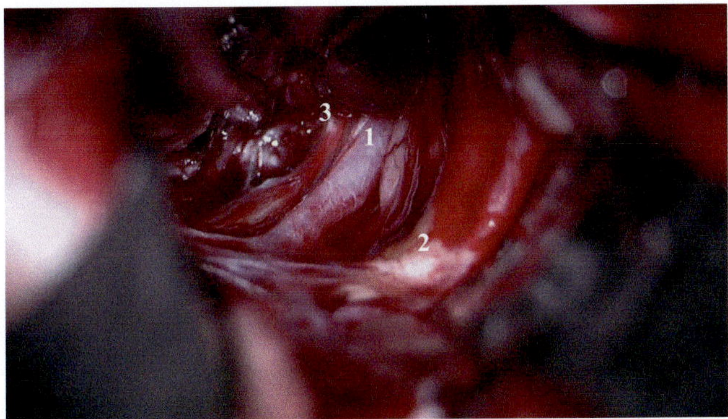

Fig. 7.46 The tumor encased the right arteria cerebri anterior, necessitating sharp dissection to release the tumor. (1) Arteria cerebri anterior (right), (2) optic chiasm, (3) tumor

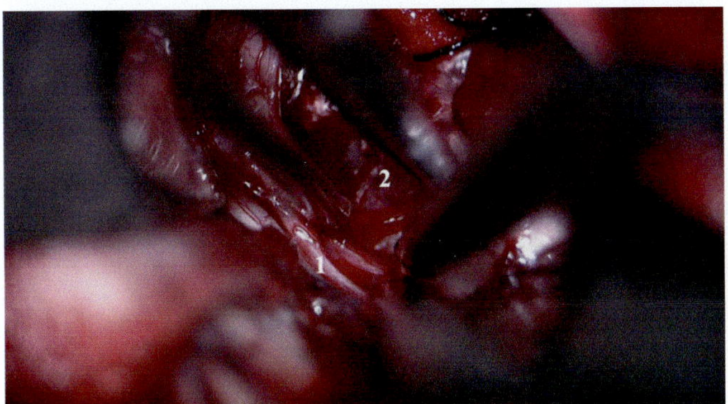

Fig. 7.45 The morphologically thin optic chiasm was pushed by the tumor. (1) Optic chiasm, (2) tumor

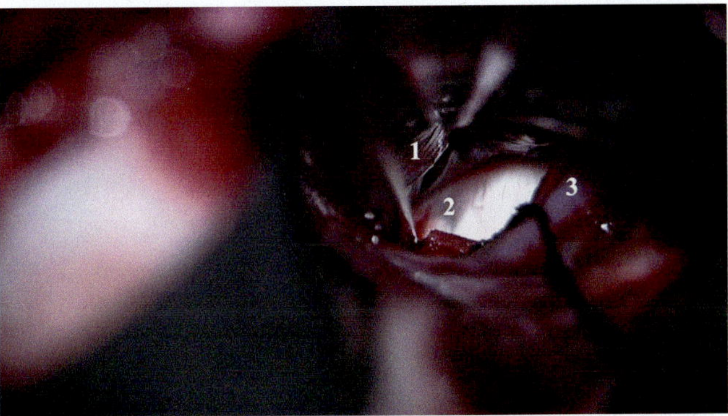

Fig. 7.47 The tumor tightly adhered to the third VF and was separated from the floor of the third VF. (1) Tumor, (2) third VF, (3) arteria cerebri anterior

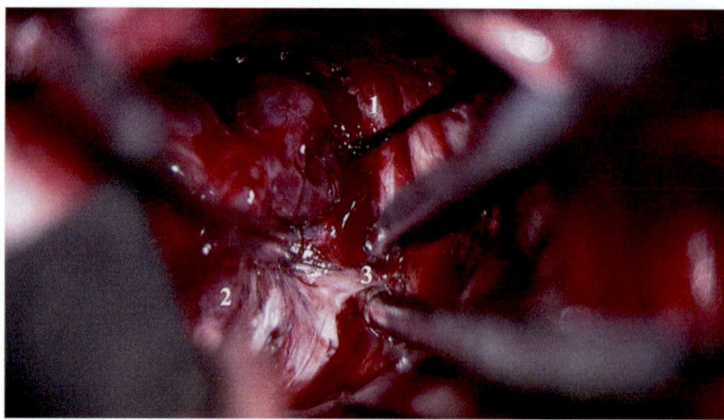

Fig. 7.48 The tumor was separated from the surrounding neurovascular structures along the suprasellar arachnoid interface. The origin site of recurrent craniopharyngioma was consistent with the first operation. The origin site of tumor was sharply dissected. (1) Pituitary stalk, (2) tumor, (3) the site of tumor origin

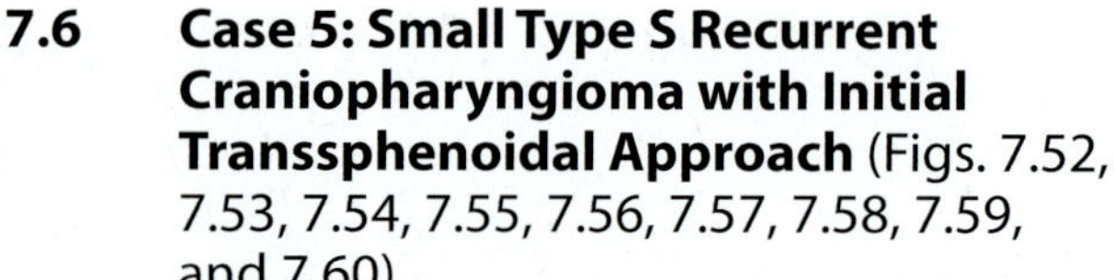

7.6 Case 5: Small Type S Recurrent Craniopharyngioma with Initial Transsphenoidal Approach (Figs. 7.52, 7.53, 7.54, 7.55, 7.56, 7.57, 7.58, 7.59, and 7.60)

The first operation was performed by the transsphenoidal approach. The transsphenoidal corridor can only provide a narrow exposure, resulting in the recurrence of craniopharyngioma. In this case, the MRI revealed the patient with recurring tumor in suprasellar region. Because of the destruction of the basal arachnoidal membrane (outer arachnoid) and other peripheral membranous structure in the first operation, the recurrent tumor has serious adhesion to the optic nerve and internal carotid artery, which restricted the application of transsphenoidal surgery in recurrent tumors. The

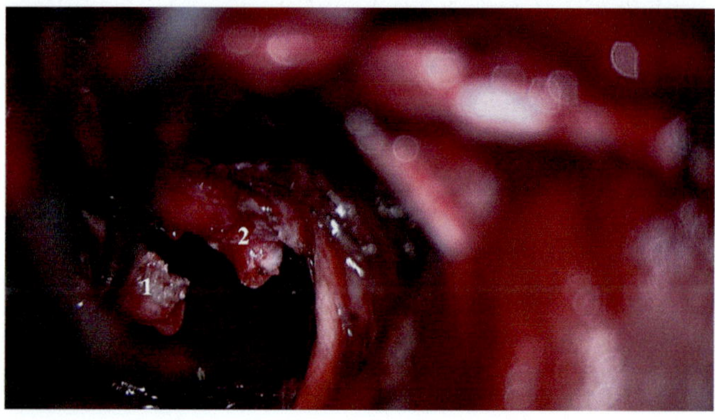

Fig. 7.49 The pituitary stalk was clearly visible; however, the pituitary stalk was sharply dissected at the origin site of the tumor to avoid tumor recurrence. (1) Tumor, (2) the pituitary stalk

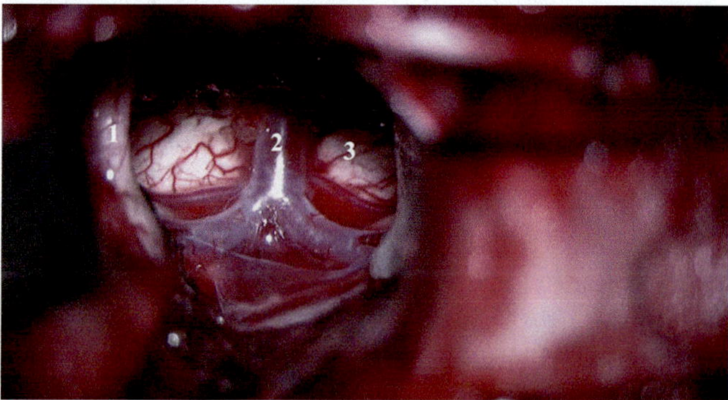

Fig. 7.50 After total tumor removal, the neurovascular structures of the sellar region were preserved. (1) Optic nerve (left), (2) basilar artery and its branches, (3) brain stem

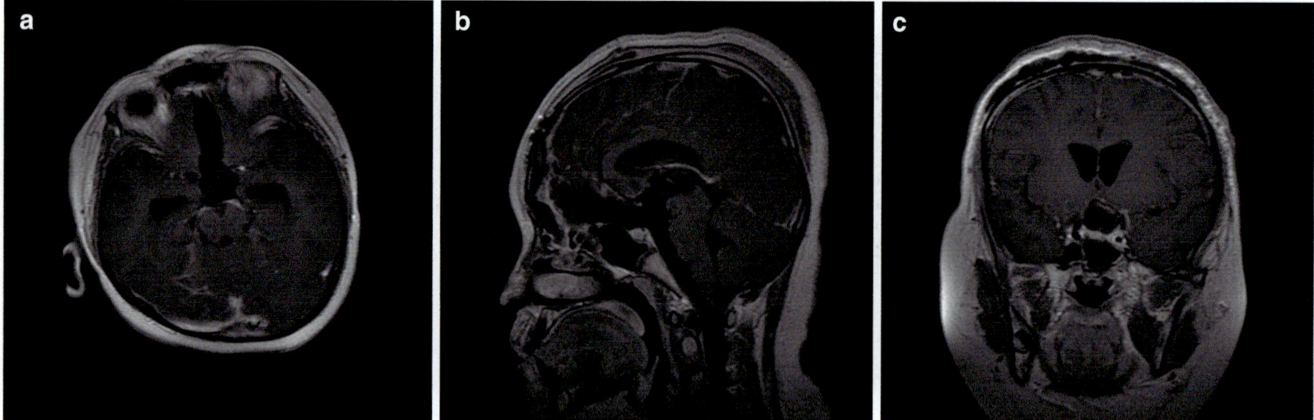

Fig. 7.51 Postsurgical radiological images. (**a**–**c**) MRI indicated that total tumor removal was achieved. The pituitary stalk was not visible. This patient returned to normal work and life through endocrine therapy after operation

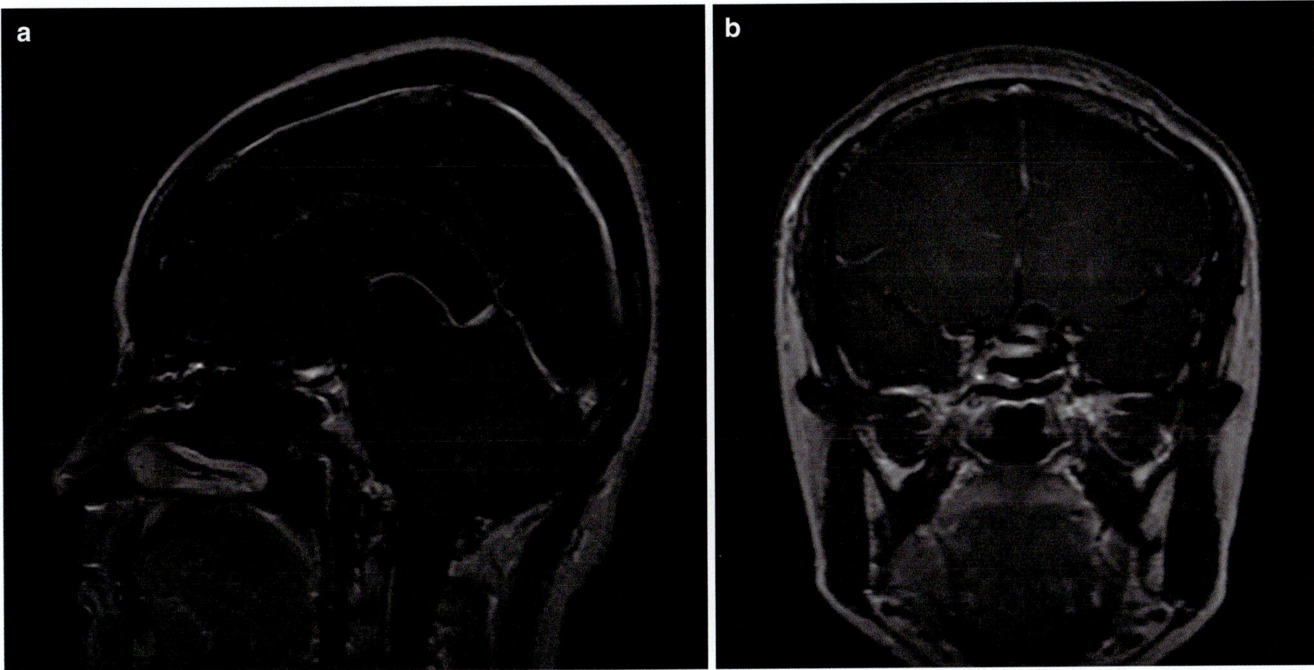

Fig. 7.52 Female, 32 years old, a type S-CP case. In June 2015, radical gross tumor removal (GTR) via the transsphenoidal approach was performed in another hospital. Postoperative radiological images. (**a**, **b**) One year after the operation, MRI showed the recurrence of the tumor

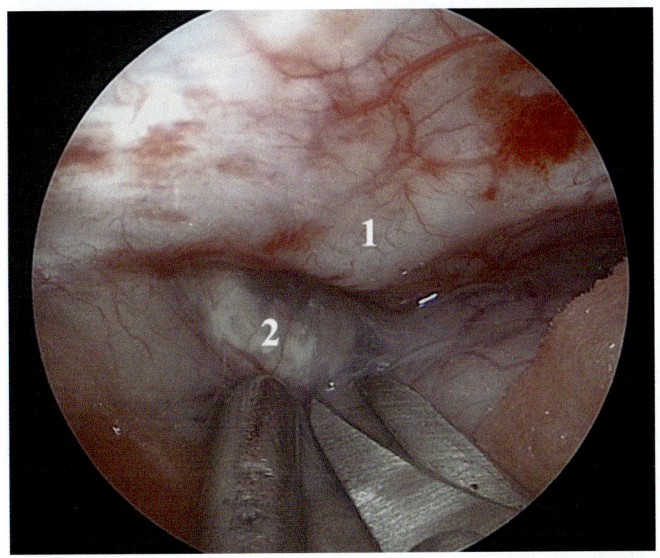

Fig. 7.53 Radical gross tumor removals (GTR) via the supraorbital eyebrow approach were performed in our hospital in July 2016. The arachnoid was dissected to release the cerebrospinal fluid from the suprasellar cistern and expose the tumor. (1) Anterior clinoid process, (2) tumor

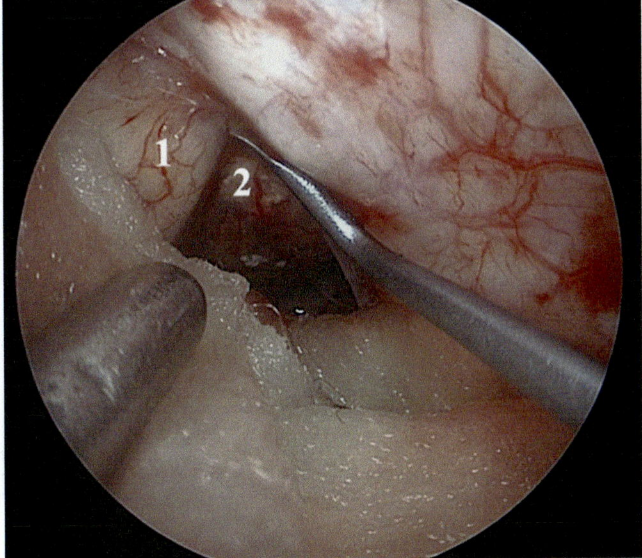

Fig. 7.54 The tumor was separated from the surrounding neurovascular structures along the suprasellar arachnoid interface. The tumor was located at the ventral aspect of the optic chiasm. The tumor tightly adhered to the optic nerve and was separated from the optic chiasm. (1) Optic chiasm, (2) tumor

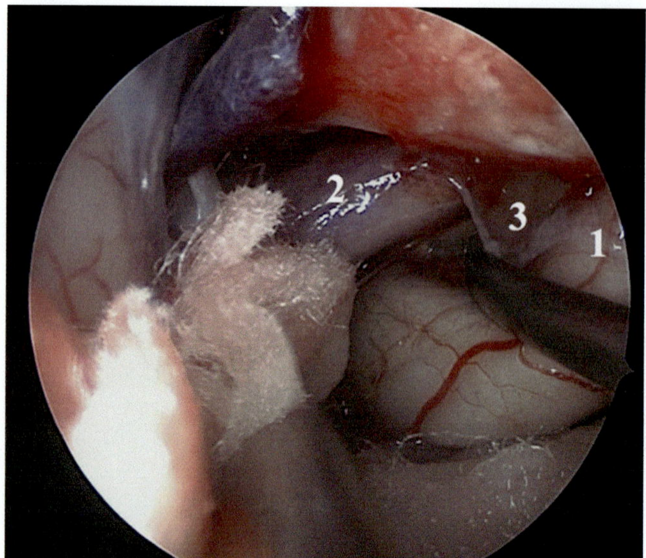

Fig. 7.55 The tumor tightly adhered to the optic nerve and internal carotid artery. (1) Optic nerve, (2) internal carotid artery, (3) tumor

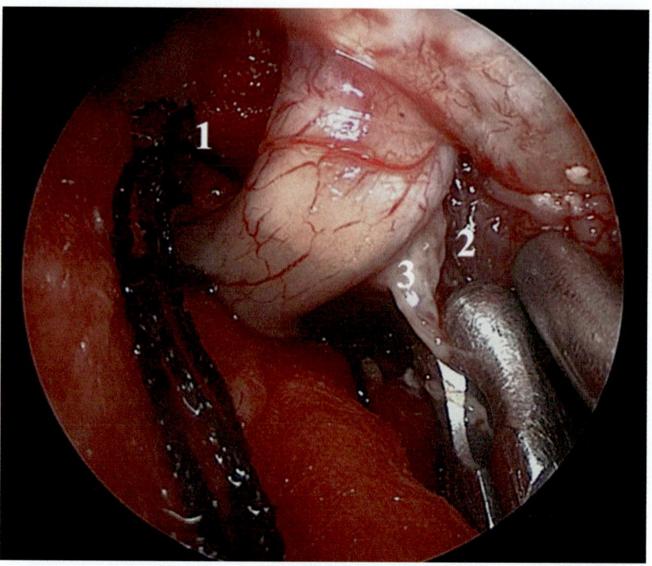

Fig. 7.57 The brain cotton piece was placed into the pre-chiasmatic space to push the tumor to the optic-internal carotid artery space. The tumor tightly adhered to the arachnoid and pia mater around the optic nerve. (1) Pre-chiasmatic space, (2) optic-internal carotid artery space, (3) tumor

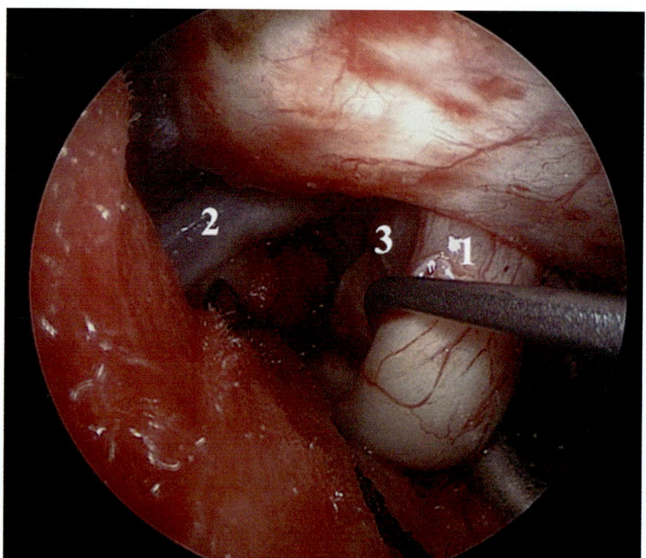

Fig. 7.56 The tumor tightly adhered to the ventral aspect of the right optic nerve and optic chiasm, necessitating sharp dissection to release the tumor through the pre-chiasmatic space. (1) Optic nerve, (2) internal carotid artery, (3) tumor

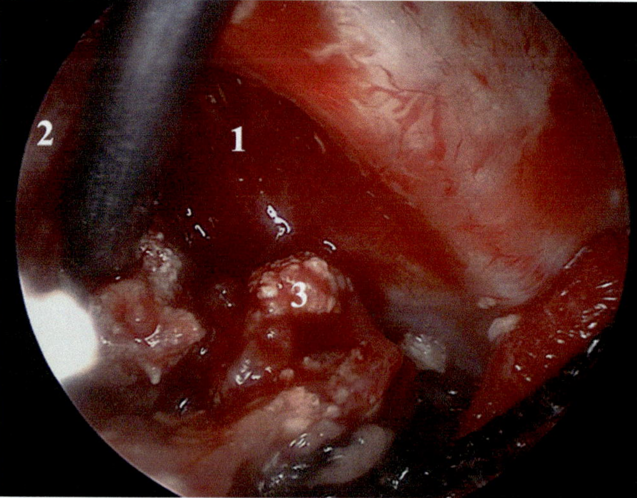

Fig. 7.58 The origin site of tumor was located in the arachnoid sleeve segment of the pituitary stalk. (1) Pituitary stalk, (2) optic nerve, (3) tumor

supraorbital eyebrow approach could achieve satisfactory exposure of the structure in the saddle region and provide a wide operative space. If the tumor grows into the intrasellar region, the tumor and the normal pituitary gland could be exposed after drilling the tuberculum sellae.

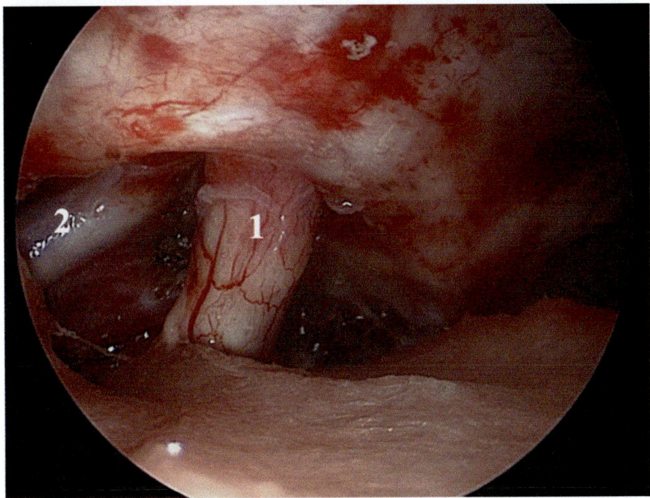

Fig. 7.59 After total tumor removal, the neurovascular structures of the sellar region were preserved. The pituitary stalk exhibited severe tumor involvement, and it was sacrificed to avoid tumor recurrence. (1) Optic nerve, (2) internal carotid artery

7.7 Case 6: Giant Type T Craniopharyngioma Recurred After Radical Tumor Resection (Figs. 7.61, 7.62, 7.63, 7.64, 7.65, 7.66, 7.67, 7.68, 7.69, 7.70, 7.71, 7.72, 7.73, 7.74, and 7.75)

Radical gross tumor removal was performed in the first operation and the tumor was en bloc removed. The tumor was originated from the pars distalis of adenohypophysis and neighbored to infundibulo-tubular part of the hypothalamus. For postoperative endocrine function retention, the pituitary stalk of the child was preserved during the first operation, resulting in postoperative tumor recurrence. The tumor recurrence may be related to tumor cytological residue. However, patients with RGT usually relapse late. The patient relapsed 6 years after the first GTR. Once the tumor recurs, it is recommended to perform surgery as soon as possible.

The surgical classification of recurrent craniopharyngioma is consistent with the preoperative classification.

Due to the peripheral arachnoid membrane structural destruction in the first operation, the recurrent craniopharyngioma could have involved several subarachnoid spaces. In this case, the tumor spread into the lateral fissure cistern, the middle fossa, and the left temporal lobe. The transsphenoidal

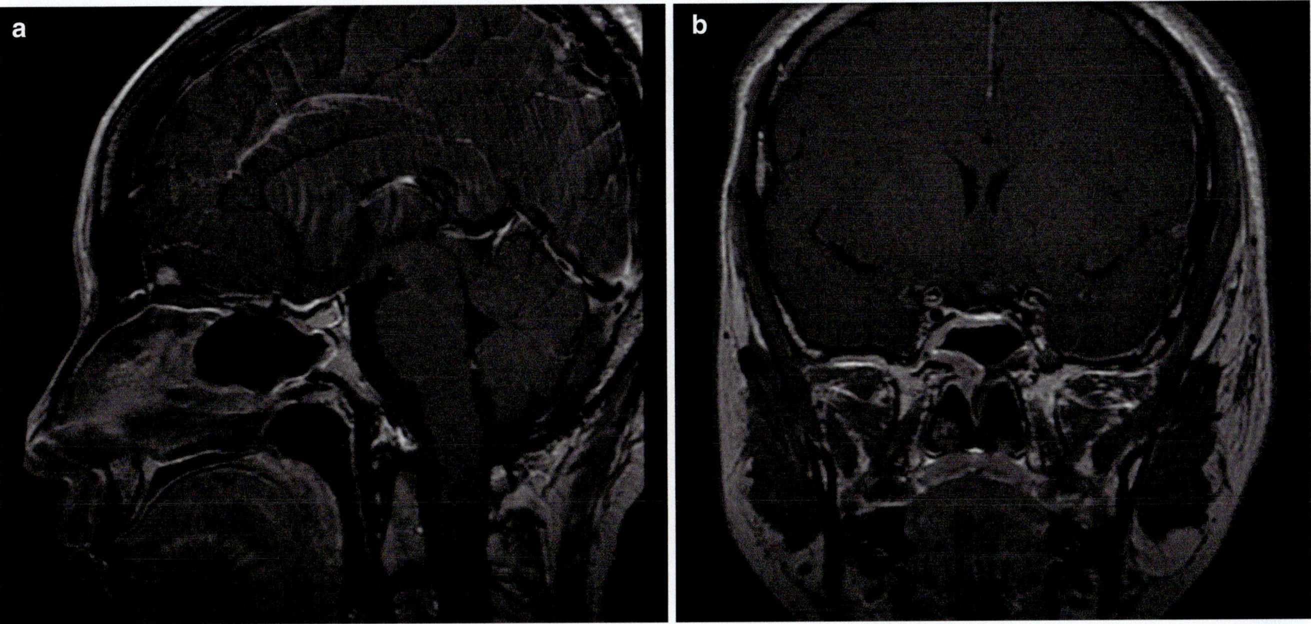

Fig. 7.60 Postsurgical radiological images. (**a**, **b**) MRI indicated that total tumor removal was achieved; the third VF remained intact

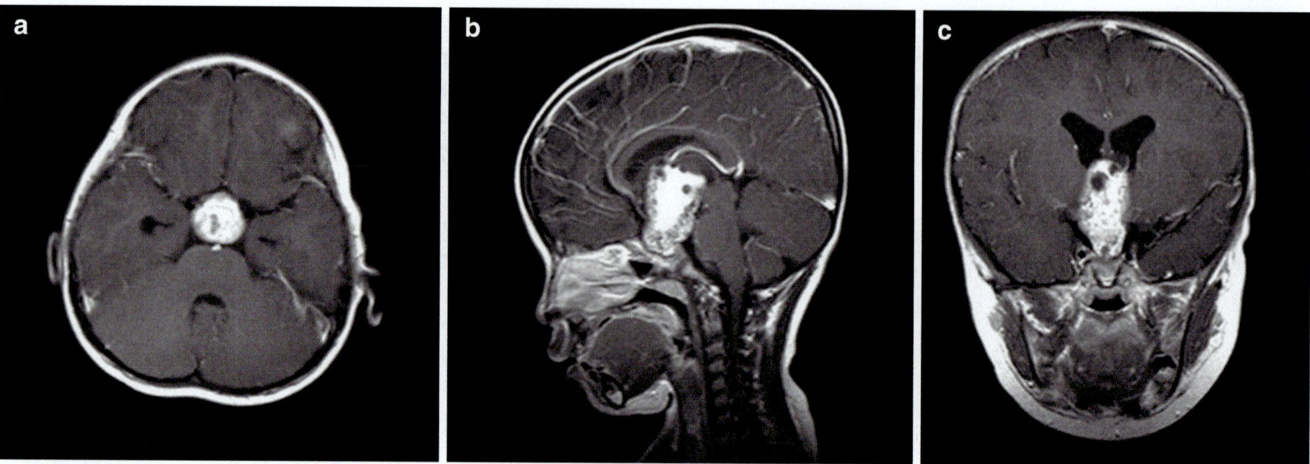

Fig. 7.61 Female, 3 years old. A type T-CP case. Preoperative radiological images were obtained in November 2010. (**a–c**) MRI revealed a tumor in the sellar region

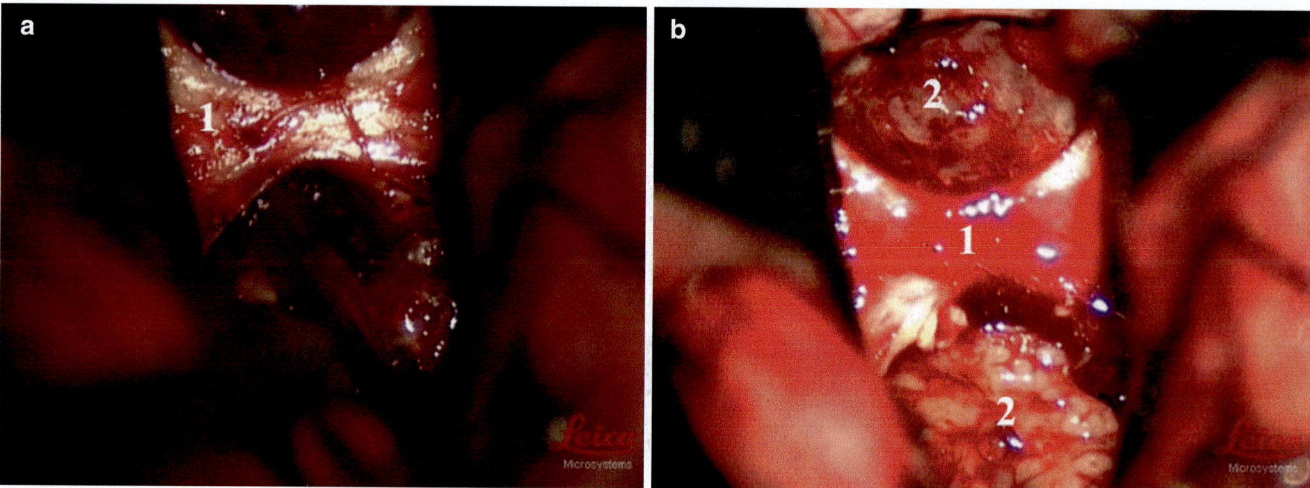

Fig. 7.62 Radical gross tumor removal (GTR) by the fronto-basal interhemispheric approach was performed in our hospital in November 2010. (**a**, **b**) Intraoperative findings. The tumor was dissected through the pre-chiasmatic space and lamina terminalis space. (1) optic chiasm, (2) tumor

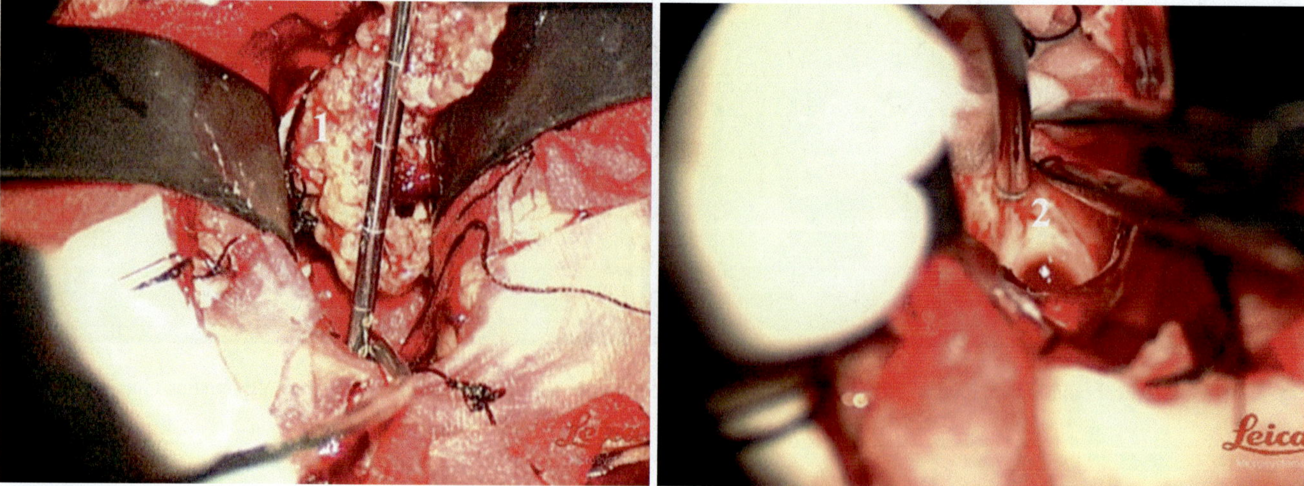

Fig. 7.63 The tumor was originated from the pars distalis of the adenohypophysis and neighbored to infundibulo-tubular part of the hypothalamus and grew toward the third VF. The tumor had an intimate relationship with the third ventricle. We opened the ventral third VF to ensure radical gross tumor removal. The tumor was en bloc removed. (1) tumor, (2) third VF

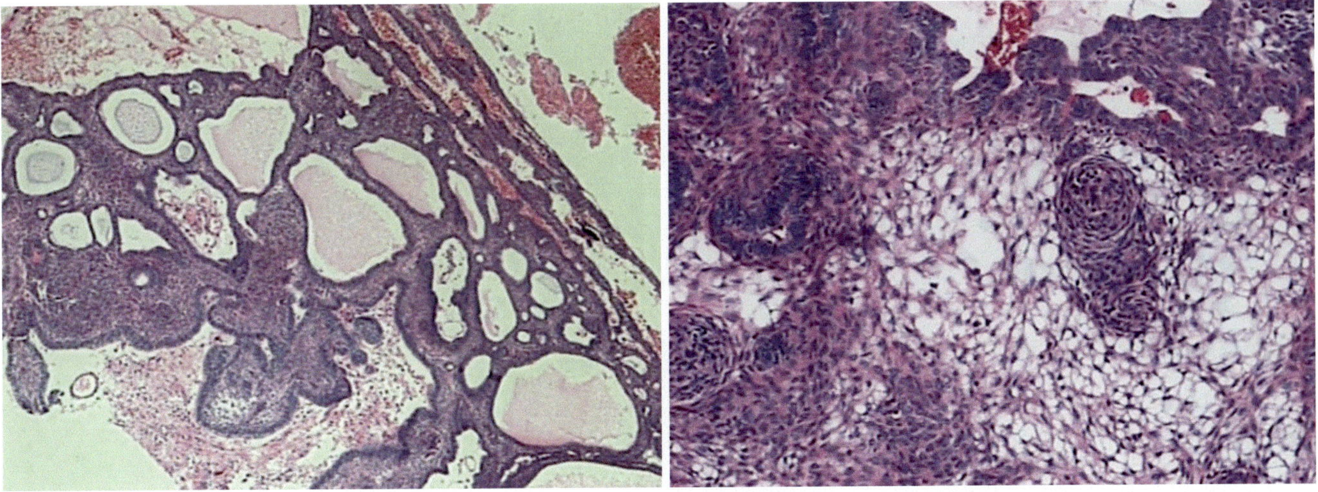

Fig. 7.64 The pathological findings indicated adamantinomatous craniopharyngioma

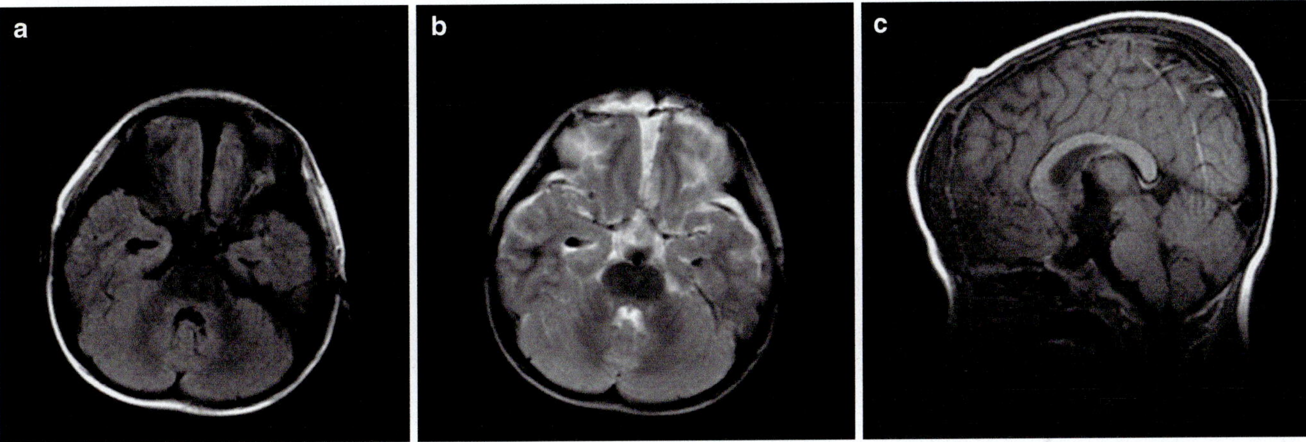

Fig. 7.65 Postoperative radiological images. (**a–c**) MRI indicated that total tumor removal was achieved

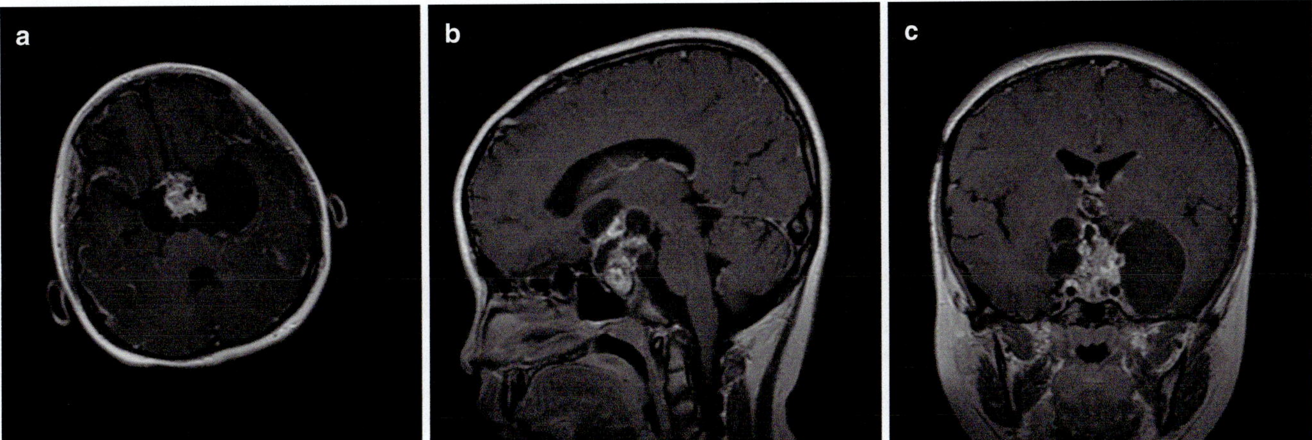

Fig. 7.66 In June 2016, MRI had proved the recurrence of the tumor; MRI (**a–c**) showed that the tumor had recurred, in the form of a predominantly cystic tumor in the suprasellar region. Tumor was originated from the pars distalis of the adenohypophysis and neighbored to infundibulo-tubular part of the hypothalamus and grew toward the third VF. Tumor mainly spread to the lateral fissure cistern, the middle fossa, and the left temporal lobe

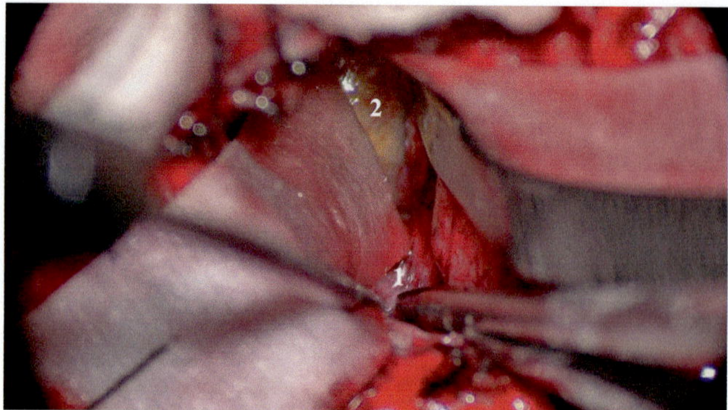

Fig. 7.67 Radical gross tumor removal (GTR) by the fronto-basal interhemispheric approach was performed in our hospital in June 2016 (6 years after the first operation). Intraoperative findings. Dissection of the arachnoidal trabecula and membrane between the two lobes to expose the sellar region. (1) Arachnoidal trabecula and membrane, (2) tumor

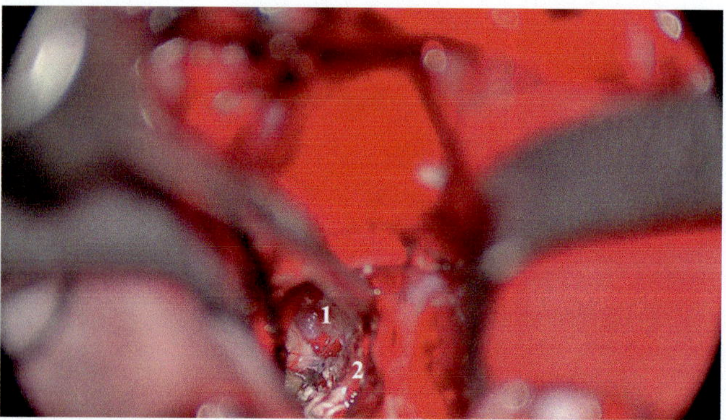

Fig. 7.68 The tumor tightly adhered to the left anterior cerebral artery, necessitating sharp dissection to release the tumor. (1) Tumor, (2) anterior cerebral artery (left)

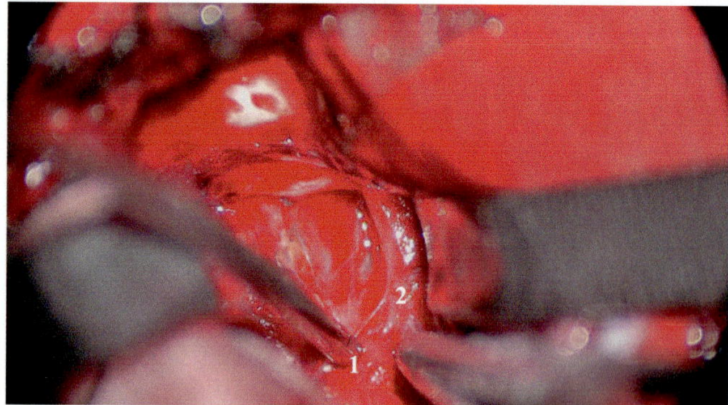

Fig. 7.69 The tumor tightly adhered to the right optic nerve, necessitating sharp dissection to release the tumor. (1) Tumor, (2) optic nerve (right)

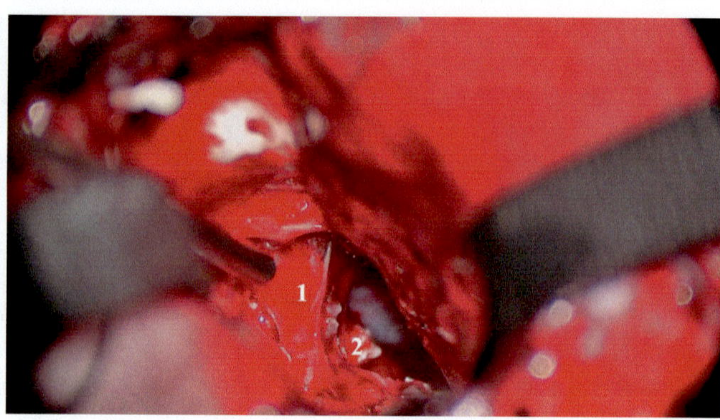

Fig. 7.70 The tumor grew through the arachnoidal sleeve segment of pituitary stalk. (1) Pituitary stalk, (2) tumor

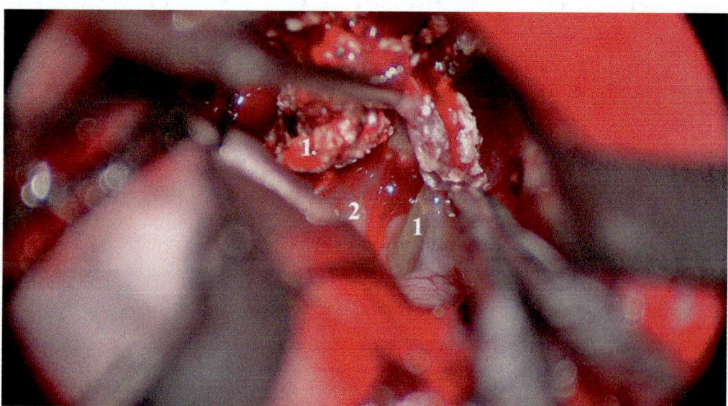

Fig. 7.71 The tumor was originated from the pars distalis of adenohypophysis and neighbored to infundibulo-tubular part of the hypothalamus. The tumor tightly adhered to the third VF and was separated from the third VF. (1) Tumor, (2) third VF

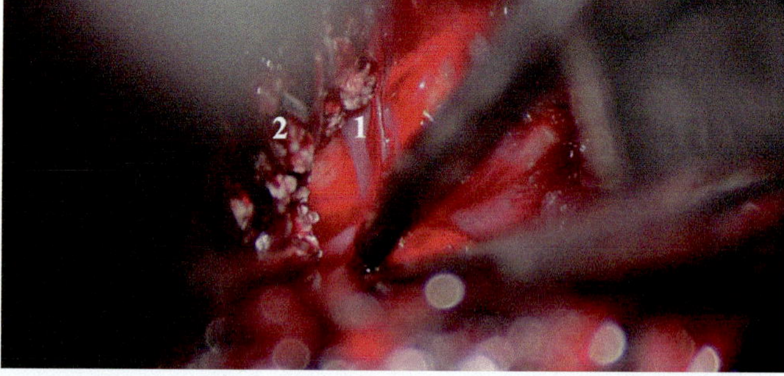

Fig. 7.72 The tumor had an intimate relationship with the basilar artery and its branches, necessitating sharp dissection to release the tumor. (1) Basilar artery and its branches, (2) tumor

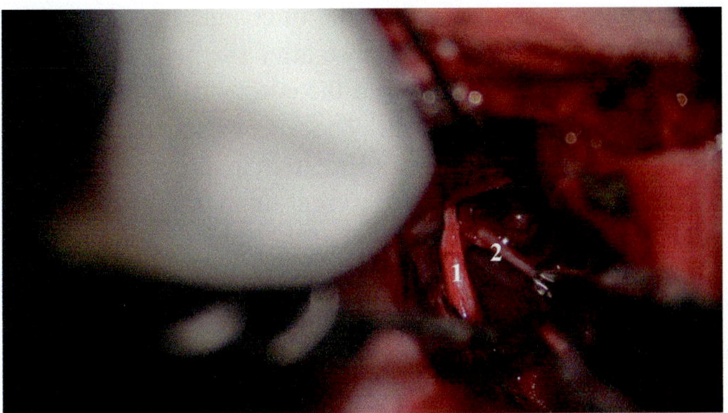

Fig. 7.73 The tumor which had spread into the left temporal lobe was separated from the ventral aspect of the left internal carotid artery. (1) Internal carotid artery (left), (2) tumor

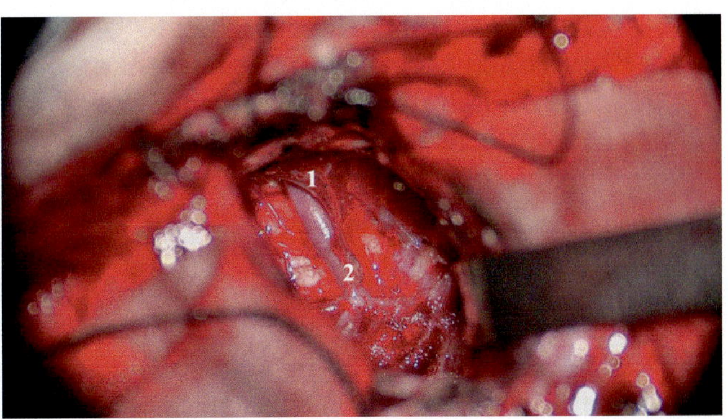

Fig. 7.74 The pituitary stalk exhibited severe tumor involvement, and it was sacrificed to avoid tumor recurrence. After total tumor removal, the neurovascular structures of the sellar region were preserved. (1) Pituitary stalk, (2) basilar artery and its branches

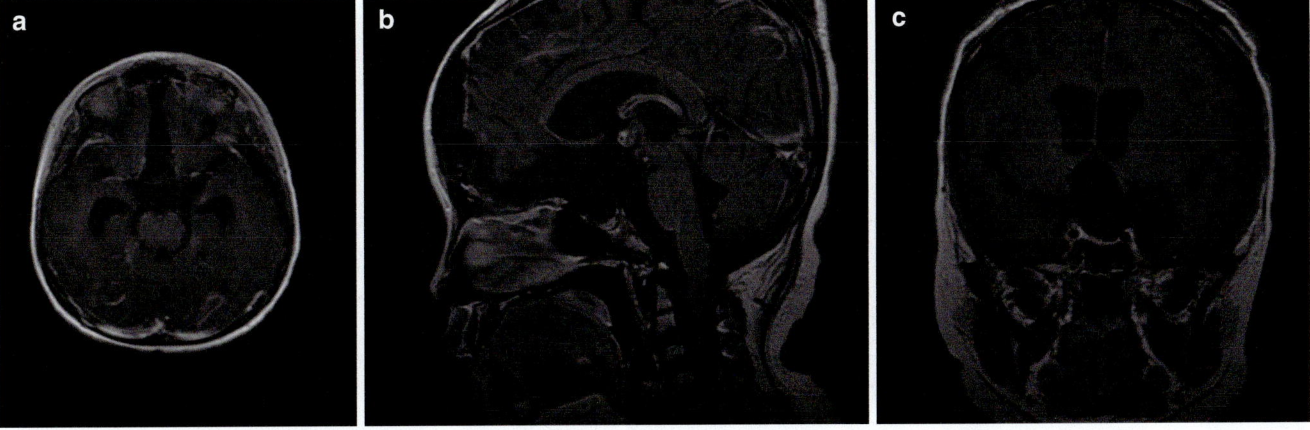

Fig. 7.75 Postoperative radiological images. (**a**–**c**) MRI indicated that total tumor removal was achieved

corridor can only provide a narrow exposure, restricting the application of transsphenoidal surgery in recurrent tumors.

For huge expanding tumors, there must be some surgical blind point; the branches of vessel might have close relationship to the tumor walls, especially in patients who relapse after a long time and when the tumor is huge. In this case, the tumor had an intimate relationship with the basilar artery and its branches, necessitating sharp dissection to release the tumor. Blindly dragging or pulling could cause vital bleeding. It was difficult to stop the bleeding under the ETS approach, and we still support the use of the transcranial approach.

For T-type CP, as the tumor grows toward the nervous tissue layer of third ventricle floor, the main nerve nucleus might be displaced downward. In such cases, opening the ventral third VF will cause severe injury to the hypothalamic function. Opening the lamina terminalis and attempting to protect the residual nervous tissue of third VF was the first choice.

However, as the surgical corridor and space were narrow, surgical manipulation was difficult at the superior part of the optical chiasm under ETS approach. Especially when the CP expanded posteriorly to a great extent, the operator might have to pull and drag the cystic wall with the results of residual partial tumor. Therefore, in our opinion, for type T recurrent CP, especially a posteriorly expanding tumor, we prefer the transcranial approach.

The origin of the tumor and surrounding membranous structure are the bases of the QST classification. Identification of different classifications of craniopharyngiomas is essential to selecting the appropriate surgical procedure and can predict operation difficulty and outcome.

7.8 Case 7: Inappropriate Surgical Approach Leads to the Recurrence of Type T Craniopharyngioma After Incomplete Tumor Resection (Figs. 7.76, 7.77, 7.78, 7.79, 7.80, 7.81, 7.82, 7.83, 7.84, 7.85, and 7.86)

From the origin of the embryo, the craniopharyngioma belongs to the tumor that originates and grows outside the pia mater. Therefore, selection of a proper approach to achieve satisfactory exposure for tumor removal is very important. In this case, the neurosurgeon mistakenly chose the transcallosal approach in the first operation. It may not be able to expose the origin site of the tumor through the transcallosal approach. Therefore, the tumor may not be totally removed, so it is easy to relapse after surgery. It is easy to damage the hypothalamus and the corpus callosum through the transcallosal approach. The recurrent tumor tightly adhered to the third VF and restricted the application of transsphenoidal surgery in recurrent tumors. The upper pole of the tumor exceeded the level of the anterior communicating artery complex, and total tumor resection by the pterional approach may be very hard to expose the tumor; therefore we selected the fronto-basal interhemispheric approach. Total tumor removal was achieved; the third VF and pituitary stalk remained intact. The patient's postoperative endocrine status was good, and no obvious hypothalamic-pituitary dysfunction happened.

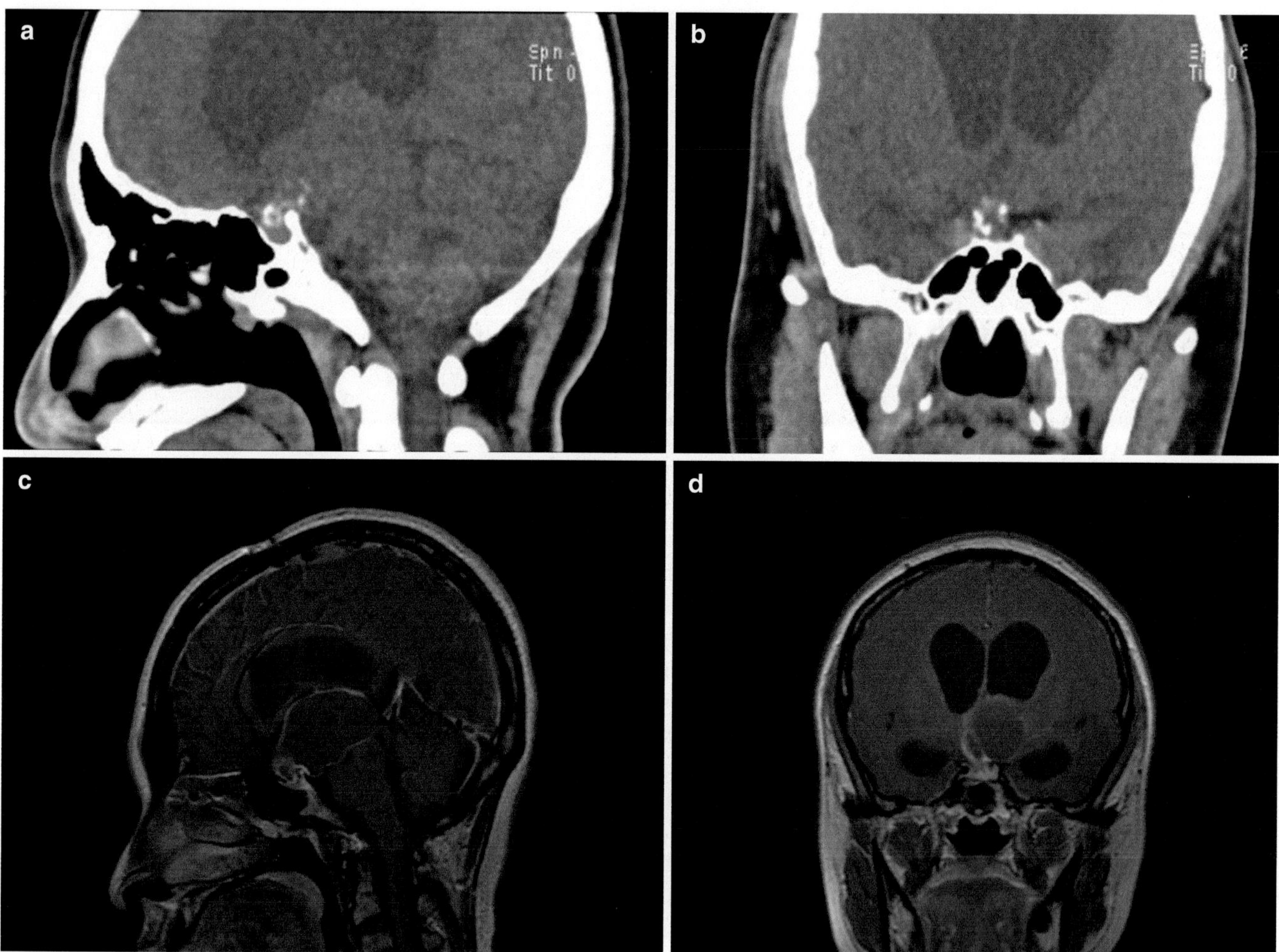

Fig. 7.76 Female, 33 years old, a type T-CP case. In March 2015, partial tumor resection by the transcallosal approach in another hospital. Postsurgical radiological images. (**a**–**d**) Two years after the operation, computed tomography and magnetic resonance imaging revealed no significant reduction in tumor volume after surgery. Tumor originated from the pars distalis of the adenohypophysis and neighbored to infundibulo-tubular part of the hypothalamus and protruded to the third VF

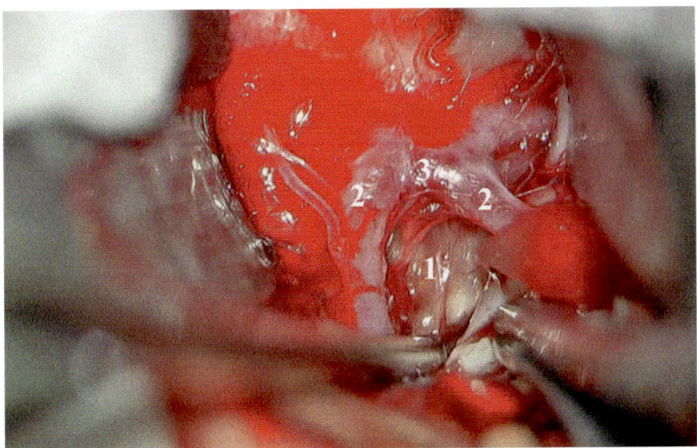

Fig. 7.77 Radical gross tumor removals (GTR) by the fronto-basal interhemispheric approach were performed in our hospital in March 2017. Intrasurgical findings. Dissect the arachnoidal trabecula and membrane between the two lobes to expose of the sellar region. The upper pole of the tumor exceeded the level of the anterior communicating artery complex (ACOAC) over more than 2 cm. (1) tumor, (2) anterior cerebral artery, (3) anterior communicating artery

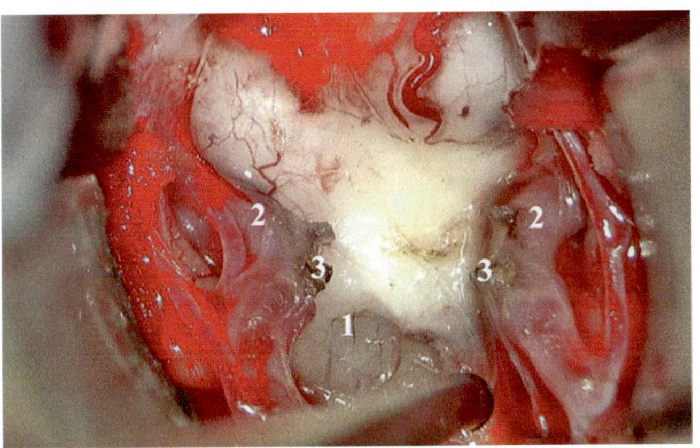

Fig. 7.78 The anterior communicating artery was divided to enhance tumor exposure. (1) Tumor, (2) anterior cerebral artery, (3) anterior communicating artery

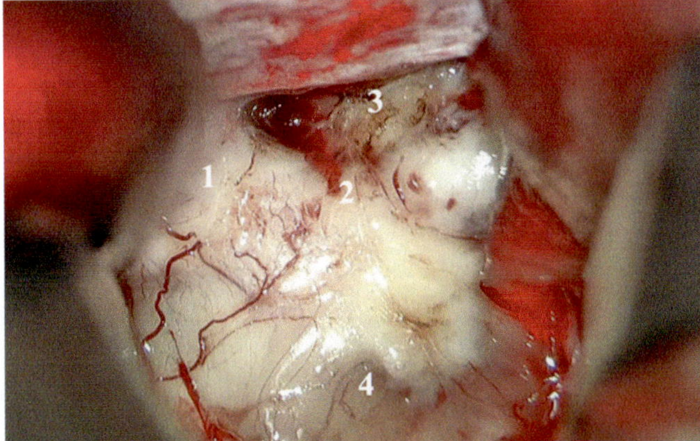

Fig. 7.79 The tumor was dissected through the pre-chiasmatic space. The tumor tightly adhered to the optic nerve and optic chiasm, necessitating sharp dissection to release the tumor. (1) Optic nerve, (2) optic chiasm, (3) tumor, (4) lamina terminalis

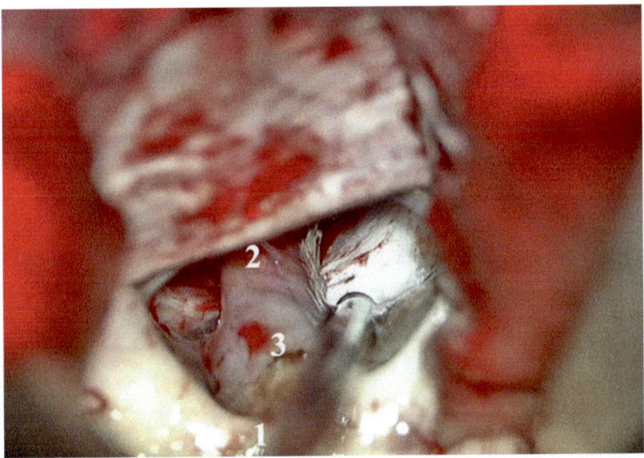

Fig. 7.80 The shape of the pituitary stalk was obviously thickened. The tumor originated from the intra-arachnoidal segment of the pituitary stalk, expanded into the arachnoidal sleeve segment, and protruded to the third VF. (1) Optic chiasm, (2) expanded arachnoidal sleeve segment of pituitary stalk, (3) tumor

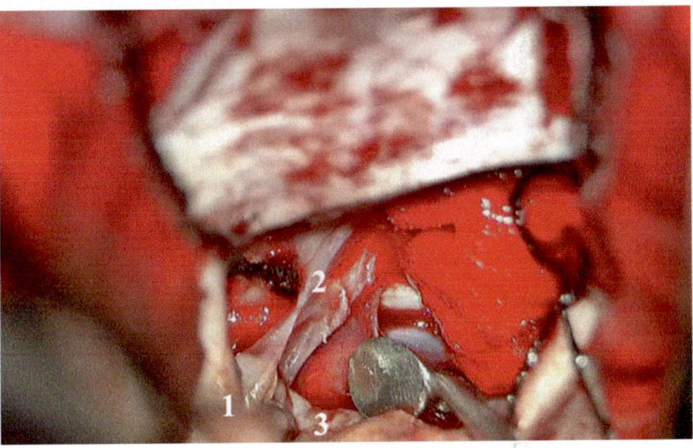

Fig. 7.81 Tumor protrudes into the arachnoidal sleeve segment of the pituitary stalk. The shape of the pituitary stalk was smooth and intact. (1) Optic nerve, (2) pituitary stalk, (3) tumor

7.9 Case 8: Small Type T Recurrent Craniopharyngioma with Severe Adhesion to Adjacent Structures (Figs. 7.87, 7.88, 7.89, 7.90, 7.91, 7.92, and 7.93)

Like the former case, although it was also a type T craniopharyngioma and the recurrent tumor was small, according to the preoperative radiological images, the tumor closely adhered to the surrounding structure, so we chose the transcranial approach. Due to the peripheral arachnoid membrane structural destruction in the first operation, the branches of the right anterior cerebral artery had close relationship

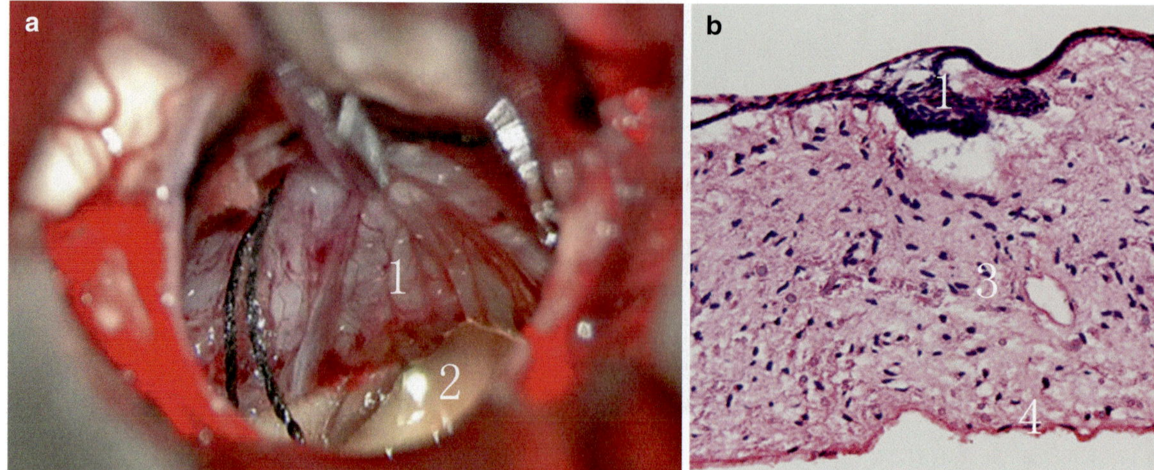

Fig. 7.82 (a) Intrasurgical findings. Open the lamina terminalis and try to separate the tumor which grew toward the nervous tissue layer of the third ventricular floor. (b) The pathological findings. The tumor tightly adhered to the third VF; the neuronal layer and the ependymal layer of the third VF were stripped together with the tumor. (1) Tumor, (2) third VF, (3) neuronal layer of the third VF, (4) ependymal layer of the third VF

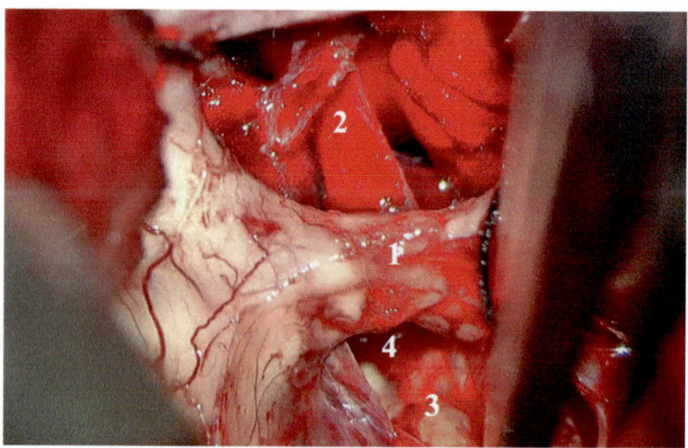

Fig. 7.83 The pituitary stalk was pushed and squeezed which shaped like a sheet by the tumor, and the tumor was pushed by brain cotton piece from the pre-chiasmatic space to the lamina terminalis space to remove the tumor. (1) Optic chiasm, (2) pituitary stalk shaped like a sheet, (3) tumor, (4) lamina terminalis space

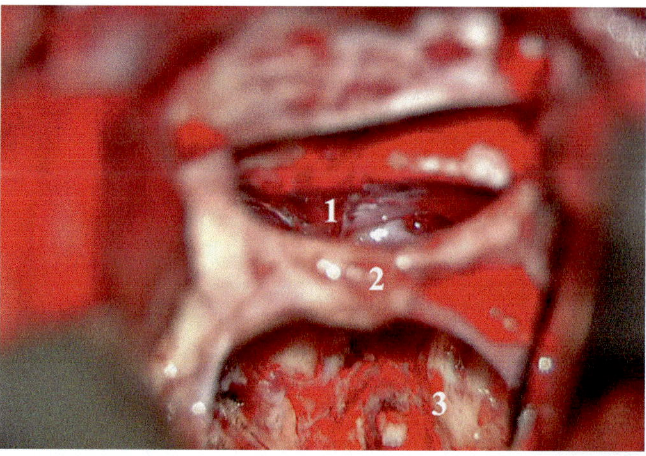

Fig. 7.84 After total tumor removal, the neurovascular structures of the sellar region were preserved. The third VF, mammillary body, and pituitary stalk were preserved. (1) Pituitary stalk, (2) optic chiasm, (3) mammillary body

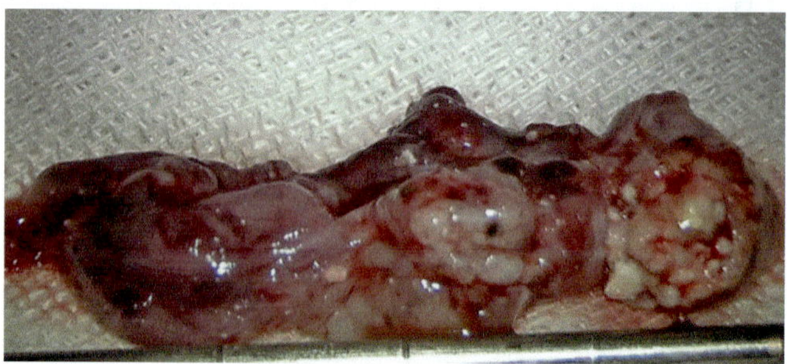

Fig. 7.85 The tumor sample showed that the tumor was en bloc removed

with the tumor, necessitating sharp dissection to release the tumor; even small recurrent tumors required complex procedures and thus blindly dragging or pulling could cause vital bleeding. It was difficult to stop the bleeding under ETS approach. Because the tumor adheres closely to peripheral structures, transsphenoidal surgery is more likely to damage the hypothalamus and pituitary. Therefore, the transcranial approach is suitable for most cases of T-type recurrent CP and is the only option.

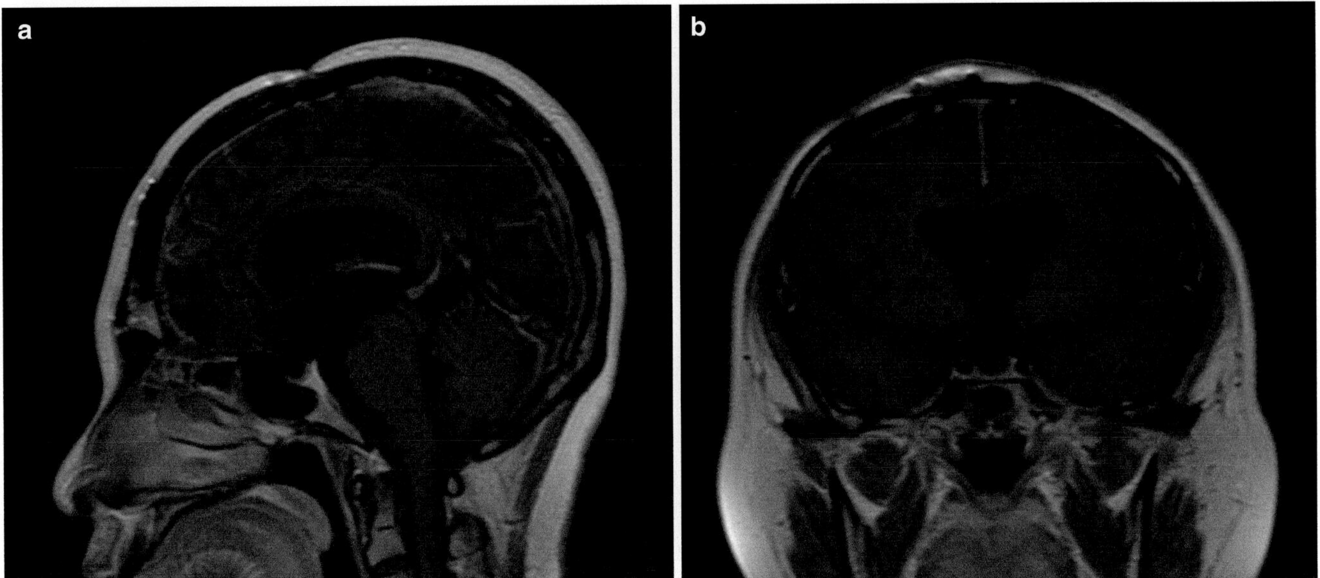

Fig. 7.86 Postsurgical radiological images. (**a**, **b**) MRI indicated that total tumor removal was achieved; the third VF and pituitary stalk remained intact

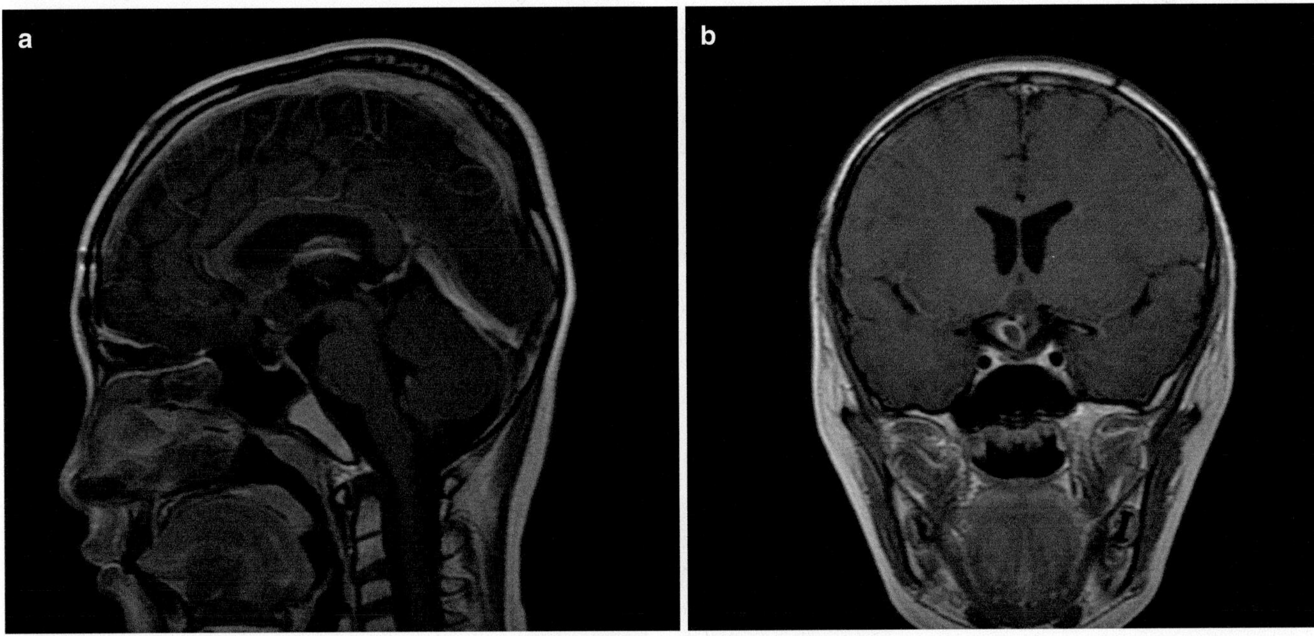

Fig. 7.87 Male, 8 years old, a type T-CP case. Radical gross tumor removals (GTR) by the fronto-basal interhemispheric approach were performed in another hospital in 2016. In June 2017, MRI (**a**, **b**) showed the recurrence of the tumor

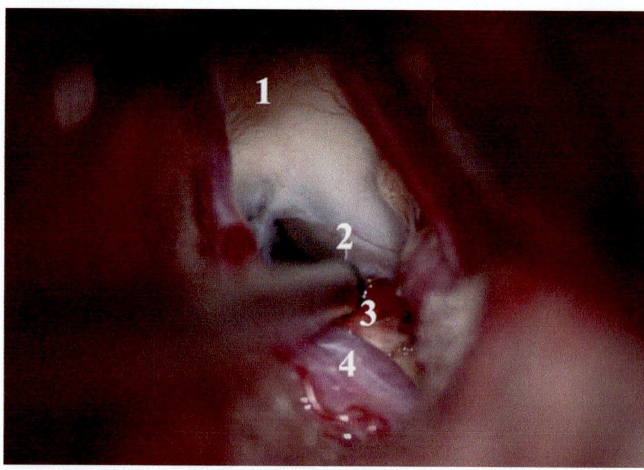

Fig. 7.88 Radical gross tumor removals (GTR) by the fronto-basal interhemispheric approach were performed in our hospital in June 2017. Intraoperative findings. The tumor mainly expanded from the lamina terminalis space. (1) Optic chiasm, (2) lamina terminalis, (3) tumor, (4) anterior cerebral artery

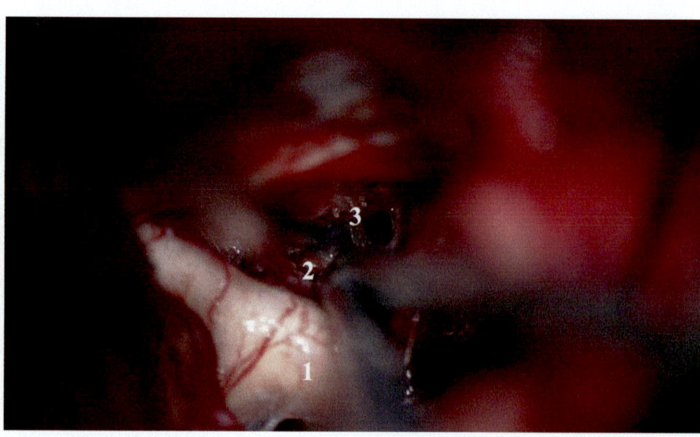

Fig. 7.91 The tumor was dissected through the pre-chiasmatic space. (1) Optic chiasm, (2) pre-chiasmatic space, (3) pituitary stalk

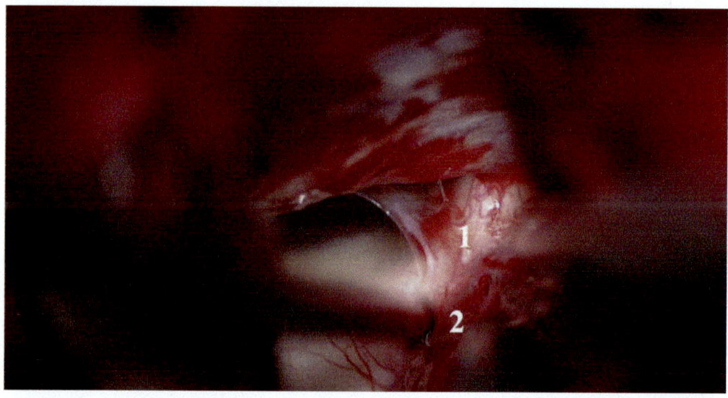

Fig. 7.89 The tumor tightly adhered to the right optic nerve and optic chiasm, necessitating sharp dissection to release the tumor. (1) Optic nerve (right), (2) tumor

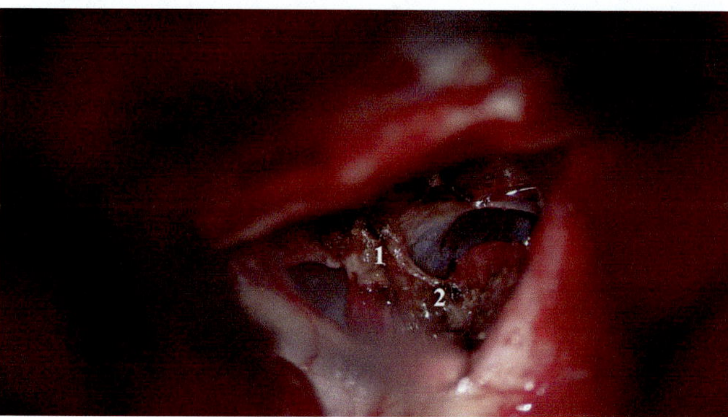

Fig. 7.92 The pituitary stalk was split vertically to expose the tumor. The right side of the pituitary stalk exhibited severe tumor involvement, and it was sharply dissected; the left side of the pituitary stalk remained intact. (1) Pituitary stalk, (2) tumor

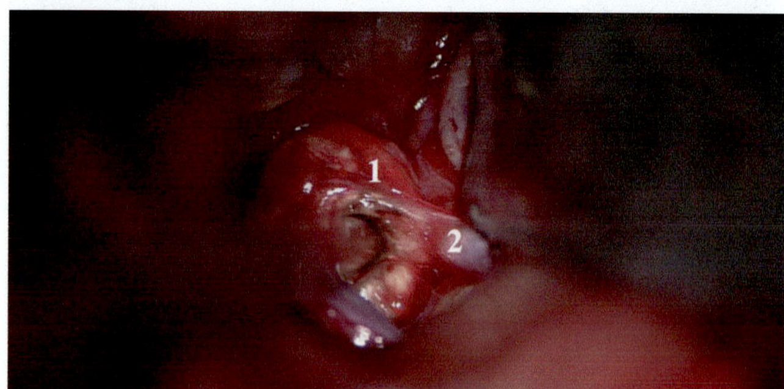

Fig. 7.90 The tumor tightly adhered to the right anterior cerebral artery, necessitating sharp dissection by multiple directions to release the tumor. (1) Tumor, (2) anterior cerebral artery

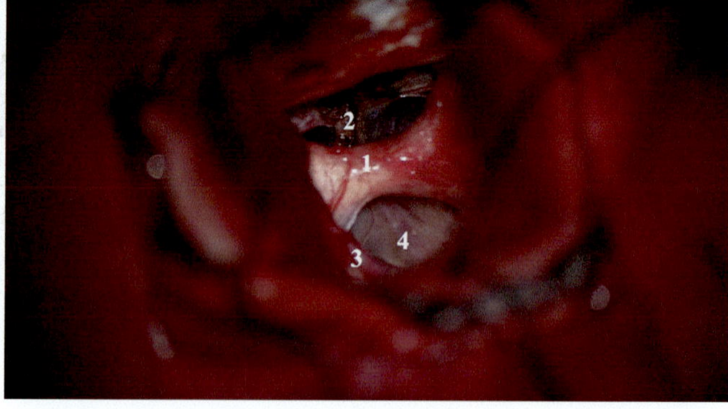

Fig. 7.93 After total tumor removal, the neurovascular structures of the sellar region were preserved. (1) Optic chiasm, (2) pituitary stalk, (3) anterior cerebral artery, (4) third VF

7.10 Case 9: Resection of Type T Recurrent Craniopharyngioma by the Extended Transsphenoidal Approach (Figs. 7.94, 7.95, 7.96, 7.97, 7.98, 7.99, 7.100, and 7.101)

It is difficult to radical gross remove of type T recurrent craniopharyngioma by the expand the transsphenoidal approach. In this case, by reviewing the patient's first surgical procedure and preoperative and postoperative imaging data, we learned that the patient had only received partial tumor resection and biopsy in the first operation, the peripheral membrane structure basically remained, and the patient's tumor recurrence interval was short; therefore, we selected the extended transsphenoidal approach (ETS). For T-type CP, without extreme expansion to the frontal and temporal lobes or posterior cranial fossa, we could select the extended transsphenoidal approach (ETS). The ventral anterior exposure provided easy exposure to the ventral aspect of the optic chiasm and pituitary stalk. As the tumor was located ventrally to the optic chiasm, ETS could avoid the retraction of nerves.

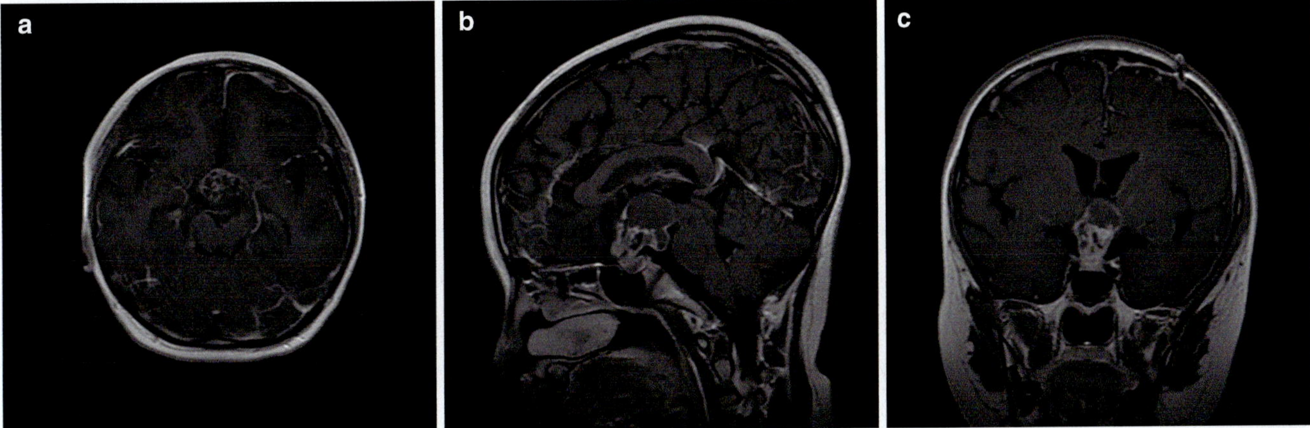

Fig. 7.94 Male, 10 years old, a type T-CP case. In March 2018, partial tumor resection and biopsy by the left-side pterional approach was performed in another hospital. Preoperative radiological images. (**a–c**) MRI revealed a patient with a tumor in the intrasellar and suprasellar regions. Figure **c** showed the surgical incision of the left-side pterional approach

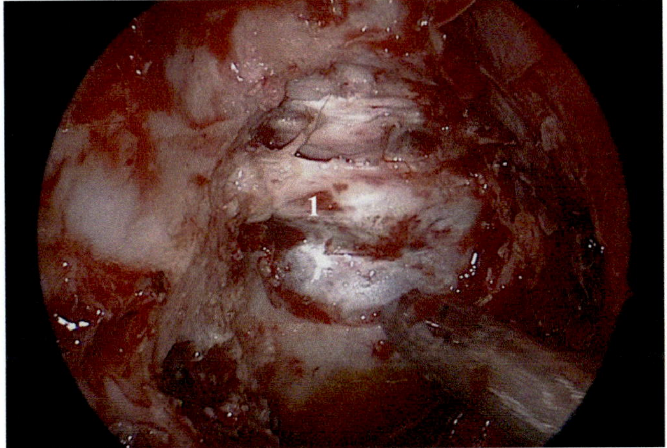

Fig. 7.95 Radical gross tumor removal by the extended transsphenoidal approach (ETS) was performed in our hospital in June 2018 (3 months after the biopsy). Intraoperative findings. The ETS approach for type T-CP removal requires extensive exposure of the sellar region, especially the anterior extension of the tuberculum sellae. (1) Dura

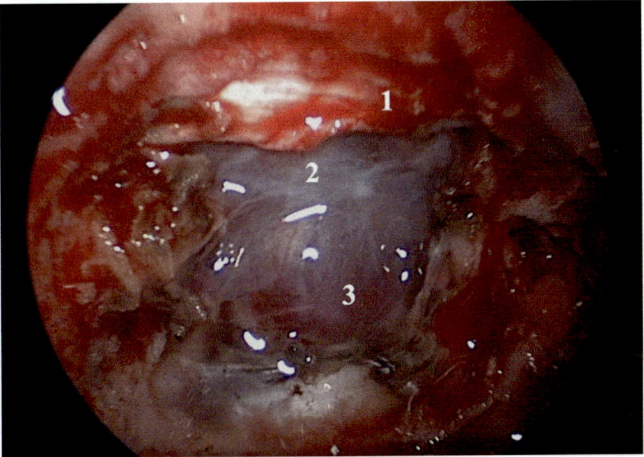

Fig. 7.96 The basal membrane was intact; it showed that the tumor was in the arachnoidal sleeve segment of the pituitary stalk. (1) Dura, (2) basal arachnoidal membrane (outer arachnoid), (3) pituitary stalk

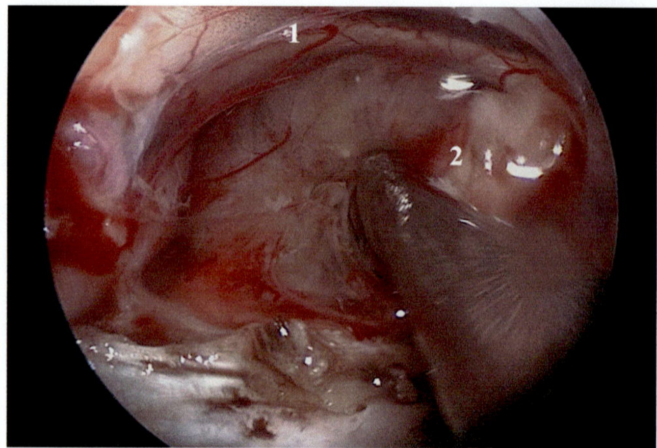

Fig. 7.97 The tumor was separated from the surrounding neurovascular structures along the suprasellar arachnoid interface. (1) Optic chiasm, (2) tumor

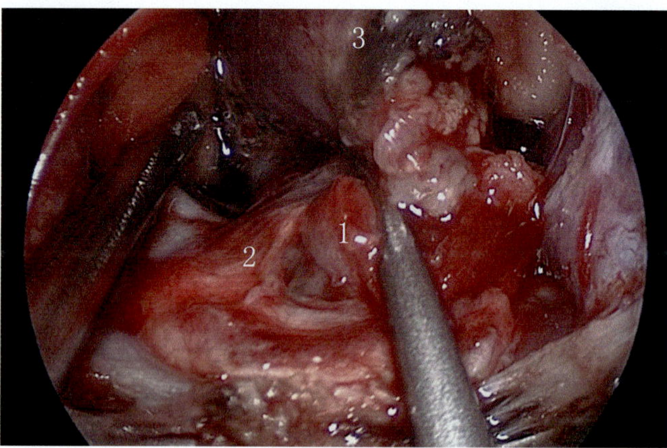

Fig. 7.98 The tumor grew along the arachnoidal sleeve of the pituitary stalk and broke through the foramen of the diaphragma sellae from the suprasellar region to the intrasellar region. (1) Tumor, (2) diaphragma sellae, (3) origin site of the tumor

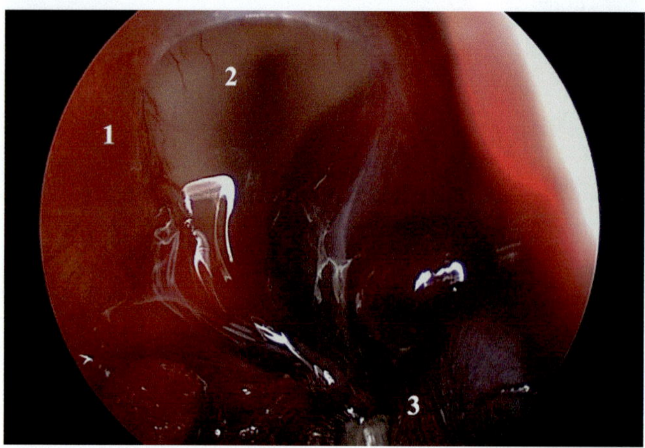

Fig. 7.99 Opened the thinner third VF to ensure radical gross tumor removal. (1) Third VF, (2) the third ventricle, (3) tumor

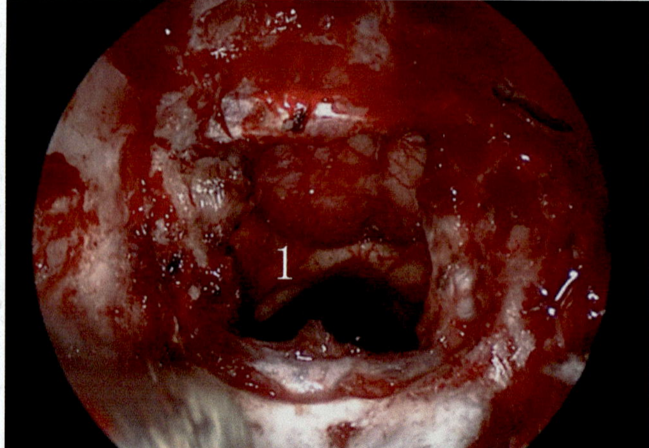

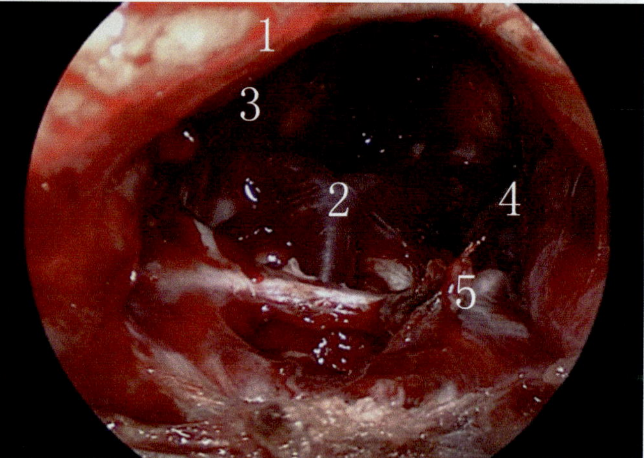

Fig. 7.100 Tumor was originated from the pars distalis of the adenohypophysis and neighbored to infundibulo-tubular part of the hypothalamus. After total tumor removal, the neurovascular structures of the sellar region were preserved. The pituitary stalk exhibited severe tumor involvement, and it was sacrificed to avoid tumor recurrence. (1) Optic nerve and optic chiasm, (2) basilar artery and its branches, (3) third VF, (4) internal carotid artery, (5) residual pituitary stalk

7.11 Case 10: The Treatment of a Type T Craniopharyngioma Which Continued to Progress and Could Not Be Controlled Without Operation After Repeated Radiotherapy, Cystic Fluid Aspiration, and Internal Irradiation (Figs. 7.102, 7.103, 7.104, 7.105, 7.106, and 7.107)

Radiotherapy, cystic fluid aspiration, and internal irradiation remain in common use for treatment of craniopharyngioma. However, the recurrence is inevitable for patients with long-term survival, and radiotherapy might induce disturbances in hypothalamic-pituitary function, which lead to a poor life quality. Direct neuronal damage caused by ionizing radiation followed by degeneration and death is the current pre-

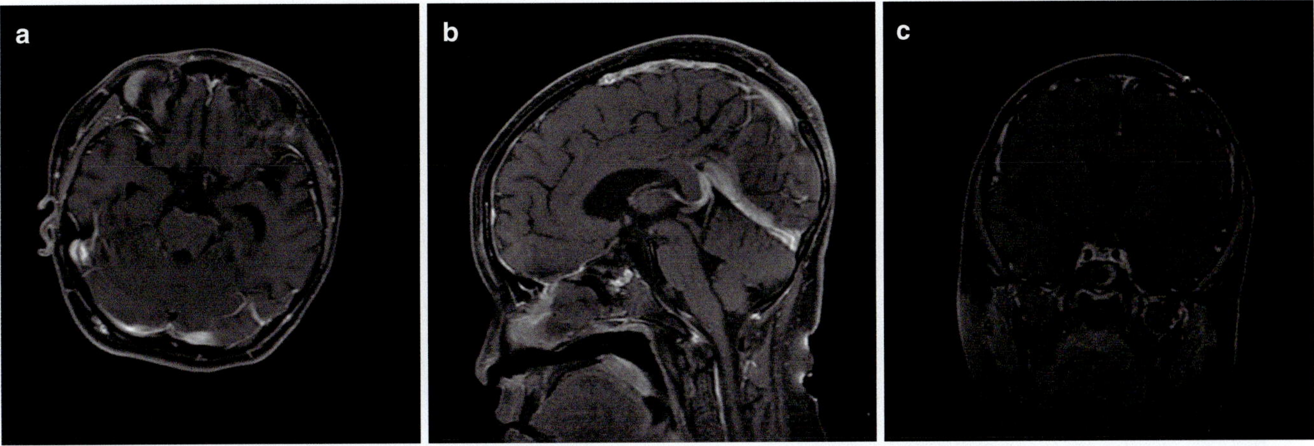

Fig. 7.101 Postoperative MRI (**a**, **b**) showed that total tumor removal was achieved. The neurohypophysis and partial adenohypophysis were preserved

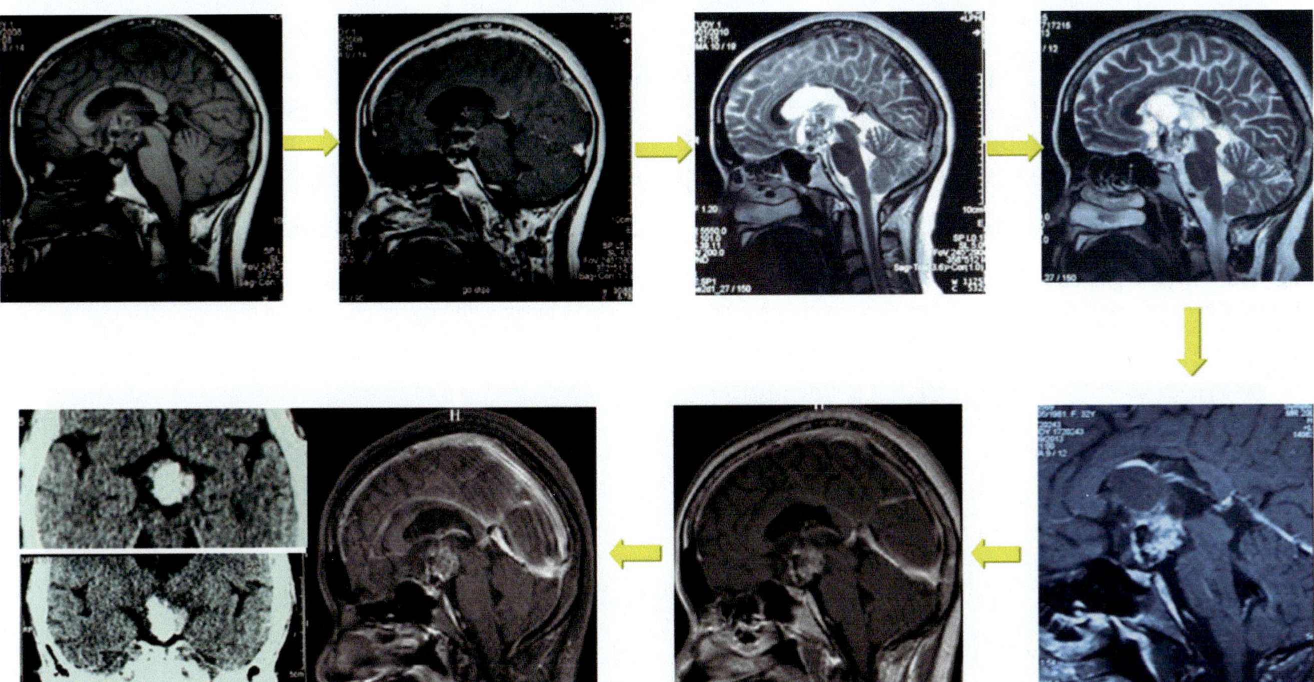

Fig. 7.102 Female, 23 years old, a type T-CP case. The patient had received treatments ten times including radiotherapy, cystic fluid aspiration, and internal irradiation before surgery in another hospital, but the tumor continued to progress, and the patient suffered from behavioral, cognitive, endocrine, and visual disturbances. The patient was bedridden and lost consciousness due to the hypothalamic-pituitary dysfunction. Preoperative radiological images revealed the tumor continued to progress in suprasellar region

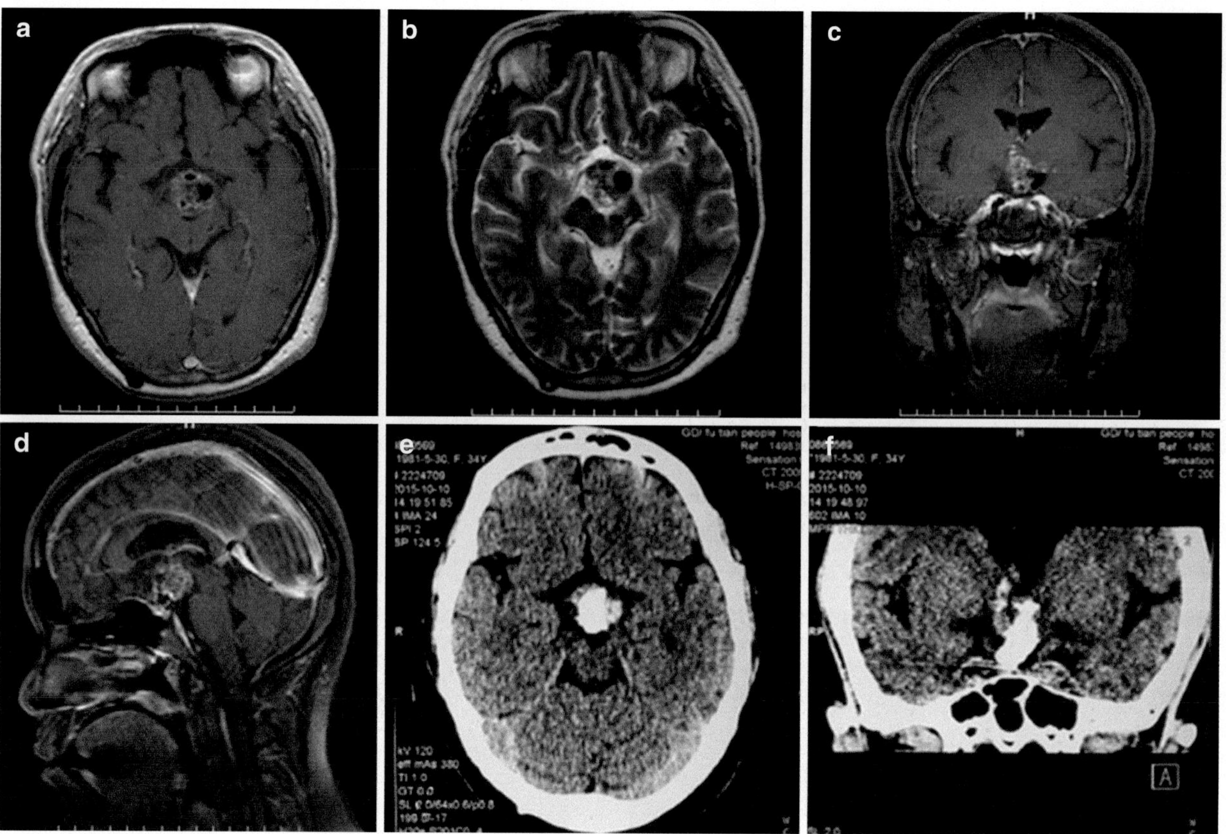

Fig. 7.103 Radical gross tumor removal (GTR) via the fronto-basal interhemispheric approach was performed in our hospital in January 2016. Preoperative radiological images. (**a**–**f**) Computed tomography and MRI revealed a tumor with large calcification in the suprasellar region

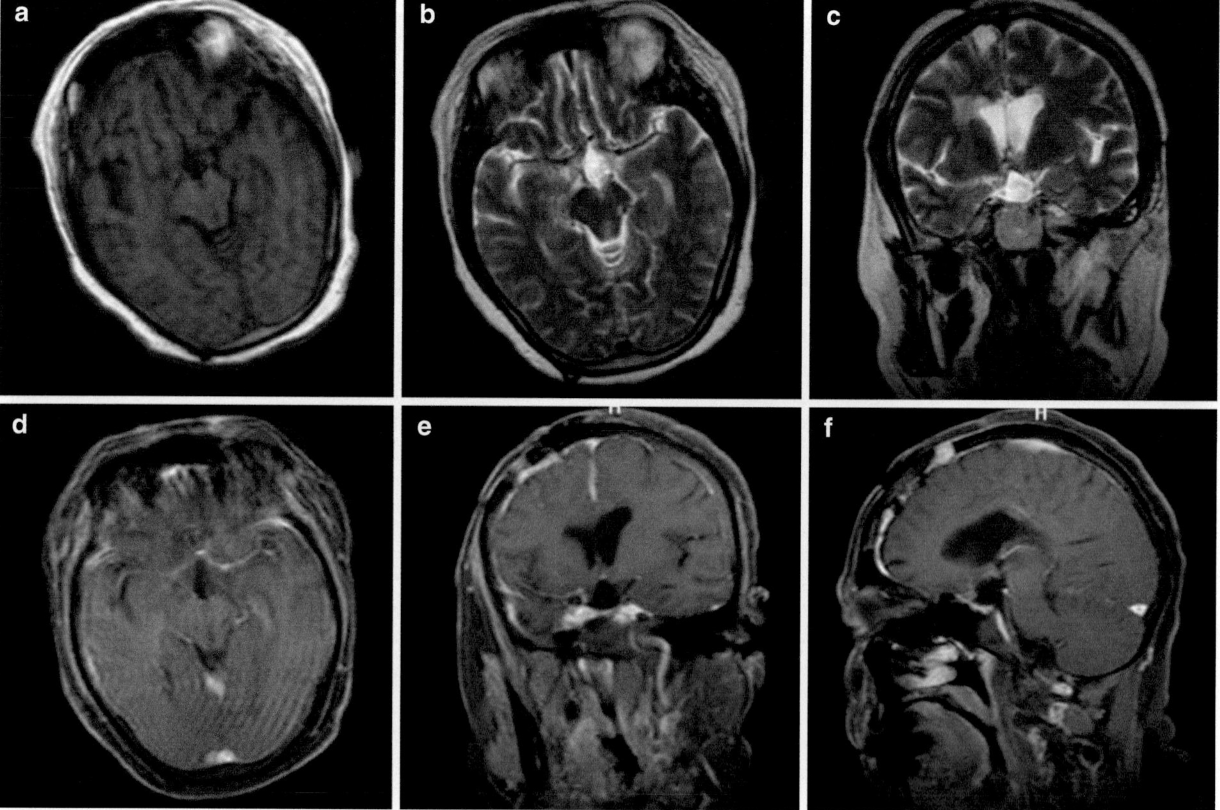

Fig. 7.104 Postoperative radiological images. (**a**–**f**) MRI indicated total tumor removal

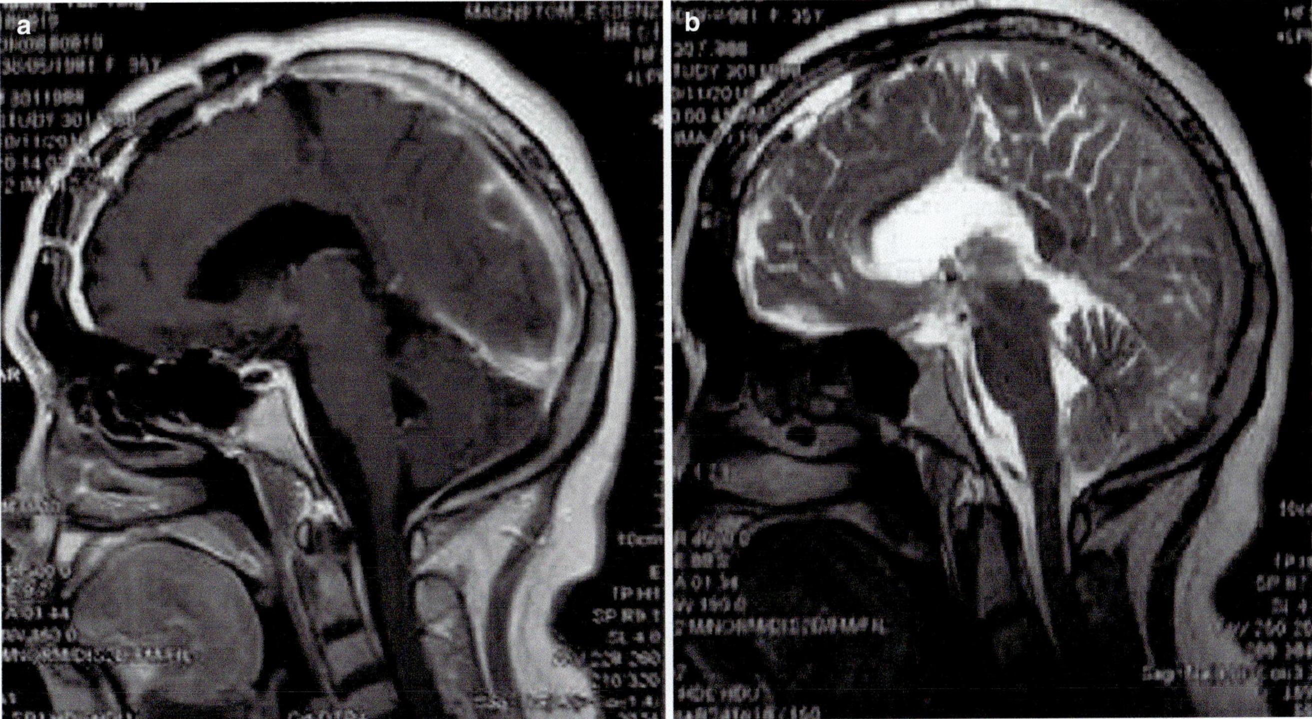

Fig. 7.105 Postoperative radiological images (1 year after the operation). (**a**, **b**) MRI indicated that total tumor removal was achieved and no recurrence of the tumor

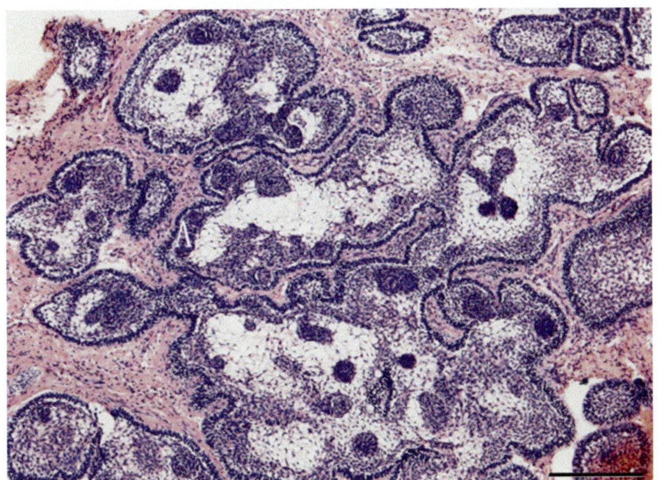

Fig. 7.106 The pathological findings. Radiotherapy caused the tumor to exhibit a typical morphological change: a large number of whirl-like cells appeared, which might cause tumor retaliatory growth

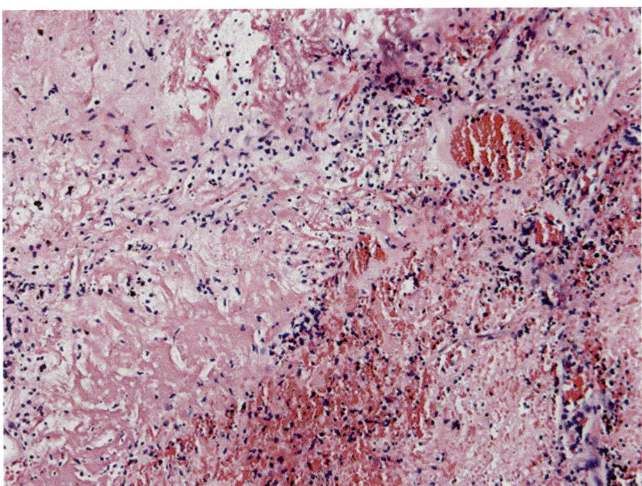

Fig. 7.107 The pathological findings. Radiotherapy caused the hypothalamus around the tumor to lack normal neural structure and a large amount of necrosis occurred

ferred theory. This patient suffered from behavioral, cognitive, endocrine, and visual disturbances. The patient was bedridden and lost consciousness due to hypothalamic-pituitary dysfunction before surgery. The authors have a clear view that craniopharyngioma is a surgical disease and radical surgical resection is the only possible cure for patients.

Radiotherapy caused the tumor to exhibit a typical morphological change: a large number of whirl-like cells appeared, which might cause tumor retaliatory growth. The morphological change may explain the reason the tumor continued to progress after ten times of therapy.

Neurosurgeons need to understand that once a patient received radiotherapy and chemotherapy and cystic fluid aspiration and internal irradiation and intracapsular chemotherapy, it means that the patient has lost the possibility of true cure and high-quality survival.

Radiotherapy causes the gliotic layer around the craniopharyngioma to become sparse or even missing. The loss of gliotic layer leads to increased risk of hypothalamic damage. The operation of recurrent craniopharyngioma is more difficult, but the prognosis is not necessarily worse. This patient has survived for more than 6 years through GTR combined with postoperative endocrine therapy.

7.12 Case 11: The Treatment of an S-Type Recurrent Craniopharyngioma Which Was Treated with Ommaya Reservoir (Figs. 7.108, 7.109, 7.110, 7.111, and 7.112)

Although subtotal resection and adjuvant radiotherapy and ommaya reservoir placement surgery can delay the tumor progression, these ways are conservative treatments that can't cure tumors. The recurrence is inevitable for patients with long-term survival. The common complications of

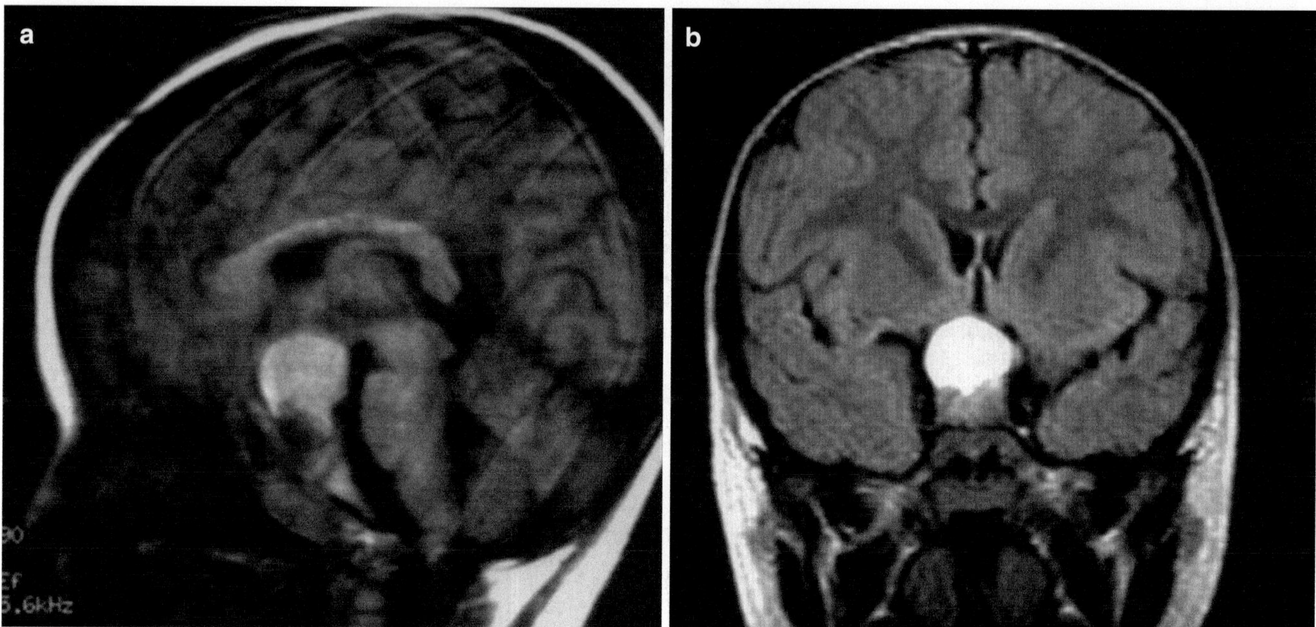

Fig. 7.108 Male, 7 years old, a type S-CP case. Preoperative radiological images (**a**, **b**) revealed a predominantly cystic tumor in the suprasellar region

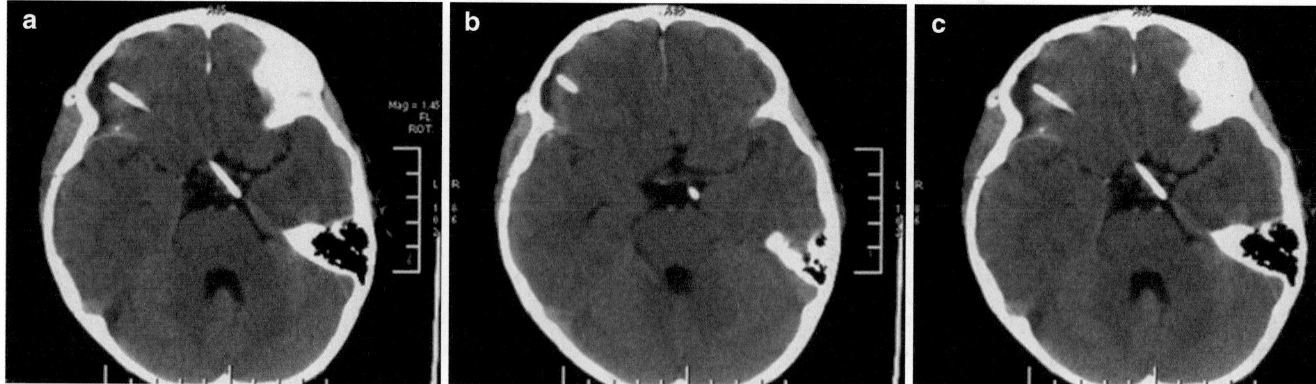

Fig. 7.109 In March 2009, partial tumor resection via the right-side pterional approach and ommaya reservoir placement surgery and cystic fluid aspiration and intracapsular chemoradiotherapy were performed in another hospital. Postoperative radiological images. (**a**–**c**) CT revealed patient with residual tumor in suprasellar region

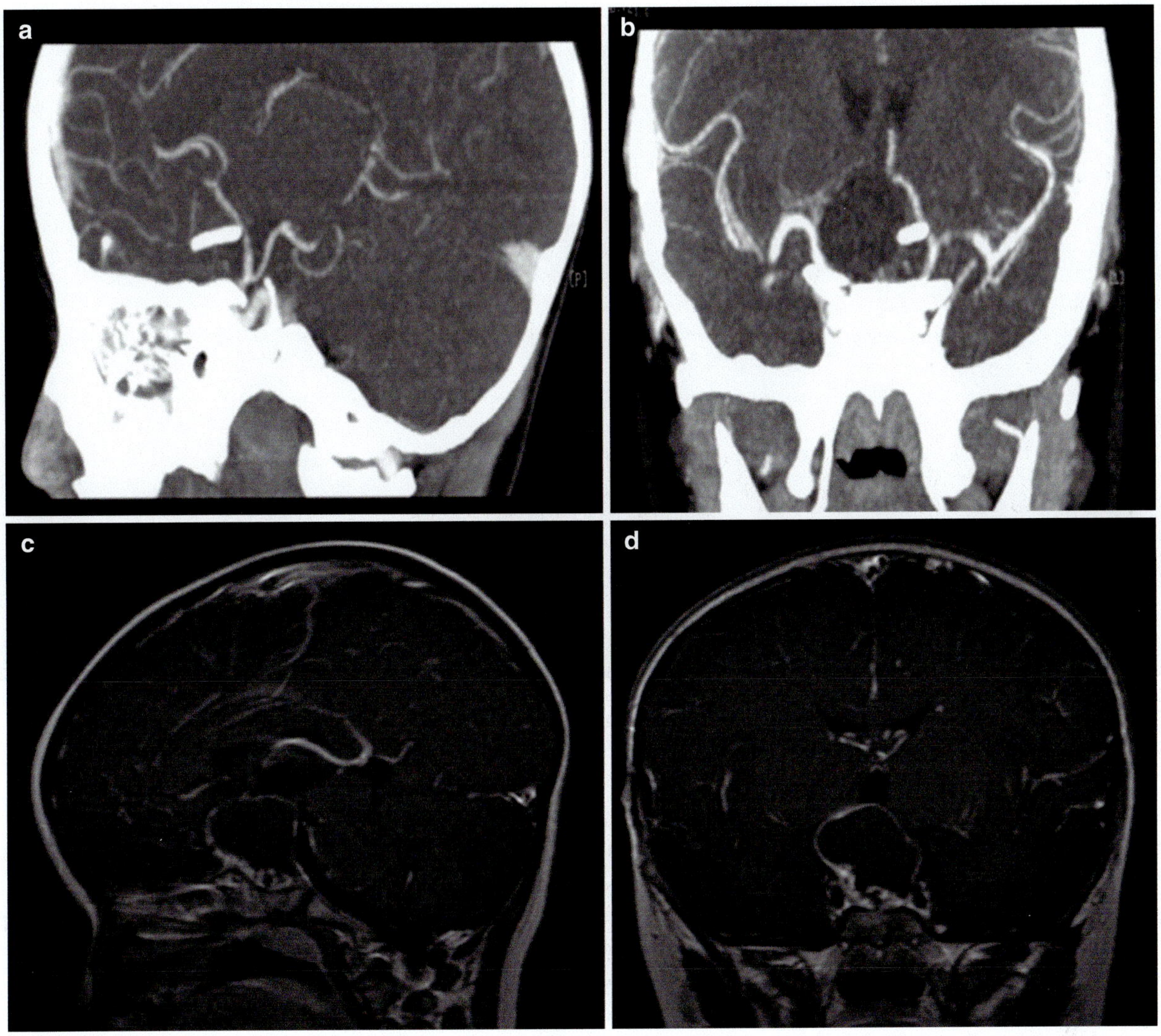

Fig. 7.110 In November 2009, the ommaya reservoir was blocked. (**a**–**d**) CT and MRI showed the tumor continued to progress

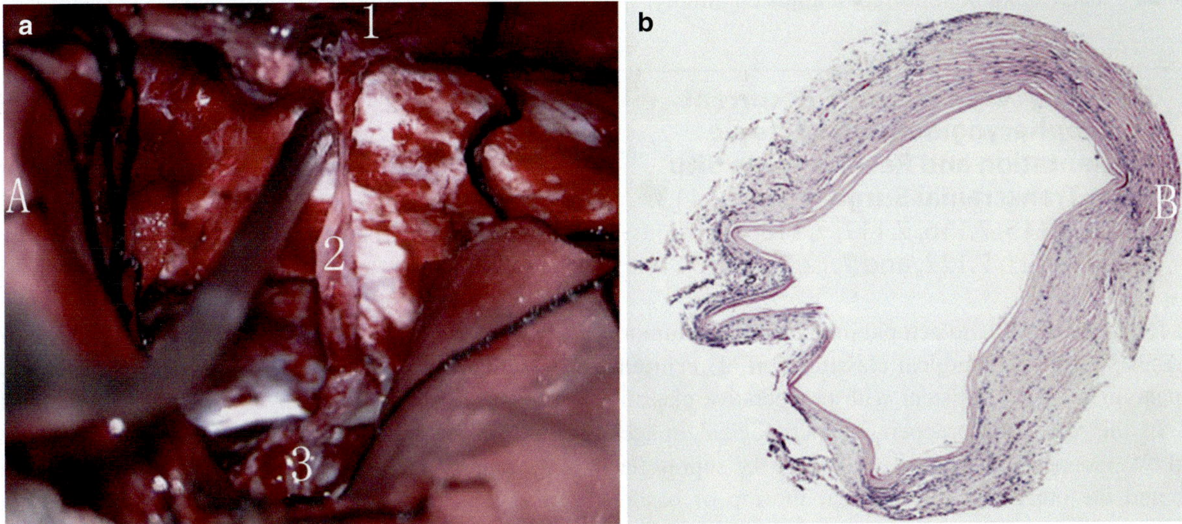

Fig. 7.111 Radical gross tumor removal via the fronto-basal interhemispheric approach was performed in our hospital in November 2009. (**a**) Intrasurgical findings. The drainage tube of the ommaya reservoir was blocked. The drainage tube was wrapped by the tubelike structure from the dura mater to the tumor and tightly adhered to the tumor and peripheral blood vessels and nerves. (**b**) The pathological findings. The fibrous connective tissue composed of the tubelike structure. (1) Dura mater, (2) the tubelike structure, (3) tumor

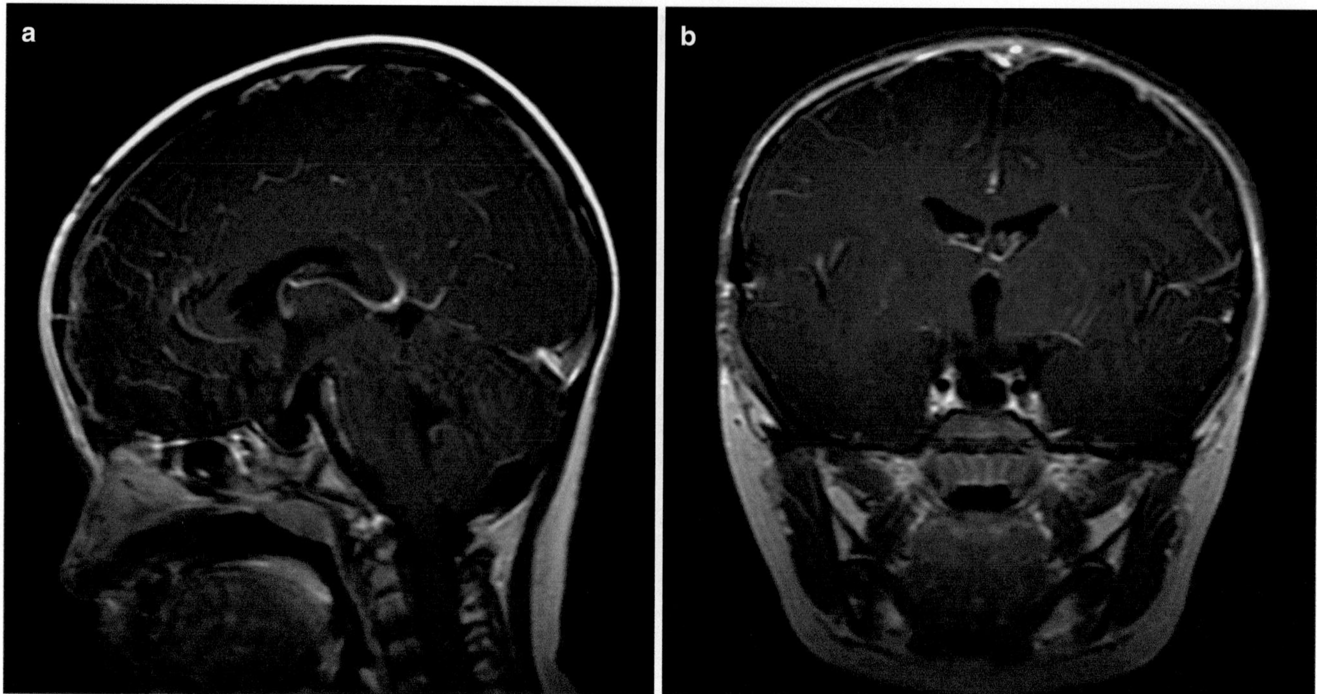

Fig. 7.112 Postsurgical radiological images (3 years after the operation). (**a**, **b**) MRI indicated that total tumor removal was achieved and no recurrence of the tumor

ommaya reservoir placement surgery and cystic fluid aspiration include block of the drainage tube, displacement of the drainage tube, etc., which may lead to surgical failure. In this case, the drainage tube tightly adhered to the tumor and peripheral blood vessels and nerves; blindly dragging or pulling could cause vital bleeding. The separation of the drainage tube and the adhesions of the surrounding structure was required to safely remove the drainage tube. We recommend that when the drainage tube is blocked or dislocated, the drainage tube cannot be removed or adjusted blindly.

7.13 Case 12: A Case of Type T Recurrent Craniopharyngioma with Ectopic Implantation and Recurrence In Situ After Transcranial Surgery (Figs. 7.113, 7.114, 7.115, 7.116, 7.117, 7.118, 7.119, 7.120, 7.121, 7.122, and 7.123)

Except for rare cases due to ectopic implantation of tumors in previous surgery, the surgical classification of recurrent craniopharyngioma is consistent with preoperative classification. In this case, the preoperative radiological images showed two independent tumors; one was in the suprasellar region, and the other was located near the top of basilar artery. By reviewing the patient's preoperative and postoperative imaging data of the previous four operations, we learned that the tumor near the top of basilar artery was ectopic implantation in the first operation. We believed that ectopic implantation was related to the doctor's improper operation and the tumor should be completely removed along the tumor boundary and repeated washing of the surgical field to prevent tumor cell residue can avoid ectopic implantation.

The origin site of the recurrent tumor in the suprasellar region was consistent with the preoperation.

The first operation was performed via the right-side pterional approach. Radical gross tumor removal via the frontobasal interhemispheric approach was selected in order to avoid adhesion of the surrounding structure caused by the previous three surgical approaches. The arachnoidal sleeve segment of the pituitary stalk was destructed in the previous operation. The pituitary stalk exhibited severe tumor involvement in recurrent tumor, and it was sacrificed to avoid tumor recurrence. After total tumor removal, the neurovascular structures of the sellar region were preserved.

Radiotherapy, cystic fluid aspiration, and internal irradiation remain in common use for treatment craniopharyngioma. The aim of radiotherapy is to achieve long-term disease control in patients lacking complete removal or with recurrent tumors. However radiotherapy might induce disturbances in hypothalamic-pituitary function. The nature of radiation-induced damage to the hypothalamic-pituitary axis is not fully understood. Direct neuronal damage caused by

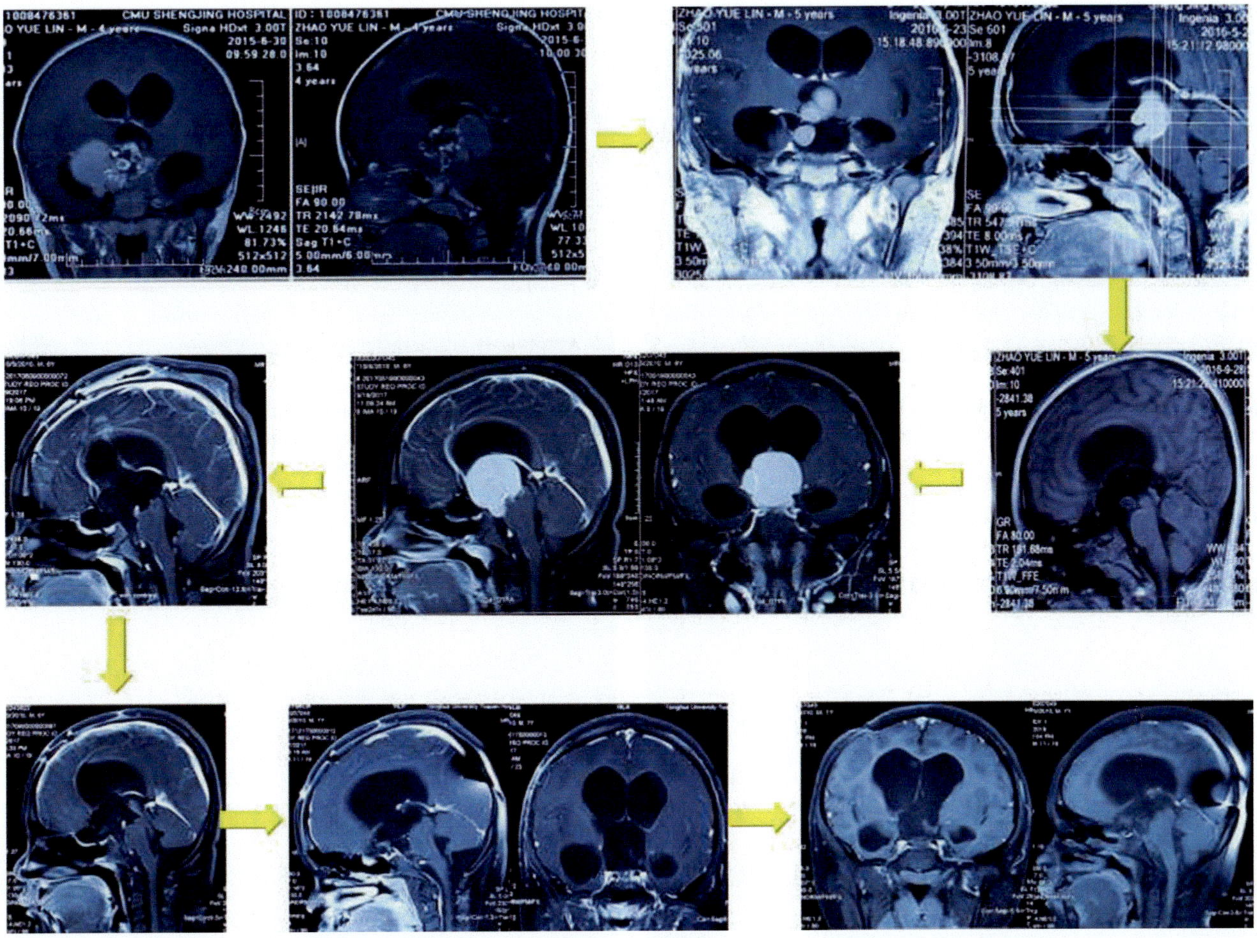

Fig. 7.113 Male, 8 years old, a type T-CP case. Partial tumor resection via the right-side pterional approach was performed in May 2015 in another hospital. Due to repeated recurrence of the tumor, three more operations were performed in the following 3 years, but the tumor continued to progress, and the vision decreased. The patient was unable to take care of herself due to hypothalamic-pituitary dysfunction. Preoperative radiological images revealed the tumor continued to progress in suprasellar region

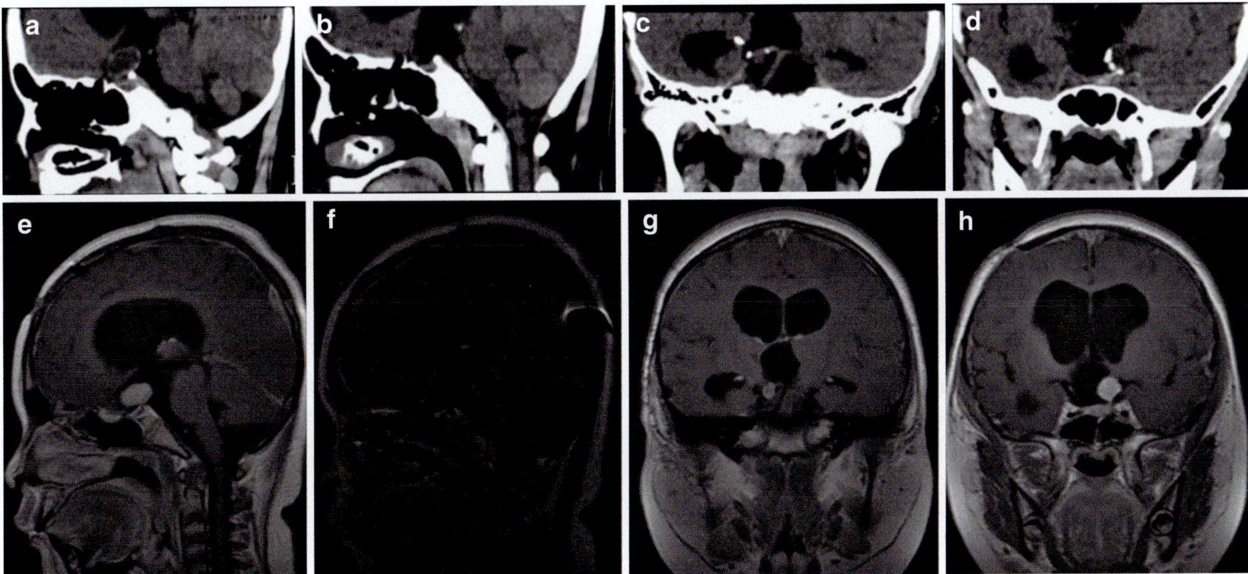

Fig. 7.114 Radical gross tumor removal (GTR) via the fronto-basal interhemispheric approach was performed in our hospital in October 2018. Preoperative radiological images (**a**–**h**) CT and MRI showed two independent tumors; one was in the suprasellar region, and the other was located near the top of basilar artery

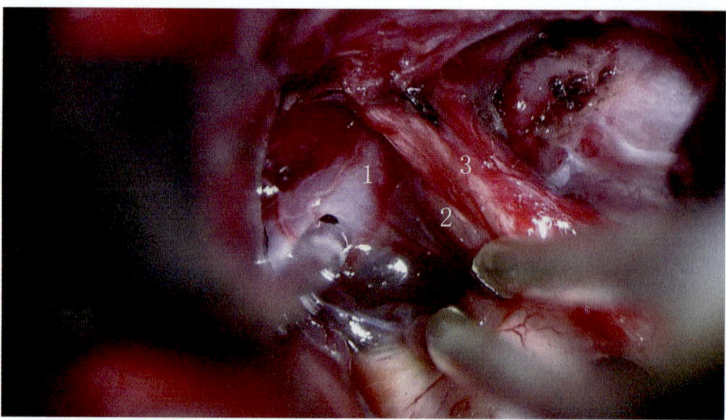

Fig. 7.115 The tumor tightly adhered to the optic nerve, internal carotid artery, and its branches. (1) Internal carotid artery and its branches, (2) tumor, (3) optic nerve

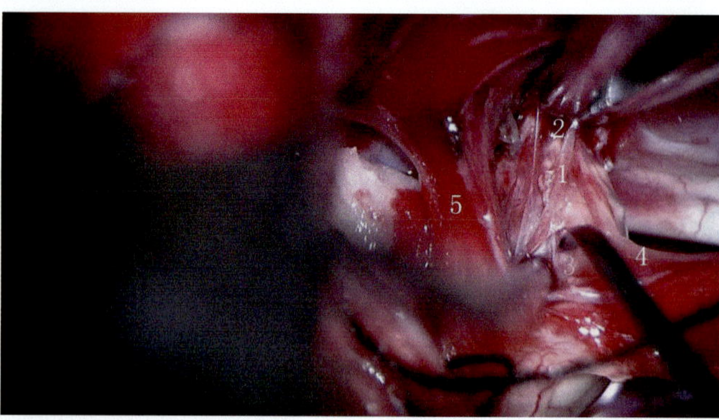

Fig 7.118 The tumor grew through the arachnoidal sleeve segment of pituitary stalk. The pituitary stalk exhibited severe tumor involvement and it was sacrificed to avoid tumor recurrence. (1) The arachnoidal sleeve of pituitary stalk, (2) tumor, (3) origin site of the tumor, (4) third VF, (5) optic nerve (left side)

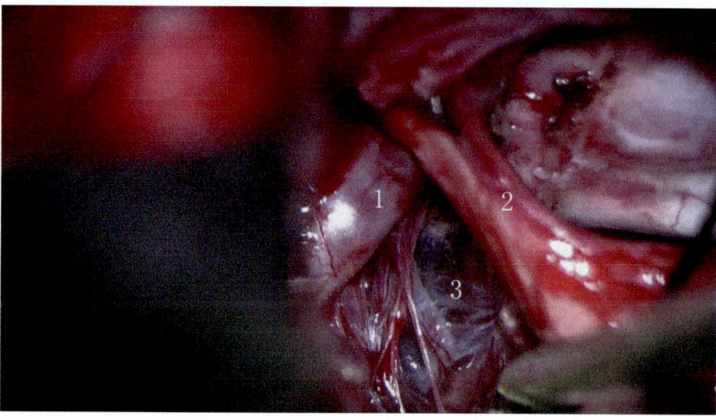

Fig. 7.116 The tumor was dissected through the optic-internal carotid artery space. (1) Internal carotid artery, (2) optic nerve, (3) Liliequist membrane

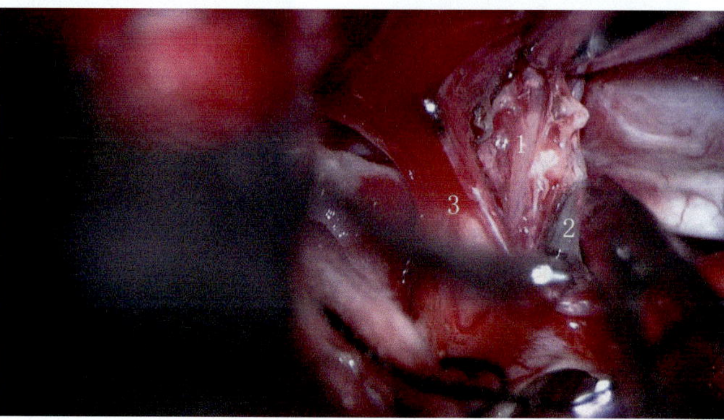

Fig. 7.119 The tumor tightly adhered to the third VF. (1) Tumor, (2) third VF, (3) optic nerve

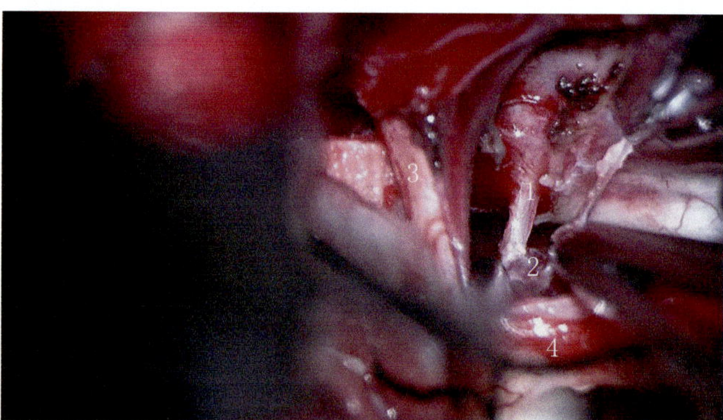

Fig. 7.117 The tumor was dissected through the pre-chiasmatic space. (1) Pituitary stalk, (2) tumor, (3) optic nerve, (4) optic chiasm

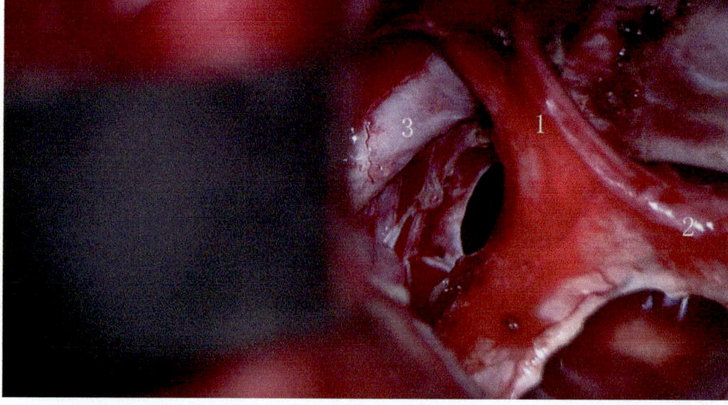

Fig. 7.120 The tumor was totally removed; the neurovascular structures of the sellar region were preserved. (1) Optic nerve, (2) optic chiasm, (3) internal carotid artery

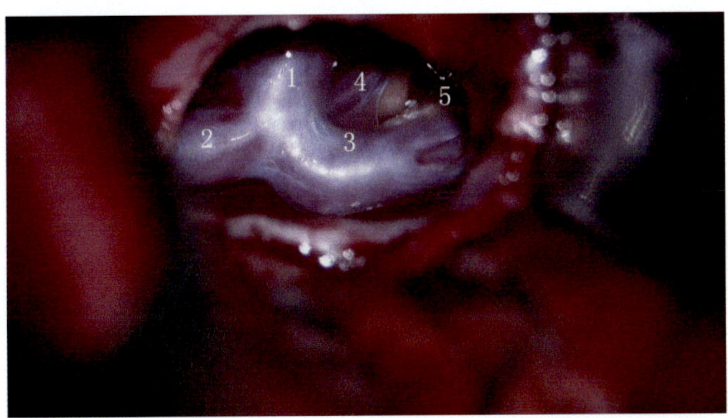

Fig. 7.121 Partial tumor resection via the right-side pterional approach was performed in the first operation. We believed that this tumor belonged to ectopic implantation, because the craniopharyngioma could not originate from this region. The ectopic implantation of tumor was located behind the right side of the basilar artery and between the right superior cerebellar artery and the right posterior cerebral artery. (1) Basilar artery, (2) left posterior cerebral artery, (3) right posterior cerebral artery, (4) right superior cerebellar artery, (5) tumor

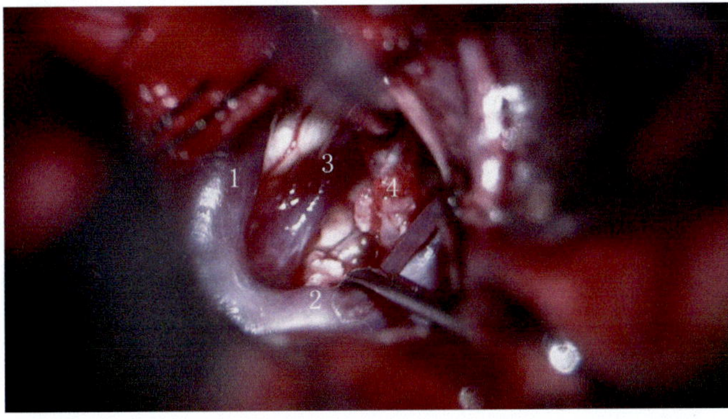

Fig. 7.122 The tumor tightly adhered to the basilar artery and its branches and was separated from the right superior cerebellar artery and the right posterior cerebral artery. (1) Basilar artery, (2) right posterior cerebral artery, (3) right superior cerebellar artery, (4) tumor

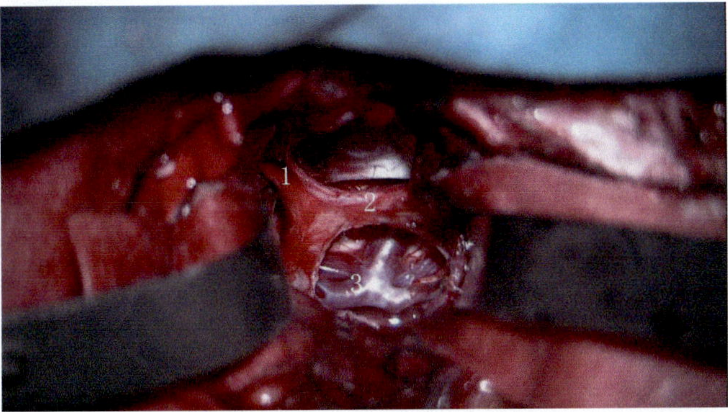

Fig. 7.123 After total tumor removal, the neurovascular structures of the sellar region were preserved. (1) Optic nerve, (2) optic chiasm, (3) basilar artery and its branches

ionizing radiation followed by degeneration and death is the current preferred theory. Radiation-induced dysfunction may occur in approximately 80% of patients subjected to long-term follow-up and is associated with unfavorable effects on growth, skeletal health, fertility sexual function, and physical and psychological health. Moreover stereotactic radiotherapy for pituitary tumors does not appear to reduce the long-term risk of hypopituitarism. Neurosurgeons need to understand that once a patient received chemoradiotherapy and cystic fluid aspiration and intracapsular chemoradiotherapy, it means that the patient has lost the possibility of true cure and high-quality survival.

Radical tumor resection is the best option for treating recurrent craniopharyngiomas, even the re-recurrent craniopharyngiomas. Radiotherapy, p32 therapy, and ommaya reservoir placement surgery are conservative treatments that cannot cure this kind of tumors.

Profound understanding of the arachnoidea around the pituitary and the growth pattern of CPs is very important. The origin of tumor and surrounding membranous structure are the bases of QST classification. Identification of different classifications of craniopharyngiomas is essential to selecting the appropriate surgical procedure and can predict operation difficulty and outcome.

The real radical tumor resection is the only possible and effective cure for CPs; however, the surgical treatment and the perioperative management of recurrent CPs are difficult; a professional medical team is needed. Therefore, in our opinion, the surgical management key points for recurrent CP are (1) knowing the origin and growth pattern of the first primary tumor, (2) understanding the first operation process and how much the neurosurgery perspectives are about craniopharyngiomas and membrane structures, and (3) different treatments being based on the growth pattern of the recurrent tumor.

Part IV

Other Aspects of Craniopharyngioma

8 Retreatment of Craniopharyngioma After External Radiotherapy and Intracapsular Radiochemotherapy

Jun-xiang Peng, Yun Bao, and Songtao Qi

8.1 Introduction

To control tumor growth and recurrence, radiation therapies are suggested as alternatives for patients with craniopharyngiomas who could not tolerate surgery. Radiation therapy may delay or prevent recurrence; however, the side effects of radiotherapy were underestimated. This section presents a review of literature on radiological treatment of craniopharyngiomas. We discuss the issue of radiotherapy, their efficacy, and prognosis according to complications and quality of life. Based on pathology and QST classification, we aim to explain the difficulties of reoperation after radiotherapy.

Craniopharyngioma (CP) is a type of common benign tumor that originates from Rathke's pouch remnants. CP is usually cystic, occasionally solid, and sometimes mixed (solid and cystic). It accounts for 2–5% of primary intracranial tumors and 5.6–15% of intracranial tumors in children. Although nearly a century of exploration has passed, the best treatment for craniopharyngioma, which is of multi-point origin and a complicatedly and variably growing tumor, remains controversial, especially for craniopharyngioma in children. According to the results from a large number of clinical studies, based on long-term follow-up, there is significant benefit in a 10-year recurrence-free survival rate after total resection. Most patients with CP after radiotherapy had worse tendency toward hypopituitarism and impairment of hypothalamic function. Nowadays, it has been documented that hypopituitarism and diabetes insipidus caused by total resection is more acceptable compared to continuous impairment of endocrine function caused by tumor recurrence. Radical excision should be the aim when possible in order to prevent tumor recurrence and to avoid radiotherapy.

To control tumor growth and recurrence, radiation therapies such as external radiotherapy, proton beam therapy, stereotactic radiotherapy, intracavitary β-irradiation, and instillation of sclerosing substances for cystic tumors are suggested as options for patients who could not tolerate surgery. Undeniably efficacy of radiation therapy has been documented for delaying or preventing recurrence in patients with subtotal removal of the tumor. However, the side effects of radiotherapy after partial resection of craniopharyngioma were underestimated. First, patients with CP are associated with higher risk of neurological and neuropsychological complications. It is more difficult to control neuroendocrine disorders after radiotherapy, as different cumulative range and different radiation dose have different radiotherapeutic effects on the tumor. Second, although subtotal resection adjuvant radiotherapy and chemotherapy can delay the recurrence of tumors, the recurrence is almost inevitable for patient with long-term survival; even smaller recurrent tumors require complex procedures. Compared with total resection, the 10-year local control rate of partial resection was worse. Third, after radiotherapy, adhesion between tumor and vital stellar structures will greatly increase the difficulty of the operation, and it also increases the risk of operational complications. Finally, it is noted that radiotherapy plays an important role in malignant transformation from benign CP.

The QST classification of craniopharyngiomas based on the relationship between the location of tumor origin and the surrounding membrane structures is important for the choice of treatment methods. Because of the destruction of the peripheral membranous structure, the peripheral blood vessels and nerves might have serious adhesions to the tumor, especially in patients who relapse after a long time and when the tumor is larger, which renders protection of vital structures more difficult. The general rules of endocrine disorders after radiotherapy of CP are described briefly below:

1. According to the QST classification of craniopharyngioma, almost all Q-type tumors are adamantinomatous craniopharyngiomas. After radiotherapy of Q-type CP, due to destruction of the peripheral membranous

J.-x. Peng (✉) · Y. Bao · S. Qi
Department of Neurosurgery, Nanfang Hospital of Southern Medical University, Guangzhou, Guangdong, China

© Springer Nature Singapore Pte Ltd. 2020
S. Qi (ed.), *Atlas of Craniopharyngioma*, https://doi.org/10.1007/978-981-13-7322-0_8

structures, the peripheral blood vessels and nerves might have severe adhesions to the tumor. Using H&E staining, it can be observed that the boundary between the tumor and the adenohypophysis was broken, and the tumor mainly involved the pituitary gland, a finger-like structure can be seen between the tumor and neurohypophysis (Fig. 8.1). The degree of pituitary function worsens, and new neurohypophysis dysfunction may occur, with most patients showing panhypopituitarism. In addition, the types and dosage of hormone replacement therapy for patients with CP are significantly increased compared to those of patients who do not undergo radiotherapy.

2. S-type tumors mainly involve the pituitary stalk. After radiotherapy of S-type CP, the arachnoid between the CP and the pituitary stalk is unclear (Fig. 8.2), which renders protection of the pituitary stalk more difficult. Furthermore, tumor recurrence led to more severe hypopituitarism and hypothalamic dysfunction.
3. T-type tumors mainly involve both the third ventricle floor (hypothalamus) and the pituitary stalk. Using H&E staining, it can be observed that the tumor may break through the pia mater and involve the nerve tissue of the third ventricle floor; the moat-like and beach-like types are more common after radiotherapy of T-type CP (Figs. 8.3 and 8.4). Severe hypothalamic obesity (HO), insulin resistance, overeating, and other symptoms may develop due to endocrine dysfunction, and it may be accompanied by complex hypothalamic syndromes such as mental abnormalities, abnormal circadian rhythms, and diabetes insipidus without thirst, which are difficult to control and seriously impair the quality of life of patients.

In conclusion, total resection may be acceptable for patients with CP to avoid repeated procedures. Radiotherapy was suggested as an alternative method only for patients who could not tolerate surgery. Hypopituitarism caused by total resection is secondary because it can be well supplemented by hormonal therapy. Most patients can resume normal activities after total resection with the help of individualized and precise hormone replacement therapy.

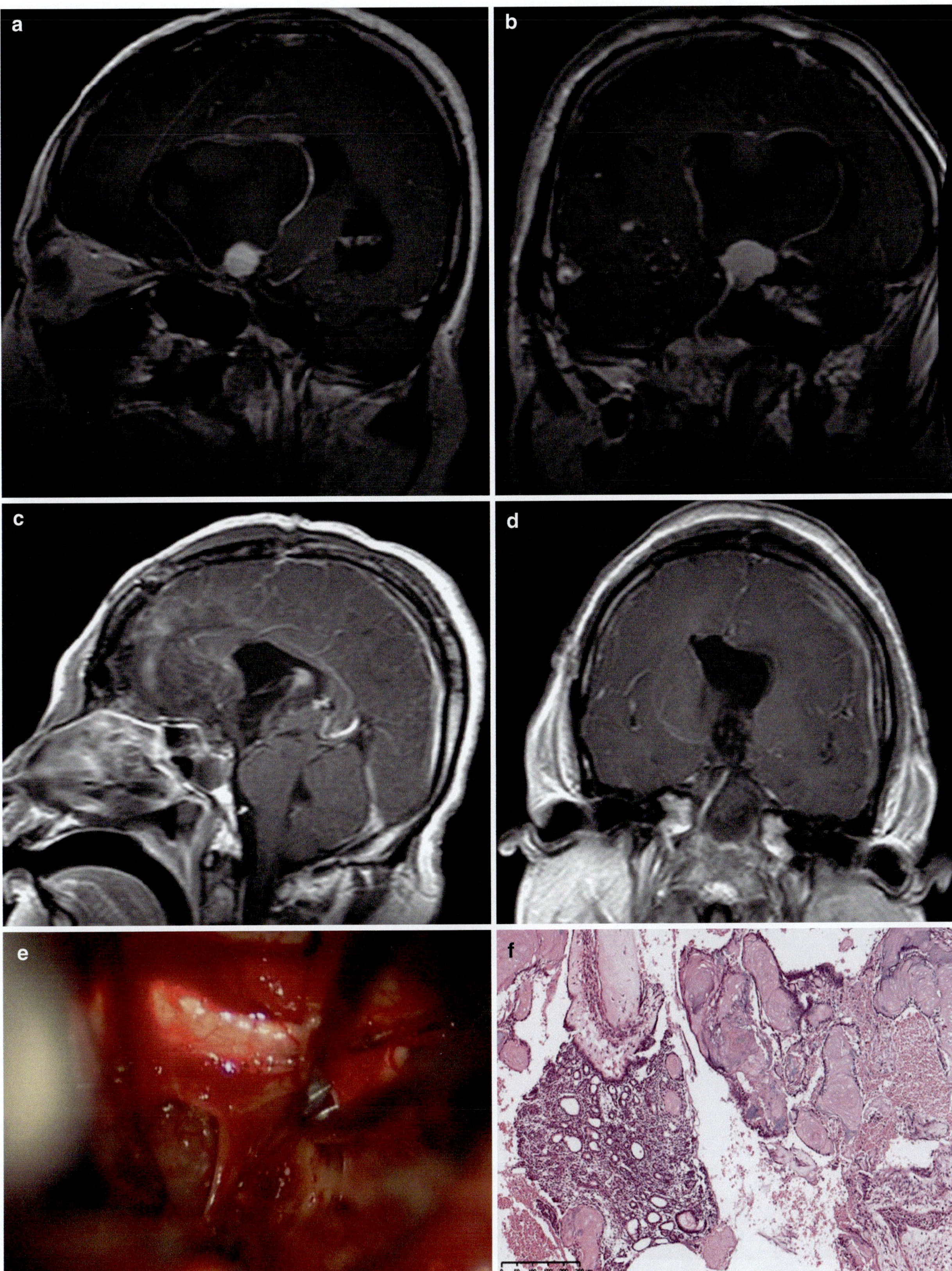

Fig. 8.1 This is the case of a patient with Q-type craniopharyngioma who had received intra-cyst irradiation therapy after subtotal resection surgery at a local hospital. Tumor recurrence was found 18 months after the first surgery, and preoperative examination revealed severe hypothalamic obesity and panhypopituitarism. During the operation, we found that the tumor adhered to the pituitary and hypothalamus severely. Tissue section confirmed vast infiltration of inflammatory cells. (**a, b**) Preoperative radiological images. (**c**) Intraoperative images showing tumor's adhesion to the neural tissue. (**d, e**) Postoperative MRI images confirm the gross total resection. (**f**) Tissue section of the tumor (H&E stain, 20 × 20). The invasion of the pituitary could be observed at the boundary of the tumor sample, as well as the infiltration of inflammatory cells

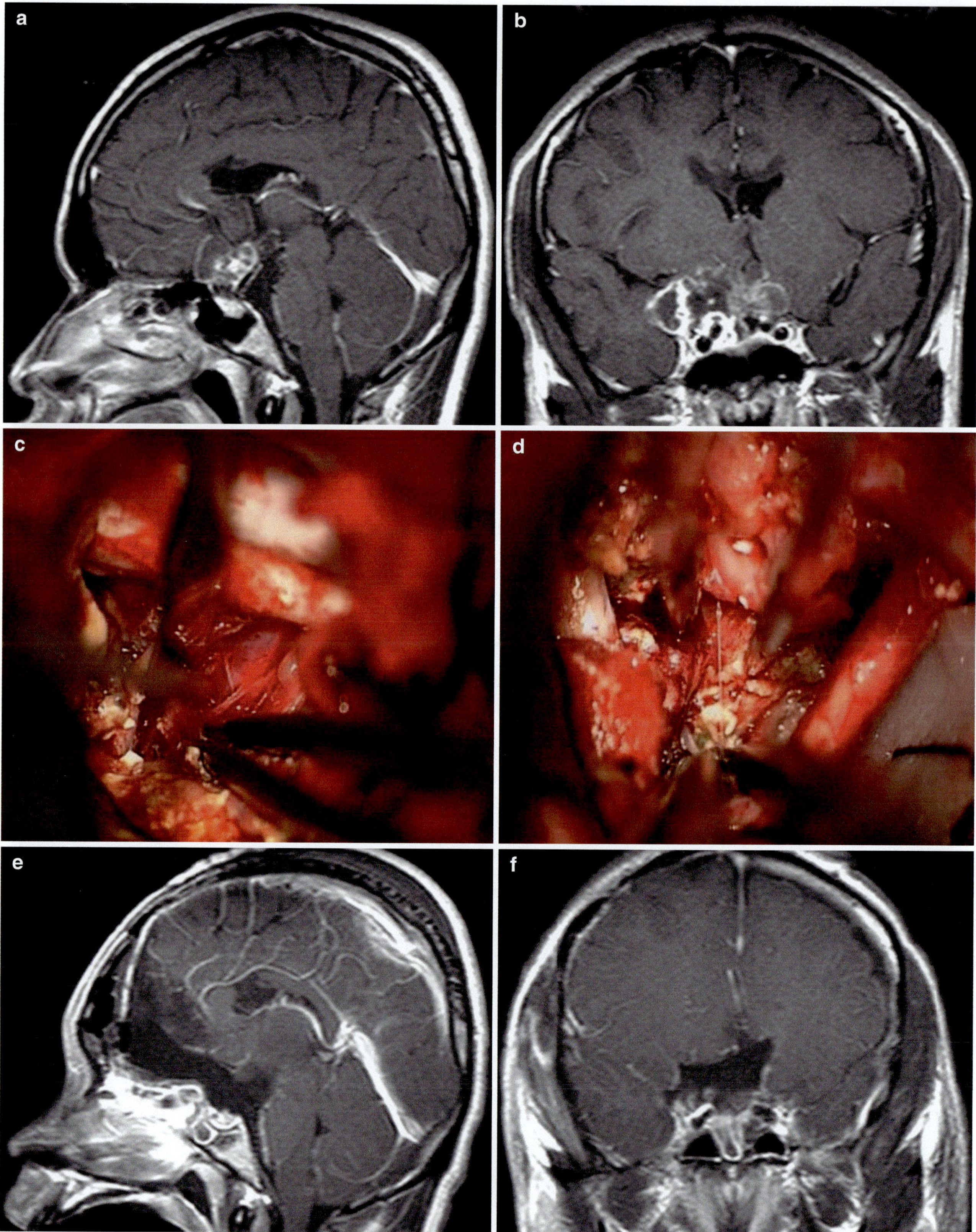

Fig. 8.2 This is the case of a patient with an S-type craniopharyngioma who had received intra-cyst irradiation therapy after subtotal resection surgery at a local hospital. Tumor recurrence was found 15 months after the first surgery and preoperative examination revealed panhypopituitarism. During the operation, we found that the tumor adhered to pituitary stalk and optic nerve severely. Tissue section confirmed vast infiltration of inflammatory cells. (**a**, **b**) Preoperative radiological images. (**c**, **d**) Intraoperative images showing the tumor's adhesion to the pituitary and optic nerve. (**e**, **f**) Postoperative MRI images confirm the gross total resection. (**g**, **h**) Tissue section of the tumor (H&E stain, 20 × 20). The invasion of the pituitary could be observed at the boundary of the tumor sample, as well as the infiltration of inflammatory cells

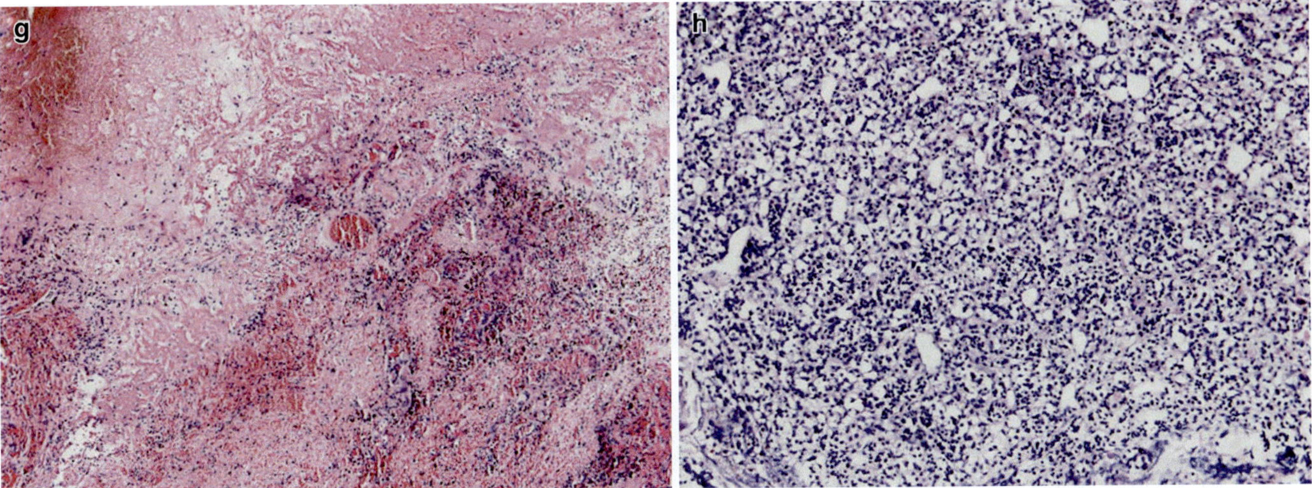

Fig. 8.2 (continued)

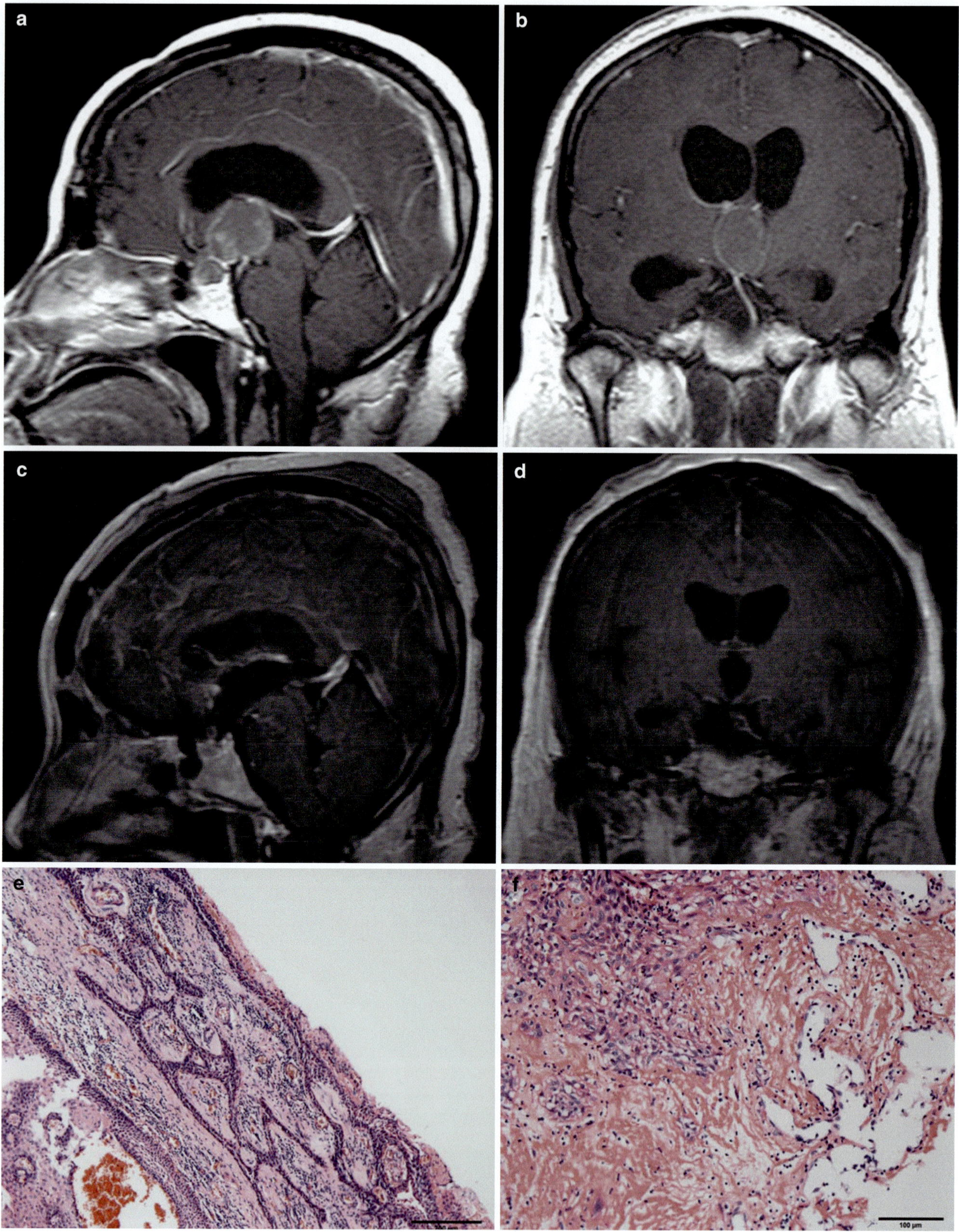

Fig. 8.3 This was the case of a patient with a T-type craniopharyngioma who had received gamma-knife treatment after subtotal resection surgery at a local hospital. Tumor recurrence was found 1 year after the first surgery and preoperative examination revealed panhypopituitarism. During the operation, we found that the tumor had escaped restriction from the arachnoid membrane and had extensively adhered to neural tissue; detachment of the tumor is very difficult under such conditions. (**a**, **b**) Preoperative radiological images. (**d**, **e**) Postoperative MRI images confirm the gross total resection. (**c**, **f**) Tissue section of the tumor (H&E stain, 10 × 20 (**c**) and 20 × 20 (**f**)). The tumor pushes the pituitary gland, and infiltration of inflammatory cells could be seen

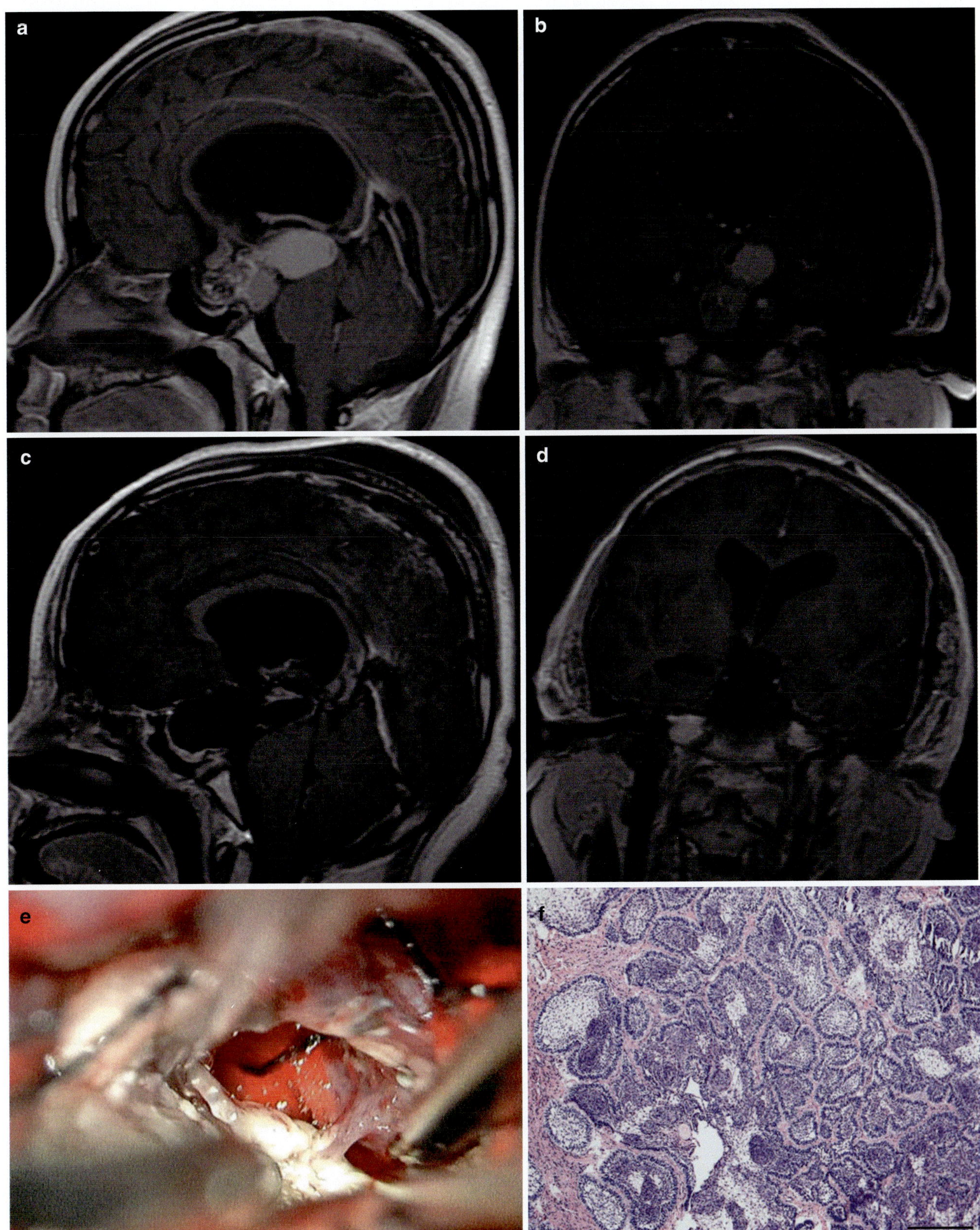

Fig. 8.4 This was the case of a patient with a T-type craniopharyngioma who had received chemotherapy after subtotal resection surgery at a local hospital. Tumor recurrence was found 18 months after the first surgery and preoperative examination revealed panhypopituitarism. During the operation, we found that the tumor adhered to the bottom of third ventricle severely. (**a**, **b**) Preoperative radiological images. (**c**) Intraoperative images showing the tumor's adhesion to the neural tissue. (**d**, **e**) Postoperative MRI images confirm the gross total resection. (**f**) Tissue section of the tumor (H&E stain, 20 × 20). The pia mater may be broken by the tumor or previous operation. The mortise and tenon structures could be observed when the tumor contacted the neural tissue directly

Basic Research in Craniopharyngioma

9

Zhan-peng Feng, Yi Liu, Chao-hu Wang, and Songtao Qi

9.1 Introduction

Although the QST classifications of craniopharyngioma are beneficial in this tumor, the perfect gross tumor resection remains difficult. Not only must the surgeon have a wealth of experience and go through long-term learning process, but also a strong perioperative management team is required, as well as accurate treatment for endocrine and pituitary function reconstruction capabilities. It is undeniable that not every doctor can become a surgeon capable of treating craniopharyngioma. Similarly, not everyone can train to achieve a performance of 100 m within 10 s. A special training process and special talent plus luck are required.

Therefore, the basic research for benign embryonic craniopharyngioma should focus on reducing the difficulty of surgery and improving the quality of the patient's life with long-term survival. In the long term, of course, specific targeted drug therapy is the ultimate goal of craniopharyngioma research, which may remove the requirement for surgical treatment. Because craniopharyngioma is more serious and complicated than the other tumors arising in the sellar region, it is not only difficult to perform and the surgery, but also the pituitary, pituitary stalk, third ventricle, and hypothalamus may be disturbed and damaged.

Based on this fact, therefore, the content of this chapter only covers two aspects that the author has explored. First, are composition and growth pattern of craniopharyngioma different in the presence of stem cell-like tumor cells? If a craniopharyngioma cell, as a benign tumor, can establish an immortalized cell line, it may lay a solid foundation for basic research in craniopharyngioma. Second, is there a possibility of regeneration and repair of the hypothalamic brain tissue in the third ventricles? If there is regeneration, what role may it play in the treatment of craniopharyngioma?

9.2 Craniopharyngioma Stem-Like Cells (CSLCs) and Immortalized Craniopharyngioma Cell Lines

Craniopharyngioma (CP) is a rare epithelial tumor that occurs in the sellar region. Pathology can be divided into adamantinomatous craniopharyngioma (ACP, Figs. 9.1 and 9.2) and papillary craniopharyngioma (PCP), the former accounted for more than 90% of craniopharyngioma. Therefore, ACP is recognized as a "benign pathological feature and a malignant clinical outcome." It is imperative to reveal the etiology of tumor calcification and tumor-associated cysts, and the molecular mechanism of tumor impact on hypothalamic structure explores potential therapeutic targets. Therefore, it is of great clinical significance to control tumor growth, reduce surgical damage, and improve patient survival rate and quality of life.

Adult stem cells maintain some markers expressed by embryonic stem cells and express other specific markers depending on the organ where they reside. Recently, stem/progenitor cells in the humans have been characterized as expressing GFAP and stem cell markers such as CD133 and CD44. Our results indicate tumor stem cell-like characteristics of CD133- and CD44-accumulating cell clusters in ACP, which may represent a tumor stem cell niche and might contribute to tumor recurrence. The potential impact of these special cell groups regarding future CP management, including postoperative follow-up and additional treatment, remains to be explored (Fig. 9.3).

Compared with malignant tumors, craniopharyngioma cells have a slow proliferation and a decrease in cell activity and phenotypic changes after multiple passages of primary cells, making them no longer suitable for in vivo and in vitro studies. Therefore, there is a need for a cell line that does not

Z.-p. Feng (✉) · Y. Liu · C.-h. Wang · S. Qi
Department of Neurosurgery, Nanfang Hospital of Southern Medical University, Guangzhou, Guangdong, China

© Springer Nature Singapore Pte Ltd. 2020
S. Qi (ed.), *Atlas of Craniopharyngioma*, https://doi.org/10.1007/978-981-13-7322-0_9

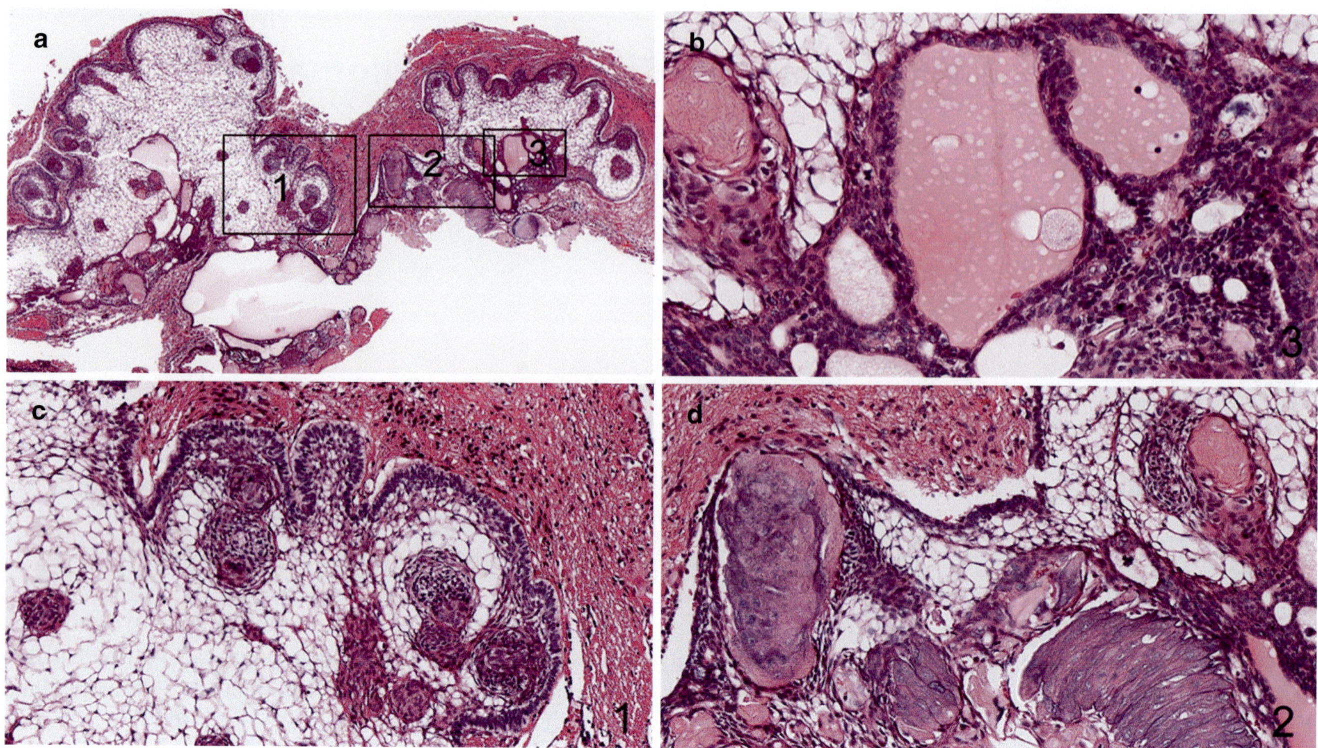

Fig. 9.1 Pathological characteristic of adamantinomatous craniopharyngioma (**a–d**). (**b–d**) are higher power view of the boxes 1–3 in (**a**), respectively. Tumor tongues surrounded by fibrosis showing "stellate reticulum," "wet" keratin, intralobular cystic degeneration, as well as cellular whorls

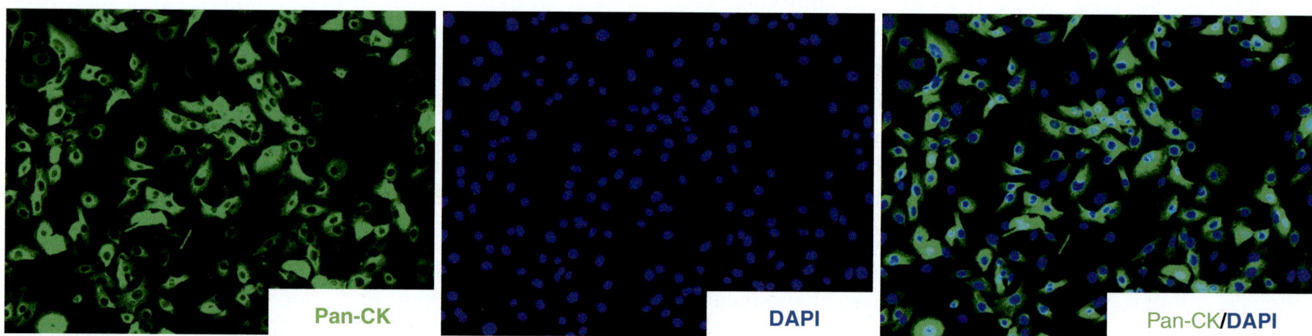

Fig. 9.2 Pan-CK sever as a classical marker of adamantinomatous craniopharyngioma

change traits during the experimental period and has a single characteristic. Therefore, the author's research center used the virus to prepare different types of immortalized craniopharyngioma cell lines. These tumor cells are the most stable and suitable for long-term experiments. As a powerful tool, it is a great advantage in benign tumor research with immortalized ACP cell line (Fig 9.4).

9.3 Neurogenesis in the Hypothalamus

Over the past few decades, with the development of progressively better tools for labeling and tracking newborn neurons, studies in multiple species have clarified that neurogenesis occurs in several brain regions in adult mammals. Initially, scientists confirmed that two main regions of active neurogenesis in the adult rodent brain occur in the

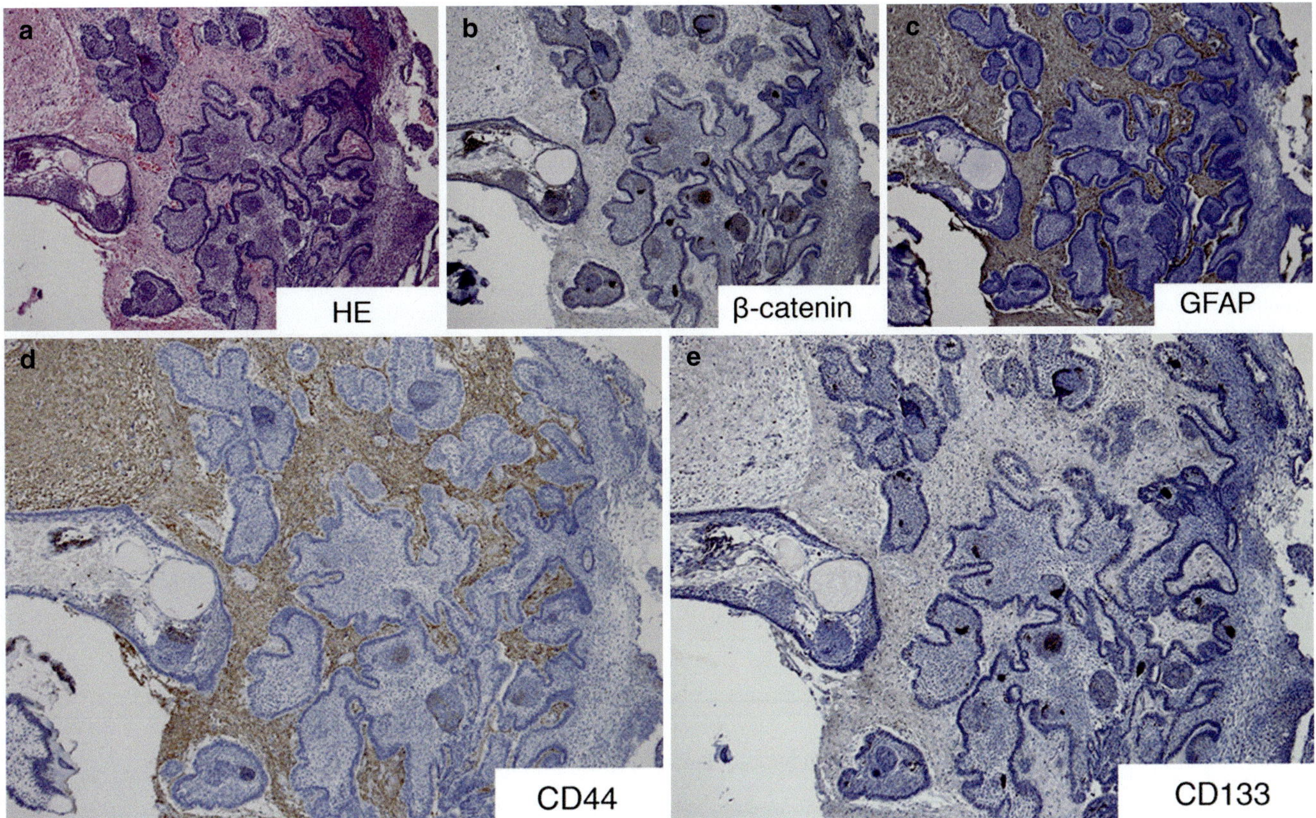

Fig. 9.3 Certain stem cell marker expressed in craniopharyngioma stem-like cells (CSLCs). (**a**) Representative image of craniopharyngioma stem-like cells by HE staining. Immunohistochemical staining of craniopharyngioma with β-catenin (**b**), GFAP (c), CD44 (**d**) and CD133 (**e**)

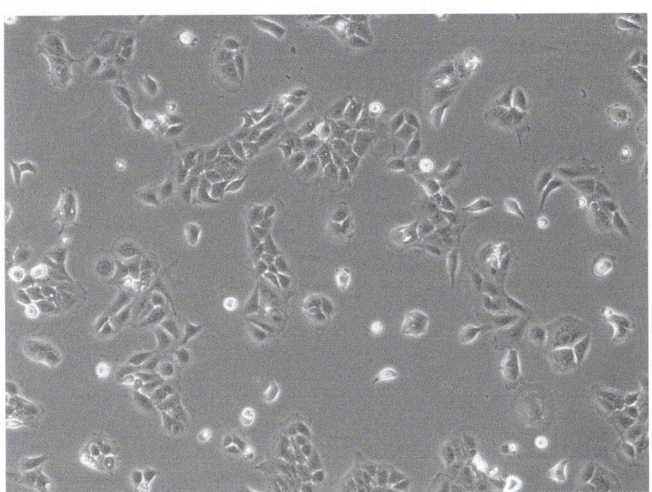

Fig. 9.4 Establishment of immortalized ACP cells. Immortalized ACP cells grew with large nuclei and plentiful cytoplasm, presenting a slab stone-like arrangement

subventricular zone (SVZ) of the lateral ventricles and the subgranular zone (SGZ) of the dentate gyrus in the hippocampus. With the development of neurogenesis research, a steady accumulation of evidence has suggested that the adult mammalian hypothalamus is not only a multifunctional center in the brain but also the third neurogenic niche in adult mammalians.

According to the recent research on adult hypothalamus neurogenesis, the third ventricle (3V), paraventricular zone, periventricular zone, and the median eminence (ME) can be the plausible candidates of the hypothalamic neurogenesis niche (Figs. 9.5 and 9.6). The ventricular zone of the mediobasal hypothalamus is largely composed of specialized radial glial-like cells called tanycytes, which line all but the most ventrally located portion of the 3V wall in this region. In contrast to the multiciliated ependymal cells that line the ventricles in most of the brain, tanycytes extend only one or two apical cilia into the ventricle and, depending on their location, project a long extended basal process either into the hypothalamic parenchyma or toward the pial surface of the hypothalamus. These radial processes are highly reminiscent of those shown by neural progenitors in the embryonic brain, which also serve as a substrate for radial migration of newly postmitotic neurons. Tanycytes express many genes that are also selectively expressed in embryonic hypothalamic progenitor cells and/or are expressed in neural stem cells of the SVZ and SGZ. These include transcription factors such as Rax, Lhx2, Sox2, and Sox9; intermediate filament proteins such as Nestin,

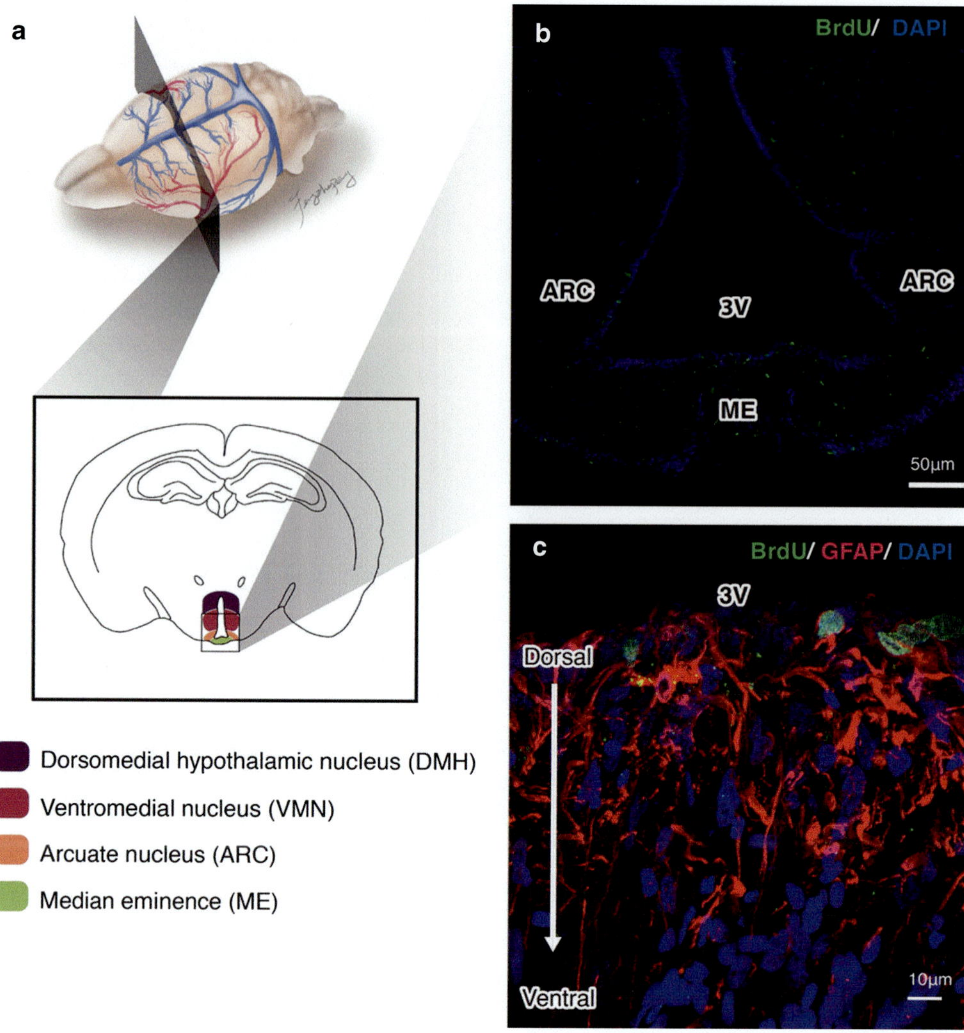

Fig. 9.5 The hypothalamic neurogenesis area is located near the third ventricle in adult rodents. (**a**) The schematic diagram shows the coronal plane through the median eminence. (**b**) Neural precursor cells (NPCs) are detected by BrdU (green) labeling, a newborn cell marker, indicating hypothalamic neurogenesis niche in the ME and around the third ventricle. (**c**) High-power image shows the GFAP (red), a NPC marker, expressed in the ME and co-staining with BrdU (green). *3V* third ventricle, *ARC* arcuate nucleus, *ME* median eminence

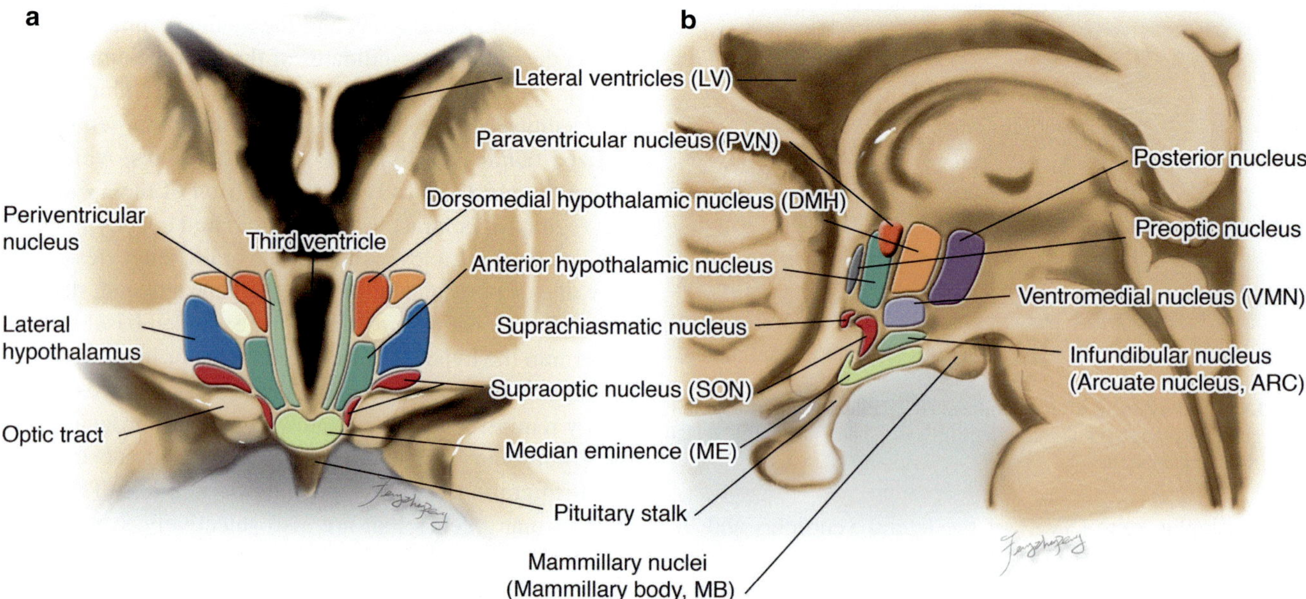

Fig. 9.6 Hypothalamic nucleus associated with craniopharyngioma. Coronal (**a**) and sagittal (**b**) views showing the location of the median eminence in human hypothalamus

vimentin (Fig. 9.7), and GFAP; growth factors such as Fgf10 and Fgf18; and Notch pathway components such as Notch1, Notch2, and Hes5.

Three different proliferative zones have been identified within the tanycytic layer. These are a subependymal region located in the dorsal α1 region, a second region in the dorsal α2 region, and a final region that has been termed the "hypothalamic proliferative region," located adjacent to the ME in the β2 region (Fig. 9.8).

Furthermore, more and more researches are focusing on the regulation and functional significance of adult hypothalamic neurogenesis. The hypothalamus is responsible for the regulation of certain metabolic processes and other activities of the autonomic nervous system. Numerous studies have shown that postnatal hypothalamic neurogenesis plays a complicated role in metabolism, body weight, reproduction, sex-specific behaviors, temperature homeostasis, aging, exercise, functional plasticity in neuronal circuits, and other processes.

Disorders of the hypothalamic or posterior pituitary usually occur after surgery of the hypothalamus and its proximal regions. A typical postoperative complication is diabetes insipidus characterized by abnormal water electrolyte balance. Despite continuous improvements in drugs and therapies targeted to maintain the homeostasis, patients still suffer from a severe situation in the perioperative period, which may cause death or develop into chronic conditions. Surprisingly, some patients were reported to recover from postoperative diabetes insipidus with routine treatment. Similarly, a self-recovery period was observed in rodents with central diabetes insipidus (CDI) induced by hypophysectomy. However, the mechanism of self-recovery remains unclear.

To assess the recovery after HNS injury in rodents, we constructed a pituitary stalk electrical lesion (PEL) model in rats with a curve head 3D printed knife (Fig. 9.9), which avoids excessive damage to the anterior pituitary. Assessment by MR and IHC showed numerous newborn cells in the supraoptic nucleus (SON) and paraventricular nucleus (PVN) after pituitary stalk lesion in rats. Such cells may originate from the median eminence (ME). Moreover, regulation of hypothalamic neurogenesis could modulate the CDI condition. Hypothalamic neurogenesis may exhibit functional diversity and provide a possibility to target this specific dysfunction (Fig. 9.10).

In craniopharyngioma weight gain can principally occur from the disruption of the normal homeostatic function of the hypothalamic centers responsible for controlling satiety and hunger and regulating energy balance.

In physiological conditions, the hypothalamic arcuate nucleus (ARC), located in the median eminence, where the

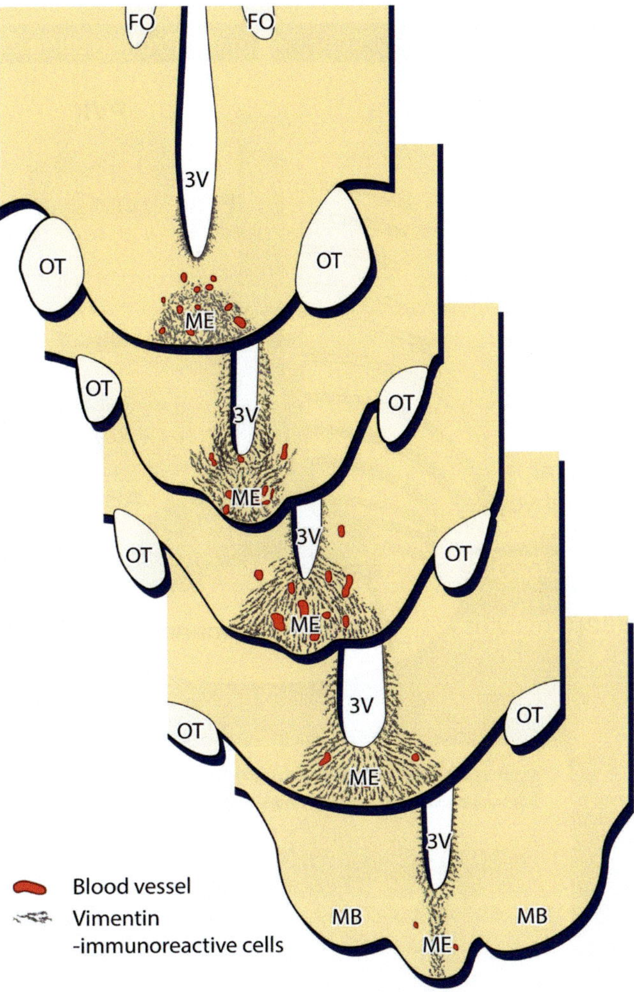

Fig. 9.7 Schematic diagram from the anterior to the posterior in the adult hypothalamic median eminence. Vimentin-immunoreactive cells are represented by gray lines around the border of the third ventricle. The red circles represent capillaries. *3V* third ventricle, *FO* fornix, *MB* mammillary body, *OT* optic tract

brain barrier is freely permeable, senses nutrient and hormonal signals from the periphery and is the primary site of two sets of neurons that form part of the central melanocortin system, a key regulator of energy balance.

The previous findings suggest that, at least in animal models, primary neurodegeneration may not be the proximate cause of obesity and altered feeding behavior in response to an HFD. However, these findings do suggest that altered hypothalamic neural stem cell homeostasis, ultimately resulting in a failure to replace neurons that degenerate or undergo apoptosis in the hypothalamus, is an important step in adapting to diet and the onset of obesity.

What remains unclear is the function of these cells under physiological conditions, when the organism is not maintained on an HFD. Furthermore, there are indications from

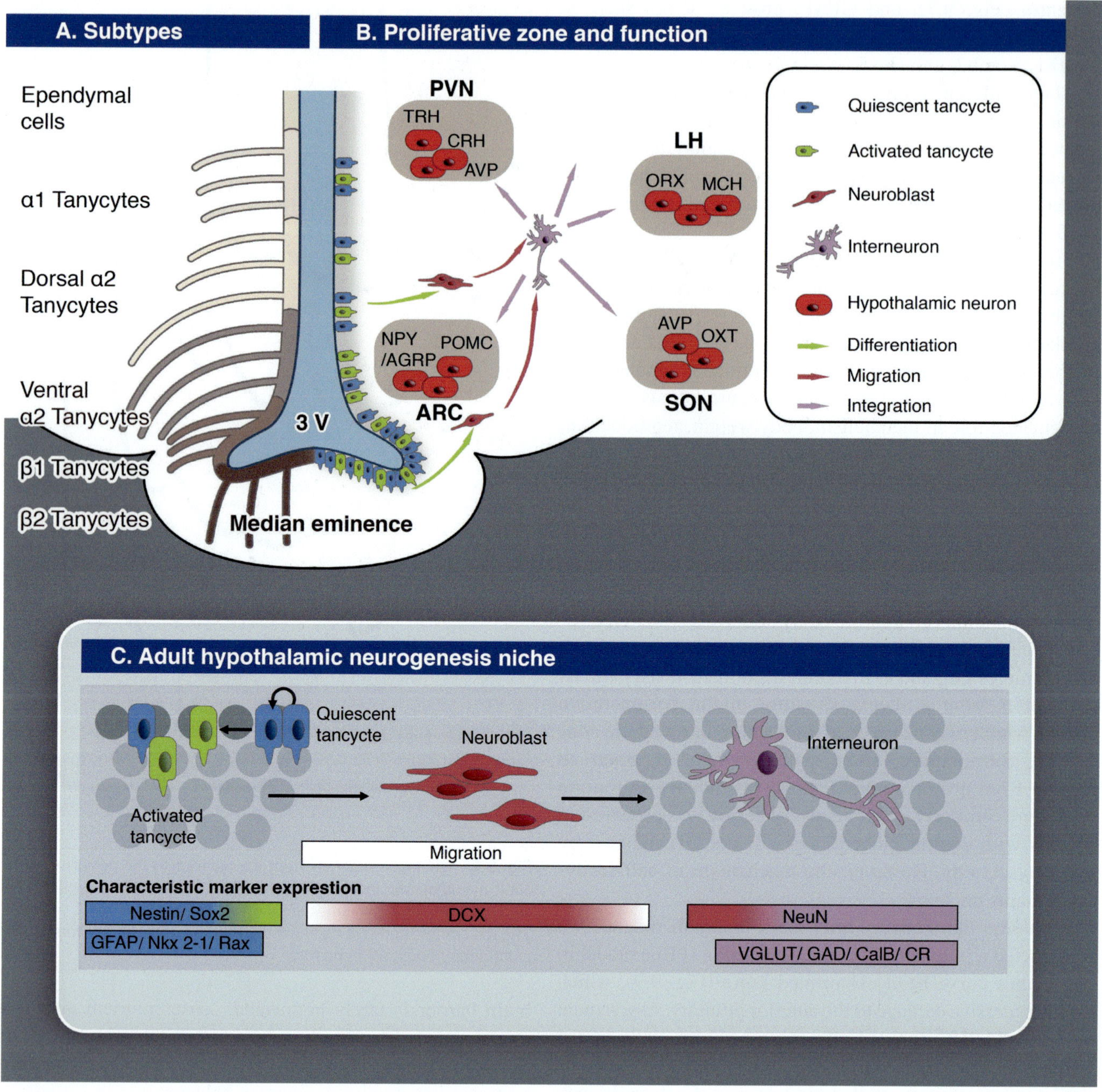

Fig. 9.8 Tanycytes as neural progenitors in the adult mammalian brain. (**a**) Schematic illustration of tanycyte subtypes. From top to bottom: ependymal cells, α1, dorsal and ventral α2, β1 and β2 tanycytes. (**b**) Proliferative zones in the tanycytic layer. These tanycytes give rise to neurons and possibly astrocytes; newly born neurons may interact with hypothalamic neurons. (**c**) Differential gene expression in different neurogenesis processes. *3V* third ventricle, *Arc* arcuate nucleus, *DMH* dorsomedial hypothalamus, *ME* median eminence, *VMN* ventromedial nucleus

the complexity of the functional outcomes of manipulating hypothalamic neural stem cells (Fig. 9.11).

The comprehension of the natural history and etiology of obesity in craniopharyngioma survivors as well as the identification of modifiable risk factors should facilitate preventive interventions in the future. In fact, the management of obesity and eating disorders remains difficult, especially in patients with hypothalamic lesions. Such view of hypothalamic neurogenesis should be helpful in obesity prevention, but could also have a wide range of additional benefits in the prevention or amelioration of other late effects of cancer treatment As far as we know, patients with craniopharyngioma have a variety of hypothalamic dysfunction during the perioperative period, most of which are caused by tumor

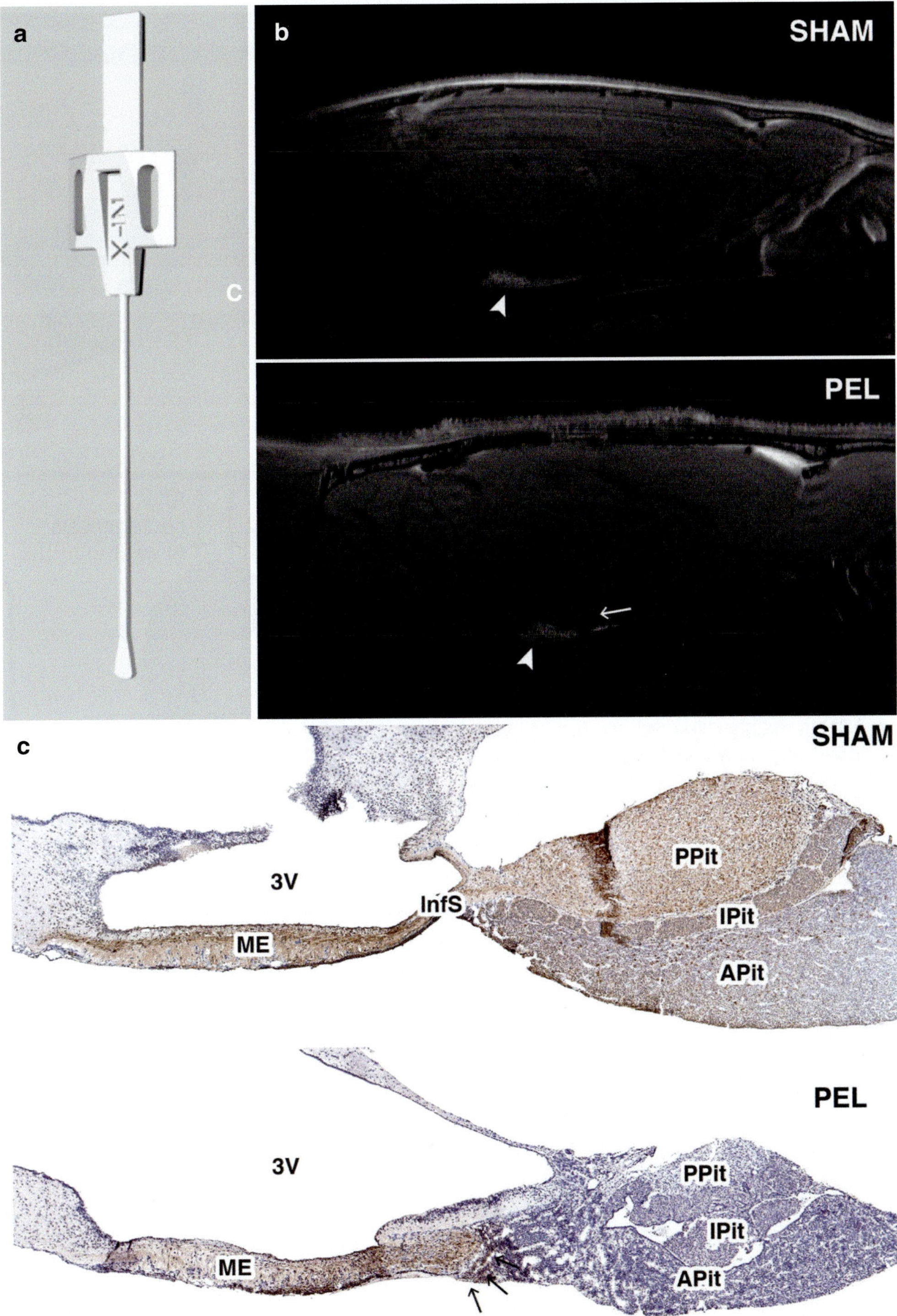

Fig. 9.9 A knife with a curved head that was applied to the lesion in the pituitary stalk of rats and MR and IHC assessment. (**a**) The layout of the lesion knife. (**b**) MR images of control and PEL rats in vivo. T1-weighted images of the middle sagittal plane in control rats (upper panel) and PEL rats 28 days after the operation (lower panel). After Gd-DTPA administration, the signal in the hypothalamic-neurohypophysis axis was interrupted in PEL rats (arrow head). (**c**) The middle sagittal plane section from the sham-operated group (upper) and the PEL group (lower) stained for AVP-ir

injury or iatrogenic injury of the hypothalamus, which includes surgical injury and excessive radiotherapy injury. The niche of neural stem cells in hypothalamus, these stem cells can be used to effectively regulate the function of the hypothalamus, so it is necessary to avoid injury or excessive damage to the tissue around the median eminence of the hypothalamus and retain its complete regeneration environment for neurons. For these endogenous neural stem cells, we suppose it is necessary to study and explore them more deeply, which may be used as a therapeutic strategy for hypothalamic neural restoration and endocrine reconstruction.

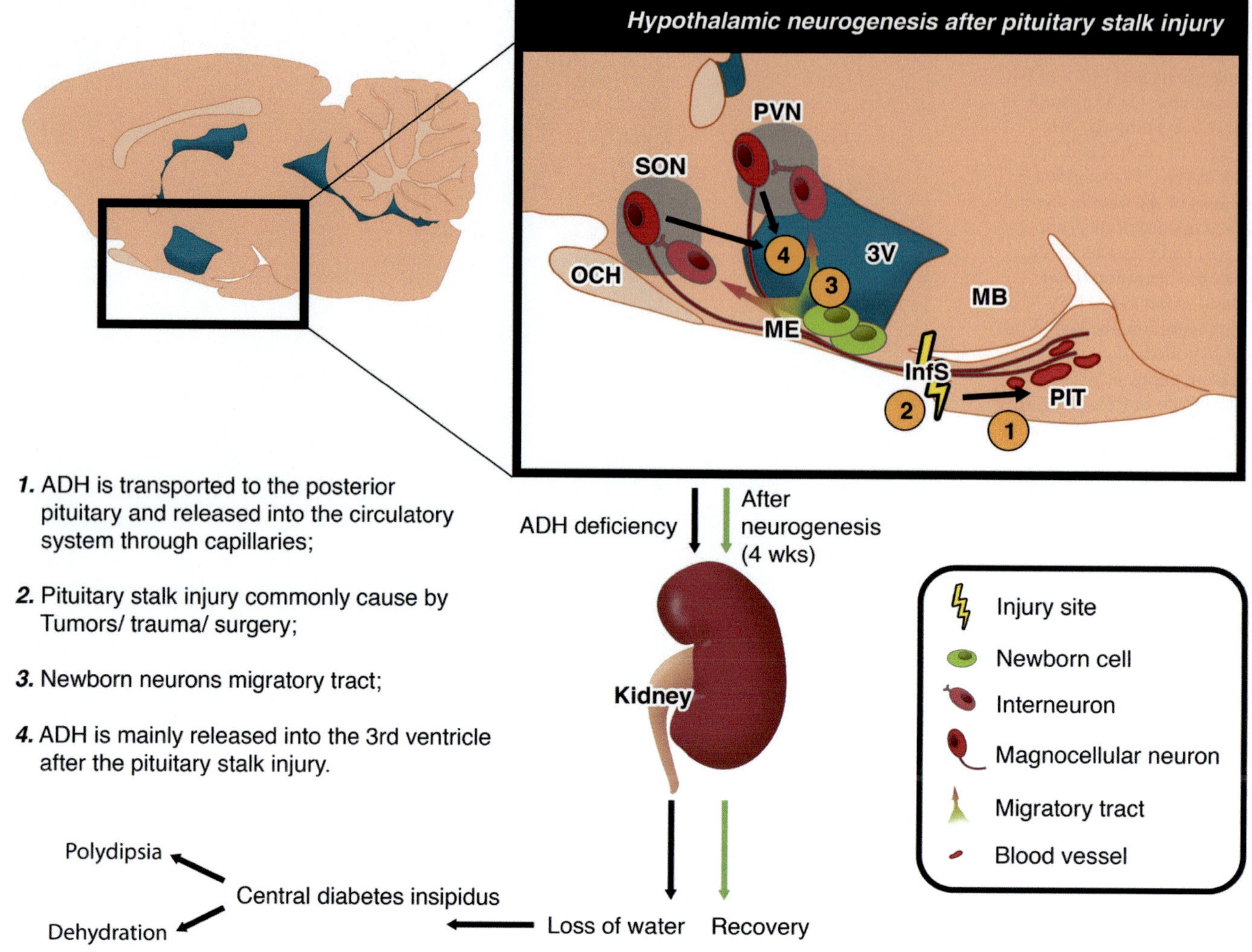

Fig. 9.10 Hypothalamic neurogenesis promotes the recovery of central diabetes insipidus after the pituitary stalk injury. *3V* third ventricle, *InfS* infundibular stem, *ME* median eminence, *MB* mammillary body, *OCH* optic chiasma, *PIT* pituitary, *PVN* paraventricular nucleus, *SON* supraoptic nucleus

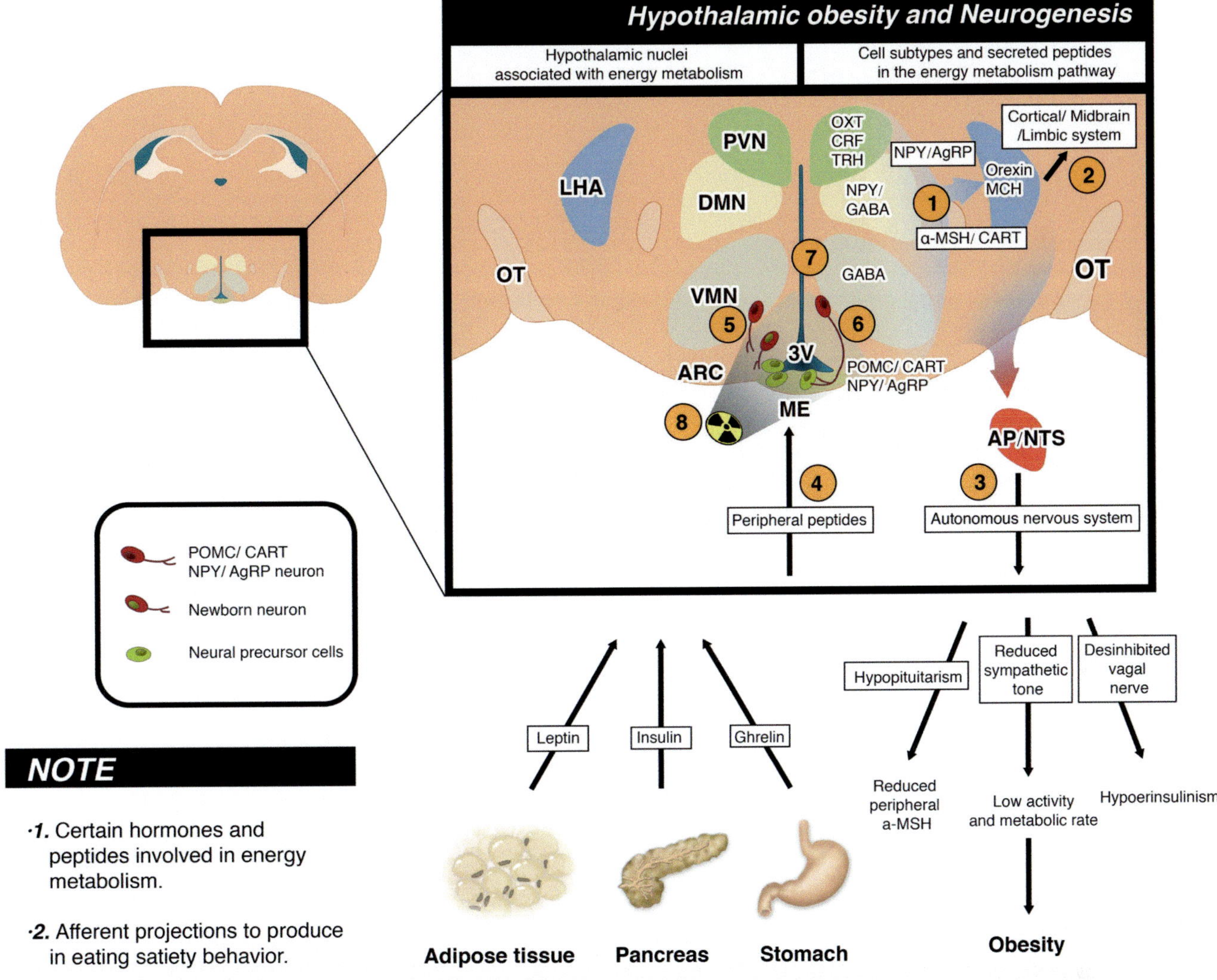

·3. Autonomous nervous control of effectors in pancreas, liver, stomach and adipose tissue.

·4. Proteins and peptides released from peripheral organs regulate the secretion activity of hypothalamic neurons

·5. Neural precursor cells (NPCs) in ME can differentiate into POMC and NPY neurons, and participate in energy metabolism pathways, involved in the regulation of obesity.

·6. The neuronal processes of the arcuate nucleus interact with the NPCs of the ME, receiving the leptin signal taken by the NPCs.

·7. Common hypothalamic nuclei damaged by craniopharyngioma: ARC, VMN, ME, (DMH, PVN)

·8. Radiotherapy also significantly reduces NPC, potentially increasing the risk of obesity and other complications.

Fig. 9.11 The role of hypothalamic neurogenesis in hypothalamic obesity. *3V* third ventricle, *AP* area postrema, *Arc* arcuate nucleus, *DMH* dorsomedial hypothalamus, *LHA* lateral hypothalamus area, *ME* median eminence, *NTS* nucleus tractus solitarii, *OT* optic tract, *PVN* paraventricular nucleus, *VMN* ventromedial nucleus

MIX
Papier aus verantwortungsvollen Quellen
Paper from responsible sources
FSC® C105338

If you have any concerns about our products, you can contact us on
ProductSafety@springernature.com

In case Publisher is established outside the EU, the EU authorized representative is:
Springer Nature Customer Service Center GmbH
Europaplatz 3, 69115 Heidelberg, Germany

Printed by Libri Plureos GmbH
in Hamburg, Germany